Clean Room Technology in ART Clinics

A PRACTICAL GUIDE

Clean Room Technology in ART Clinics

A PRACTICAL GUIDE

Edited by

SANDRO C. ESTEVES

ALEX C. VARGHESE

KATHRYN C. WORRILOW

CRC Press
Taylor & Francis Group
Boca Raton London New York

CRC Press is an imprint of the
Taylor & Francis Group, an **informa** business

CRC Press
Taylor & Francis Group
6000 Broken Sound Parkway NW, Suite 300
Boca Raton, FL 33487-2742

Printed on acid-free paper
Printed at CPI on sustainably sourced paper
Version Date: 20160426

International Standard Book Number-13: 978-1-4822-5407-5 (Hardback)

Library of Congress Cataloging-in-Publication Data

Names: Esteves, Sandro, editor. | Varghese, Alex C., editor. | Worrilow, Kathryn C., editor.
Title: Clean room technology in ART clinics : a practical guide / edited by Sandro C. Esteves, Alex C. Varghese, and Kathryn C. Worrilow.
Other titles: Clean room technology in assisted reproductive technology clinics
Description: Boca Raton : Taylor & Francis, 2017. | Includes bibliographical references and index.
Identifiers: LCCN 2016018479 | ISBN 9781482254075
Subjects: | MESH: Environment, Controlled | Reproductive Techniques, Assisted--standards | Laboratories--organization & administration | Clinical Laboratory Techniques--standards
Classification: LCC R857.M3 | NLM WA 671 | DDC 610.28/4--dc23
LC record available at https://lccn.loc.gov/2016018479

Visit the Taylor & Francis Web site at
http://www.taylorandfrancis.com

and the CRC Press Web site at
http://www.crcpress.com

Contents

Section V: Clinical outcome and new developments

Section VI: International experience: Case studies

Foreword

The quality of air surrounding us is defined by natural events and human activity. In an increasingly industrialized and populated world, controlling air quality is both a great challenge and an existential necessity. The link between human health and air quality is indisputable: while good air quality promotes health, many ailments—from respiratory to heart disease to cancer—may be caused or exacerbated by air pollution. The question we, the ART specialists, should be asking is, if humans with more than 3 trillion cells organized into highly complex organs and systems, are so profoundly affected by air pollution, what risks does air pollution pose for human gametes and preimplantation embryos? Surprisingly, and despite its obvious importance, this question has been understudied and, until recently, under-discussed in our field. The vulnerability of gametes and embryos to environmental assaults stems partly from their inability to remove or neutralize contaminants at very early stages of development. Yet, in cell and tissue cultures, concern with air quality has been minimal and largely limited to efforts to reduce infection. How contaminants and pollutants like volatile organic compounds (e.g., benzene) affect cells short term or long term, we simply do not know because the question has not been investigated in any depth. Despite this significant information gap, regulatory agencies like the Environmental Protection Agency in the United States have not become involved and professional organizations like the ASRM and ESHRE have yet to suggest guidelines on the control of air quality in ART laboratories. Though the HFEA and EU Tissues and Cell Directive have made some important suggestions, their guidelines are mostly directed to reduction of air particulates and not volatile organic compounds.

It has been nearly 20 years since the problem of air pollution in the IVF laboratory was investigated for the first time (Cohen et al. 1997). Using air sampling and analysis methodologies that are still in use today, it was found rather unexpectedly that outside air, even in major North American cities, was usually cleaner than the air inside laboratories. The most polluted air was detected in embryology incubators! A number of factors contributed to this problem, including "old-school" engineering during the construction of laboratories; design and manufacturing of incubators; unmonitored and unfiltered gas supplies; and a total lack of awareness of the importance of "off-gassing" instruments, materials, and disposables.

This book is a first of its kind. It provides the reader with a much-needed overview of the topic of air pollution in the clinical embryology laboratory. Important changes in laboratory infrastructure and quality control implemented since the mid-1990s are described and discussed. Importantly, this includes customization of new IVF laboratories and the continuous monitoring of the environment, which have become standard practice in more recent years. Environmental engineering is now an important aspect of the planning, design, and construction of new IVF facilities. The quality of building materials, allowance for an off-gassing period, and continuous filtration not just of particulates but also volatile organic compounds and biological contaminants are emphasized. Manufacturers of new tools and disposables are sensitive to these concerns and respond by reassessing and altering their manufacturing processes. This book will give those involved in ART practice an excellent start in understanding why good air quality is a prerequisite to safe laboratory practice and good clinical outcomes. It provides the basic knowledge and tools for practitioners to do what it takes to maintain a safe environment for gametes and embryos free of pollutants and contaminants.

Jacques Cohen

Reference

Cohen J, Gilligan A, Esposito W, Schimmel T, and Dale B. Ambient air and its potential effects on conception in vitro. *Hum Reprod* 1997; 12: 1742–9.

Preface

Human conception involves the coordination of a complex cascade of biochemical and molecular intracellular signaling events between human gametes, resulting in the production of viable embryos capable of implantation and the establishment of a viable pregnancy. The physiological continuum involved in the *in vitro* culture of the human embryo constitutes one of the most challenging applications of cell culture technology. The continual advancement of assisted reproductive technologies (ARTs), such as the extended culture of the genomically active human embryo, demands a more critical environment. Human embryos are largely unprotected, and it is highly likely that gametes and embryos grown *in vitro* are more sensitive to environmental influences than are complex organisms with more developed mechanisms for protection. Therefore, successful preimplantation embryogenesis is critically dependent on the culture environment provided by the IVF laboratory. New and significant data have demonstrated a significant association between environmental and airborne pathogens in the laboratory ambient air, their influence on epigenetic processes, and the role they play in preimplantation toxicology towards successful embryogenesis, implantation, and conception.

The association between the environment, preimplantation toxicology, and successful embryogenesis demands a more comprehensive evaluation of the variables that contribute to the IVF culture environment. Such variables include but are not limited to the design of the laboratory, the selection of the proper mechanisms of remediation for airborne contaminants, the location of the source of outside air, the selection of materials to use in the construction of the laboratory, the selection and placement of equipment, and personnel and operations work flow. Each variable should be considered thoughtfully and carefully, as each can be negatively impactful to the success of the *in vitro* culture environment. Laboratory and clinical operations and personnel constitute some of the greatest sources of bioburden contributing bacteria, viruses, and mold spores to the environment. The origin of the ambient air serving the IVF laboratory is often a combination of outside fresh or source air and the air recirculated from the IVF laboratory and clinical procedure rooms. Each source of ambient air is perpetually dynamic in its contribution of airborne chemical and biological pathogens to the *in vitro* culture environment. Activities occurring outside of the IVF laboratory cannot be controlled by the IVF program and contribute a significant level of embryotoxic chemical and biological contaminants to the laboratory environment. A suboptimal laboratory or culture environment will compromise preimplantation embryogenesis, the production of viable blastocysts, and therefore, successful implantation and conception.

This book, the first of its kind, is intended to provide the reader with a comprehensive and thoughtful overview of critical variables that must be considered when designing, improving, and maintaining the optimal *in vitro* culture environment. Leading and internationally recognized basic scientists and clinicians have been invited to share their

"A to Z" expertise in designing, building, and protecting the optimal IVF laboratory and clinical environment—each providing invaluable information and, therefore, a significant step toward the support of optimal human embryogenesis. Together, the invited thought leaders provide a comprehensive discussion of the critical role of the *in vitro* culture environment in successful human embryogenesis, the role of ambient air pathogens in preimplantation toxicology, existing and newer transformational mechanisms of remediation of airborne contaminants, key elements to consider in the design of the optimal IVF laboratory; variables to consider before, during, and after construction; the development and maintenance of proper standard operating procedures to ensure and maintain the *in vitro* culture environment; and, finally, experiences from colleagues, across the world, sharing varying international regulatory requirements for air quality in the IVF laboratory. The editors and contributing authors are confident that the information provided in the text will serve as both an invaluable tool and resource for the basic scientists and clinicians striving to optimize the environment provided to support the growth of their patients' embryos, and ultimately, impact the level of care offered to their patients.

About the editors

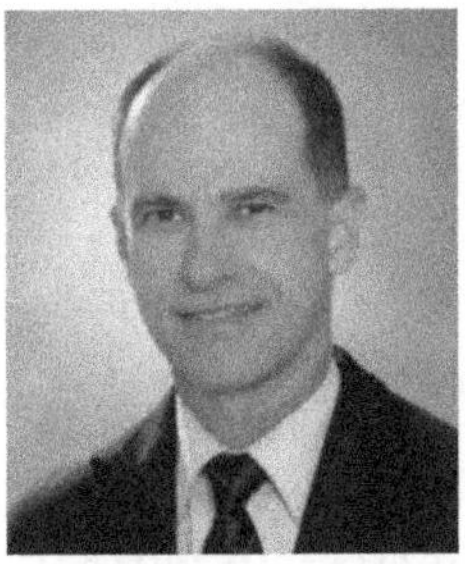

Sandro C. Esteves, MD, PhD, is the Medical and Scientific Director of Androfert—Andrology and Human Reproduction Clinic—a referral fertility center for male reproduction in Brazil. His center was the first in Brazil to obtain full ISO 9001 certifications and to implement clean room technology in its reproductive laboratories.

Dr. Esteves earned his MD in 1990 from the University of Campinas (UNICAMP), Brazil, where he did residency training in urology/andrology. He completed his training in andrology in the United States (1995–1996) as a research fellow at the Cleveland Clinic's Center for Reproductive Medicine. He earned his PhD in 2001 from the Federal University of São Paulo (UNIFESP), Brazil. Dr. Esteves is a board-certified urologist and infertility consultant with over 15 years of experience.

He is a collaborating professor in the Department of Surgery (Division of Urology) at the University of Campinas (Brazil) and research collaborator at both the Cleveland Clinic's Center for Reproductive Medicine (USA) and the Genetic Unit, Department of Biology, Universidad Autónoma de Madrid (Spain). His research/clinical interests include azoospermia-related infertility, microsurgical sperm retrieval techniques, fertility preservation, varicocele, reproductive endocrinology, clean room technology, and quality management.

Dr. Esteves has published over 130 scientific papers and review articles in peer-reviewed scientific journals, authored over 60 book chapters, and presented over 150 papers at both national and international scientific meetings. His current Hirsch index (h-index) is 26 while his citation count is more than 2000. According to ResearchGate, Dr. Esteves has an RG score of 43.37 on 241 publications. Dr. Esteves has served as an editor of four medical textbooks related to reproductive medicine and assisted reproductive technology, including the best-selling textbook *Quality Management in ART Clinics: A Practical Guide*. He is the guest editor of three special issues in scientific journals. Dr. Esteves is a member or office bearer of several professional societies and he serves on the editorial board of the *Asian Journal of Andrology, International Urology and Nephrology, Clinics* (São Paulo) and *Medical Express*. He is also associate editor of the *International Brazilian Journal of Urology*.

Dr. Esteves has been an invited guest speaker at many international meetings in over 30 countries. He is the recipient of the 2006 "Alumni of the Year" award from the Cleveland Clinic's Center for Reproductive Medicine, and the Star Award from the American Society for Reproductive Medicine since 2012.

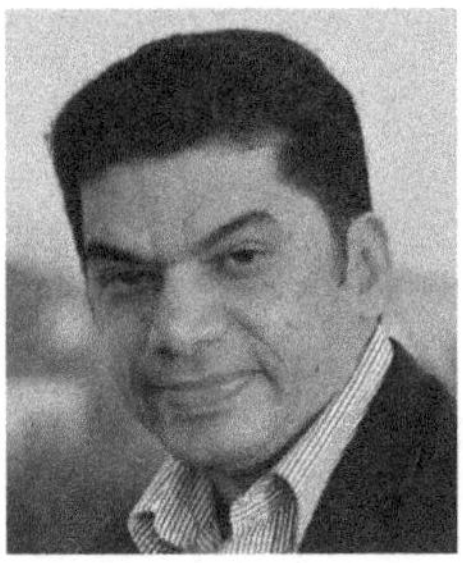

Alex C. Varghese is presently the Scientific & Laboratory Director, Astra Fertility Group of IVF Centres at Mississauga, Bolton, Brampton and Milton, Ontario, Canada. He earned his PhD in Biochemistry from the University of Calcutta, India, for his thesis based on ART. He was a Postdoctoral Research Fellow at the Center for Reproductive Medicine, Cleveland Clinic Foundation (2007–2008) and worked as Senior Embryologist at the Montreal Reproductive Centre (ORIGENELLE), Quebec, Canada.

He has been active in clinical embryology since 1997 and has initiated many successful training programs in ART and helped in designing and setting up many IVF units in rural and urban India and neighboring countries. In 2010 he founded the educational web platform for IVF professionals—www.lifeinvitro.com—which is now popular in 165 countries. Dr. Varghese has authored over 30 manuscripts and edited 8 books in assisted reproduction, including the popular and bestselling *Practical Manual of In Vitro Fertilization: Advanced Methods and Novel Devices*. He has also published 20 book chapters in the area of assisted conception.

Dr. Varghese serves on the editorial board of many journals in reproductive medicine and technology. He is also the advisory board member of C-Create, an educational program by Ferring and ISAR-India. Dr. Varghese is also a research collaborator and external preceptor at the Center for Reproductive Medicine, Cleveland Clinic, Cleveland, Ohio.

Dr. Varghese's research interests are in assisted reproductive technology, in particular, in understanding the molecular and environmental causes and prevention of male infertility, vitrification of gametes and embryos, probiotics in fertility, microbiota in health and disease associated with reproduction and developing stress-free, automated embryo culture systems for *in vitro* fertilization.

He is also the co-investigator in the research project funded by the Department of Biotechnology, Government of India and the Immediate Past President of the Academy of Clinical Embryologists–India. Dr. Varghese was the organizing chairperson of the 4th International Congress (September 18–20, 2015) of the Academy of Clinical Embryologists, India.

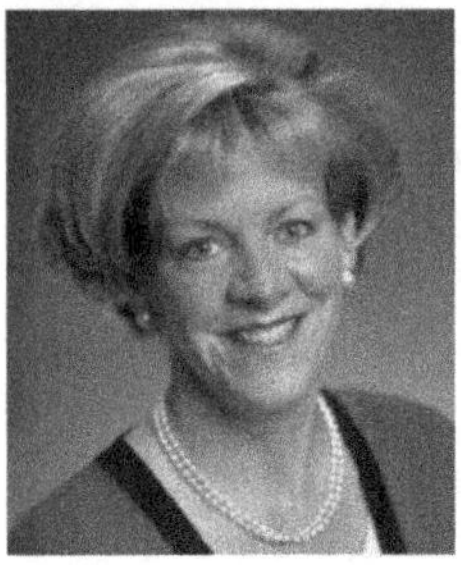

Kathryn C. Worrilow, PhD, founder and CEO of LifeAire Systems, earned her doctorate in Anatomy and Cell Physiology from the University of Virginia School of Medicine and completed her postdoctoral fellowship in Reproductive Physiology and Infertility at the University of Pennsylvania School of Medicine. She has served as the scientific director of *in vitro* fertilization programs for over 20 years and has performed extensive work specific to molecular signaling between the sperm and oocyte, the contribution of the paternal genome to the embryo, and the impact of ambient air on successful human embryogenesis and preimplantation toxicology. Her work, with that of her colleagues, led to the development and design of the LifeAire Systems' patented air purification technology and System, Aire~IVF®. The Aire~IVF System delivers the most pristine air quality available for IVF environments through an in-duct system by inactivating biologicals and eliminating embryotoxic volatile organic compounds using revolutionary and proprietary air purification technologies. One of the most unique features of the LifeAire Systems is the extensive data supporting the design, the specificity of its design toward the human embryo, and the results from nearly five years of clinical implementation. Based upon the data, Dr. Worrilow and her team were invited by the

Canadian Standards Organization to participate in the updated standards for air quality in IVF. The LifeAire Systems carries issued patents in the U.S. and internationally.

Dr. Worrilow has authored over 60 scientific papers and chapters, served as an invited reviewer for leading journals and has been invited to present and publish her research both nationally and internationally. She has been a recipient of the Star Award from the American Society for Reproductive Medicine since 2011, has been honored by the invitation to serve as a TedTalk speaker, and has enjoyed supporting and participating in a number of entrepreneurial-, women in science and engineering-, and STEM-education programs both locally and nationally.

LifeAire Systems is dedicated to improving patient care. Although the proprietary system was developed specifically for the human embryo, LifeAire Systems is excited and positioned to offer its technology to improve patient care along the continuum of care, to infants in the NICU, the child in the PICU, and the elderly in long-term care. The LifeAire Systems' proprietary technology provides a 9-log reduction of airborne pathogens responsible for hospital acquired infections in operating rooms, intensive care units, burn units, pharmacies, and long-term care facilities, thereby improving patient outcomes and healthcare economics while reducing overall cost. The team at LifeAire Systems is proud of the contribution its air purification technology is making to provide clean, contaminant-free air for health, wellness, and life.

As an advocate of science education and the role of science in our community, she also enjoyed her position on the Board of Trustees of The Da Vinci Science Center and Penn State Lehigh Valley LaunchBox in Lehigh Valley, Pennsylvania. Dr. Worrilow's career has always involved a great deal of teaching and she has enjoyed her participation as an adjunct professor with the Emerging Health Professionals Program at Pennsylvania State University Lehigh Valley.

Contributors

Charlene A. Alouf
Good Start Genetics
Cambridge, Massachusetts

Fabiola C. Bento
Androfert, Andrology and Human Reproduction Clinic
Campinas, Brazil

Normand Brais
Sanuvox
Saint-Laurent, Quebec, Canada

Benthe Brauer
Department of Gynecological Endocrinology and Reproductive Medicine
University Hospital of Schleswig-Holstein, Campus Lübeck
Lübeck, Germany

Hsin Chu
National Cheng Kung University
Tainan, Taiwan

Sandro C. Esteves
Androfert, Andrology and Human Reproduction Clinic
Campinas, Brazil

Luciano Figueiredo
Veco Group
Campinas, Brazil

John T. Fox
Lehigh University
Bethlehem, Pennsylvania

Antonia V. Gilligan
Alpha Environmental, Inc.
Emerson, New Jersey

Georg Griesinger
Department of Gynecological Endocrinology and Reproductive Medicine
University Hospital of Schleswig-Holstein, Campus Luebeck
Lübeck, Germany

Johan Guns
Quality Department, Medical Laboratories and Tissue Banks
UZ Brussel
Brussels, Belgium

Ryan J. Heitmann
Madigan Army Medical Center
Tacoma, Washington

Micah J. Hill
Eunice Kennedy Shriver National Institute of Child Health and Human Development
and
National Institutes of Health
and
Walter Reed National Military Medical Center
Bethesda, Maryland

Aidita N. James
Art Institute of Washington, Inc.
Bethesda, Maryland

Ronny Janssens
Centre for Reproductive Medicine
UZ Brussel
Brussels, Belgium

Sangita Jindal
Albert Einstein College of Medicine
Bronx, New York

and

Montefiore's Institute for Reproductive Medicine and Health
Hartsdale, New York

Lars Johansson
Reproductive Center
Academic Hospital
Uppsala, Sweden

Paul Knaggs
Wales Fertility Institute
Heath Park, Cardiff, United Kingdom

Alcir Leal dos Santos
CCL, Controle e Validação
Campinas, Brazil

Terrence D. Lewis
Eunice Kennedy Shriver National Institute of Child Health and Human Development
and
National Institutes of Health
and
Walter Reed National Military Medical Center
Bethesda, Maryland

Yi Hsing Lin
Department of Environmental Engineering
National Cheng Kung University
Tainan, Taiwan

Jayant G. Mehta
Queen's Hospital
Barking, Havering and Redbridge University Hospitals NHS Trust
Essex, United Kingdom

Dean E. Morbeck
Department of Obstetrics and Gynecology & Laboratory Medicine and Pathology
Mayo Clinic
Rochester, Minnesota

Martine Nijs
Nij Geertgen, Fertility Treatment Center
Elsendorp, the Netherlands

and

Embryolab Academy
Thessaloniki, Greece

Giles Palmer
London Women's Clinic Wales
Cardiff, Wales, United Kingdom

Adrianne K. Pope
Adrianne Pope Consulting
Brisbane, Queensland, Australia

Matts Ramstorp
BioTekPro AB
Malmö, Sweden

Raul A. Sadir
Veco Group
Campinas, Brazil

Raul I. Sadir
Veco Group
Campinas, Brazil

Tim Sandle
Bio Products Laboratory
Hertfordshire, United Kingdom

Patrick J. Traver
IPS—Integrated Project Services, Inc.
Blue Bell, Pennsylvania

Ting Ke Tseng
National Cheng Kung University
Tainan, Taiwan

Alex C. Varghese
Astra Fertility Group
Mississauga, Ontario, Canada

Cesar J. Velardez
Veco Group
Campinas, Brazil

Greta Verheyen
Centre for Reproductive Medicine
UZ Brussel
Brussels, Belgium

Adriano Villarmosa
Veco Group
Campinas, Brazil

George H. Wiker
AES Clean Technology, Inc.
Montgomeryville, Pennsylvania

Kelly Athayde Wirka
Medical & Scientific Affairs
Auxogyn, Inc.
Menlo Park, California

Kathryn C. Worrilow
LifeAire Systems
Allentown, Pennsylvania

section one

The basics

chapter one

What is a clean room?

Matts Ramstorp

Contents

Abstract

Clean rooms and clean zones are used to create a clean environment surrounding products, materials, and processes as well as other things handled, which is critical with regard to contaminants. In the health industry, clean rooms and clean zones are applied to hospitals and especially tissue banks, as well as clinics and laboratories handling tissues and cells. In this chapter we will discuss clean rooms and clean zones from a tissue bank perspective and especially within the in vitro fertilization (IVF) sector.

1.1 Short historical review on clean rooms

1.1.1 Introduction

Cleanliness and hygiene are not only of interest in industrial applications. They are also one of the fundamental cornerstones within hospitals and healthcare where people are ill and in an effort to prevent them from being ill. However, cleanliness and hygiene are words that have not been used for a long period of time in a historical point of view. Even though the old Greeks had public baths, in many cases these would not be considered a healthy place, since many of them had a business on the side, by supplying prostitutes to their customers.

In fact, the real start of the hygienic period began at the same time as microorganisms were discovered. In many cases, disease and death have often been the results of various epidemics, and furthermore, no one actually had a clue as to what caused these diseases and epidemics. When microorganisms were first discovered, the first ones to take advantage of this knowledge were hospitals and those in healthcare. Prior to the discovery of microorganisms, people who fell ill, in hospitals or in poor houses, were not separated from each other; there were no thoughts as to if they could infect other patients. In practice, this could mean that a patient with a broken leg could in fact share a bed with a person with anthrax. The outcome of this care is quite easy to understand.

When microorganisms were discovered, they was also in some cases found to be the reason behind the outbreak and spread of diseases. Hospitals reacted in a very responsible way. They started to divide their patients into different groups and also tried to separate these groups from one another. The result was that patients with broken legs, arms, and so on, were moved and received care in a separate ward, whereas patients with contagious diseases, like anthrax, were placed and got care in another ward, separate from patients with no infection. In fact, this is the same principle employed to get clean rooms and contamination-control working and which also leads to their success: to separate things that are clean from things that are less clean.

1.1.2 From Lister to clean rooms

Cleanliness and hygiene had a vast impact on improving patient care in hospitals, but even so, the separation of patients was in fact not enough. The death rates in hospitals at that time were high despite all the knowledge that was gathered and used during the first period of the microbiological era. One person who had an important impact in further minimizing death rates was Joseph Lister, who worked as a surgeon in England.[1] Lister understood quite early that microorganisms had to be taken care of in order to minimize their impact on patients. During that time, the only way to help people who had severely injured limbs, such as a leg, an arm, a finger, and so on, was to remove the damaged limb from the body, that is, by amputation. A surgical operation like an amputation was always successful. The damaged limb was removed; however, the risk of not surviving an amputation at that time was approximately 50%! Joseph Lister performed a lot of tests with chemicals that had a destructive and killing effect on microorganisms, mostly bacteria. He used his knowledge to reduce the possible risk of infection and death by washing the skin of the operation area, washing all instruments to be used during surgery, and also washing the surgeons' hands. Lister was also aware of the fact that microorganisms did not only live and exist on the skin surface; he realized that they also could be found in the air surrounding and on the patient, that is, in the operating theater. He developed a specially designed aerosol device that sprayed the air in the operating theater with a disinfectant solution.

Lister's favorite disinfectant was a phenol compound, carbolic acid, which was known to kill microorganisms. However, this disinfecting compound could also kill humans, which was not so good for the surgeons who on a daily basis were operating in this environment. Joseph Lister is stated to be the father of asepsis, which in general terms could be explained as "keep the clean, clean" or "keep the sterile, sterile." In other words, handle things and work in such a way that you do not contaminate the things with which you work.

1.1.3 From air and space to GMP—Good manufacturing practice

Even though the discovery and knowledge of microorganisms in the eighteenth and nineteenth centuries was mainly used within the hospital sector, the first real clean rooms were not developed until the 1950s and 1960s, and furthermore clean rooms were not intended for hospitals. The first clean rooms were used within the air and space industry during the space race between the United States and the former Soviet Union.[2] It was soon discovered that quite a lot of problems arose when trying to get space rockets into the atmosphere—a lot of time, money, and effort was destroyed due to microscopically small inert particles. These particles were too small to be observed by the naked human eye, and therefore became a huge problem for the air and space industry.[2]

During the 1960s, pharmaceutical manufacturers realized that the cleanliness used when producing medicines was not always good enough and furthermore they could not rely only on the analysis of statistical samples of the end product. Clean rooms as well as clean zones were therefore introduced and later followed by the use of good manufacturing practice (GMP).[3]

A clean room is a controlled environment used to give some form of protection. Normally the protection concerns a product, cells, tissues, patient, etc., but the protection can also be directed toward the production and/or handling process as well as the personnel performing the work. All of these parts are considered in this introductory chapter of this book.

The protection or protective requirements are normally directed toward an item or a patient, in order not to contaminate, destroy, or in any other way have a negative influence. In some circumstances, the protective requirements also are a government requirement, for example, when using clean rooms in the pharmaceutical or hospital sectors, especially when working with certain types of cells and tissues.

1.2 What is a clean room and why are clean rooms used?

As stated before, a clean room is a room that is used to create a clean environment for things that will take place inside the room. The definition of a clean room used today is stated in a standard, ISO 14644-1, with the title "Clean Rooms and Other Clean Environments,"[4] and looks as follows:

> A clean room is a room in which the concentration of particles in the surrounding air is controlled, and which is constructed and used in such a way to minimize the introduction, the generation as well as the retention of particles inside the room.

Further to this definition the standard also states: "In some cases it is necessary to control other parameters such as temperature, humidity and pressure." When looking at this definition, it states that we shall control the concentration (number) of particles in the room. The definition does not say anything concerning particles on surfaces, if the particles in the room are dead particles or microorganisms, if there are other types of contaminates, such as molecular ones, etc. The purpose of defining a clean room as in this document is done because the ISO 14644 standards are generic. This means that the standard is not written for a specific user, that is, it is written neither for the pharmaceutical nor the microelectronics industry nor the hospital sector. The ISO 14644 standards are written to give operations or industrial branches help when needing a controlled environment. Table 1.1 shows the clean room classes as per the ISO 14644-1 clean room classifications.

Table 1.1 Clean room classification according to ISO 14644-1

	Maximum concentration limits (particles/m^3 of air) (for particles equal to and larger than the sizes shown below)					
Class	0.1 µm	0.2 µm	0.3 µm	0.5 µm	1 µm	5 µm
ISO 1	10					
ISO 2	100	24	10			
ISO 3	1000	237	102	35		
ISO 4	10,000	2370	1020	352	83	
ISO 5	100,000	23,700	10,200	3520	832	
ISO 6	1,000,000	237,000	102,000	35,200	8320	293
ISO 7				352,000	83,200	2930
ISO 8				3,520,000	832,000	29,300
ISO 9				35,200,000	8,320,000	293,000

To give a broader perspective, it is interesting to see what types of operations use clean rooms and why. Two ways to divide different clean room users are shown in Tables 1.2 and 1.3, respectively.[5] Table 1.2 comprises what is sometimes called non-GMP activities. GMP is an operation that will be explained in greater detail later on. The non-GMP activities include industries such as microelectronics, micromechanics, optics, nanotechnology, etc. Table 1.3 comprises activities called GMP activities, and includes industries such as pharmaceutical, medical device, food and beverage, biotechnology, and the hospital sector. One of the differences when looking at these two tables is what type of contaminants they are generally trying to keep out, that is, what type of contaminants can destroy their products, processes, personnel, etc.

The industries and/or activities in Table 1.2 are generally interested in keeping particulate matter away from their products, whereas the industries and other operations in

Table 1.2 Examples of operations where particles can be harmful

Operations	Example of products or items handled
Microelectronic	Cell phones, computer processors, hard disc drives
Micromechanics	Gyroscopes, precision ball bearings, CD players
Optics	Lenses, laser equipment, LCD displays
Electronics, general	Computers, TV/computer screens, high voltage cables

Note: After production/handling the products are normally tested with function tests. These are also called non-GMP operations.

Table 1.3 Examples of operations where microorganisms can be harmful

Operations	Example of products or items handled
Pharmaceutical	Tablets, ointments, injection solutions, vaccines
Medical device	Intravenous (IV) bags, IV needles, pacemakers, artificial hips
Hospitals	Operating theaters, isolations of patients, tissue banks
Food and beverage	Food and drinks

Note: After production/handling the products are tested with destructive tests and cannot be used after testing. These are also called GMP operations.

Table 1.3 are to a certain degree also interested in keeping particles away, but here, the main focus is on living particles, the ones that we normally refer to as microorganisms.

Another difference, which to a certain extent has a much bigger impact on the various activities listed in Tables 1.2 and 1.3, is what happens in the clean room after the product and/or material is ready. The finished products produced by the industries listed in Table 1.2 are tested to 100% by functional testing. A cellular phone, for example, is tested to see if it is able to do everything a phone should do like phoning, sending text messages, playing music and games, etc. The industries listed in Table 1.3, such as those within the hospital sector, normally do not perform any function tests with regard to the so-called final products, cells, or tissues. The most common tests are instead damaging tests, for example, cleanliness tests, that is, microbiological tests, chemical tests, etc. Since these tests alter the products, cells, or tissues, and often also destroy them, we cannot deliver the tested products, cells, or tissues for use. Instead of testing 100%, we work with GMP which is a mode of operation based on instructions, routines, and equipment that has been validated, that is, proved to give the desired results, time after time after time. Even though random samples are taken and analyzed, this is not good enough for the end user of the products, cells, and tissues.

In this chapter we will only deal with clean rooms, how they work and why, from a GMP perspective.

1.3 How does a clean room work?

The easiest way to explain how a clean room works is to go back to the definition of a clean room. In this it is stated that a clean room should be built and used in such a way to minimize (1) introduction of particles, (2) generation of particles, and (3) retention of particles in the room. All these three aspects must be dealt with. First of all, before discussing the three parts stated in the standard, a clean room must be hygienic, which is best explained by stating that the room must be easy to clean to the desired cleanliness level and be able to keep this cleanliness for as long as it is needed.

Going back to the definition, a clean room is equipped with one or more airlocks. These airlocks are intended to hinder particles either to enter the clean room, by using a positive pressure inside the room, or to leave the clean room, by using a negative pressure inside the room. The second part of the definition deals with minimizing the generation of particles, which is done mainly by controlling the personnel stationed in the clean room. In this case, the number of people in addition to special clean room clothing or garments used as well as the movement pattern of the personnel has a critical impact. Third and last, the standard states that we should minimize the retention of particles in the clean room, which is taken care of by the ventilation air supplied to the room. And compared to traditional rooms, such as offices and schools, a clean room is supplied with clean ventilation air as well as a higher shift rate of the air inside the room; that is, the exchange rate of the air is described as the number of times per hour that the entire volume of air is exchanged to cleaner ventilation air.

1.4 Different cleanliness levels in clean rooms

All clean rooms do not have the same cleanliness. In order to describe the cleanliness level of clean rooms, various standards are available, such as ISO 14644, previously described (see Table 1.1). Since this standard does not separate the various particles depending on if they are dead or of microbiological origin, that is, living particles, other standards must be used.

Table 1.4 Maximum number of particles per m³ of air in accordance with EU GMP, Appendix 1 of Volume 4 (2008)

	Maximum permitted number of particles/m³ equal to or larger than stated particle size			
	At rest		Operational	
Grade	0.5 μm	5 μm	0.5 μm	5 μm
A	3520	20	3520	20
B	3520	29	352,000	2900
C	352,000	2900	3,520,000	2900
D	3,520,000	29,000	Not defined	Not defined

Table 1.5 Maximum recommended number of colony forming units (CFUs) in accordance with EU GMP, Appendix 1 of Volume 4 (2008)

	Maximum number of viable organisms			
Grade	Air sample CFU/m³	Settling plate CFU/90 mm/4 h	Contact plate CFU/55 mm	Glove print CFU/5 fingers
A	<1	<1	<1	<1
B	10	5	5	5
C	100	50	25	–
D	200	100	50	–

In order to describe the cleanliness of a clean room, different types of clean room classes or grades are used. One of the most common used norms is the European GMP.[6] In this norm, Appendix 1 of Volume 4, with the title "Manufacture of Sterile Medicinal Products," contains two tables of interest (Tables 1.4 and 1.5).[6] Table 1.4 comprises clean room grades and the maximum allowed number of particles in air suspension within a clean room, whereas Table 1.5 defines the maximum levels of microbiological contaminants stated as colony forming units (CFUs) for the same clean room grades. Even though the majority of the numbers stated in Table 1.4 are taken directly from ISO 14644-1 clean room standards, under the subtitle "Clean room Classification," the clean room class nomination in the ISO standard is not used. Instead, when working with the grades presented in the EU GMP, the correct way to state the cleanliness levels is by using Grade A, B, C, or D, respectively.

1.5 *Clean rooms for microbiological control*

The EU GMP is one of the most commonly used GMPs around the globe. The structure of the limit values, both for particles as well as for microorganisms, gives a broader perspective as compared to other documents. The various grades A, B, C, and D are used for different activities, as explained next.

Grade A is the cleanest grade and Grade D is the least clean one. Let's start with the least clean one, Grade D. A Grade D room is a clean area for carrying out less critical stages, for example, washing, drying, and packaging of goods to be used later on in Grade C, B, or A. This type of clean room is also used for the production of oral products and for bulk production.

Grade C is also a clean area for carrying out less critical stages in the manufacturing of sterile products, especially when producing sterile products through terminal sterilization, that is, when the clean product is sealed and the packaging is sterilized as a final step of the process.

Grade B is used for aseptic preparation and filling, and is the background environment for the Grade A zone.

Grade A is a local zone for high-risk operations, for example, filling zone, stopper bowls, open ampoules and vials, and making aseptic connections. Normally such conditions are provided by a laminar air flow in the workstation.

1.5.1 Why are clean rooms used for handling cells and tissues?

Since a few years back, at least in the European Union, demands were stated that when handling critical cells and tissues, the surrounding environment should be under better control. Experts within the EU decided that critical cell and tissue laboratories and clinics should follow the basic clean room demands stated within the EU GMP, Appendix 1 of Volume 4.

The directive from the EU states in short the following in the annex dealing with air quality and cleanliness[7]:

1. If the work comprises handling tissues and cells in a system that is not closed, the handling should be performed in an environment with a specifically stated air quality and cleanliness that will minimize the risk for contamination. Measures should be taken to assure that the air quality is evaluated and monitored.
2. If nothing else is stated in item 3 below, the air quality during handling should, with no subsequent inactivation of microorganisms, correspond to Grade A (Annex 1 of the European Guideline for GMP; European Guide to Good Manufacturing Practice).
3. The background environment should be suitable for handling, according to item 1. In regard to particles and microorganisms, it should at least correspond to Grade D as per Annex 1 of the European Guideline.
4. An environment that does not fulfill the demands in item 2 above is acceptable if:
    a. A validated method for inactivating microorganisms or terminal sterilization is used.
    b. It can be shown that exposure in a Grade A environment has a negative impact on the tissue and cell quality.
    c. It can be shown that the manner in which the tissues and cells are to be used means that the risk of transferring a bacterial infection or mold infection to the receiver is significantly lower compared to the transplantation.
    d. It is not technically possible to perform the handling in a Grade A environment because specific equipment is needed that is not in compliance with Grade A.

1.6 How are clean rooms constructed?

As stated before, clean rooms can be used to protect the things handled and the handling process as well as the personnel performing the work. When discussing the definition of a clean room, there are three additional parameters of interest to control. These are temperature, humidity, and pressure. Not all of these three parameters are controlled in every clean room, but one parameter that must always be used is pressure. The general rule is that if you have a need to protect the tissues and cells in a clean room, you work with a positive pressure in the room. This positive pressure will minimize the possibility of contaminants to automatically enter the clean room. If, on the other hand, you have a need to protect personnel or people in the environment outside the clean room, you work with a negative pressure, in order to contain contaminants inside the clean room. In the following context we will only consider systems used to protect tissues and cells from contaminants and, furthermore, only deal with clean rooms having a positive pressure.

Clean rooms are, as stated before, rooms in which the concentration of particles and to a certain extent other contaminants are controlled in order to allow the handling of tissues and cells without having a negative influence on the material handled. A clean room is equipped with one or more airlocks, which are used to minimize the risk of contaminants entering the clean room unopposed. For this, different systems are possible:

1. For a Grade D clean room, normally one airlock is needed (Figure 1.1). The clean room has an air quality corresponding to Grade D, whereas the airlock has an air quality corresponding to Grade CNC/D. CNC is short for Controlled Not Classified.
2. For a Grade C clean room, two systems apply, as shown in Figures 1.2 and 1.3. In Figure 1.2, the clean room has an air quality corresponding to Grade C, and the one

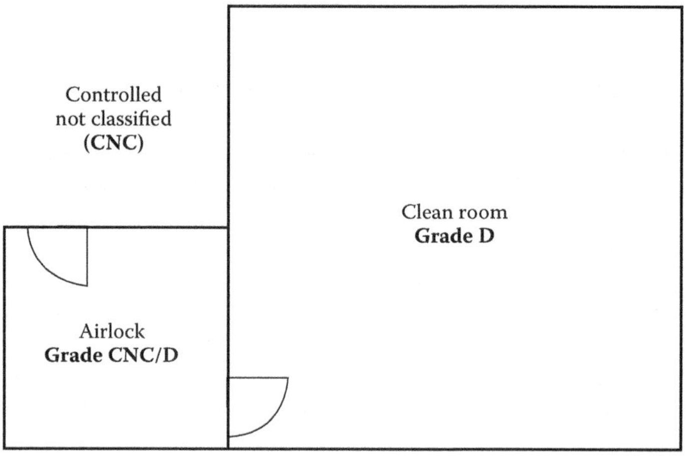

Figure 1.1 Schematic illustration of a clean room Grade D equipped with one airlock.

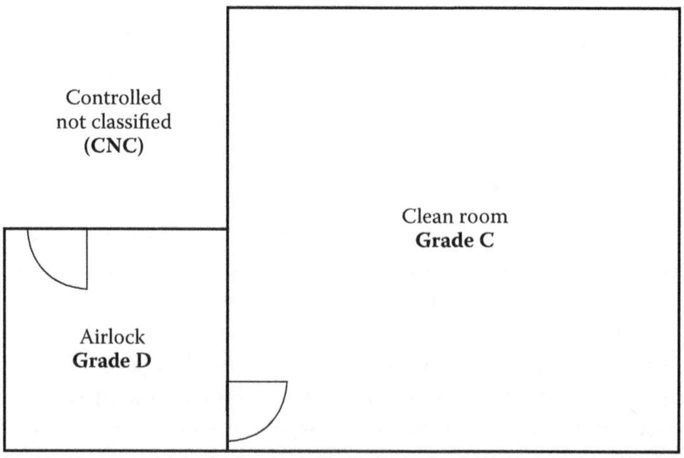

Figure 1.2 Schematic illustration of a clean room Grade C with one airlock.

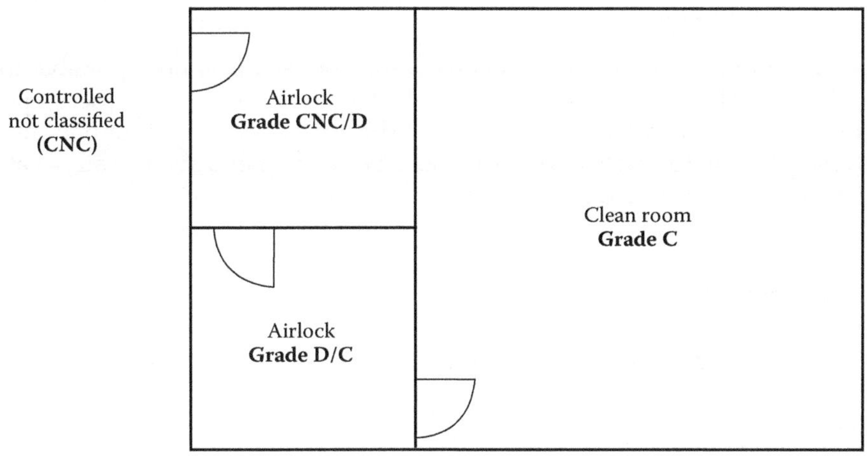

Figure 1.3 Schematic illustration of clean room Grade C with two airlocks.

and only the airlock has an air quality corresponding to Grade D. In Figure 1.3, the clean room is equipped with two consecutively placed airlocks. The clean room has a Grade C air quality, whereas airlock 2 has a Grade C/Grade D air quality. Airlock 1 has an air quality corresponding to Grade CNC/D, leading out toward either a CNC or non-controlled (NC) environment.

3. For a Grade B clean room, several system solutions are possible, similar to those discussed for Grade C clean rooms.

1.7 Clean zones

1.7.1 Introduction

When first clean rooms were first used, they normally comprised one big room only. Many different activities and work were performed in this room, all of them having different demands on cleanliness. However, the work station in that room had the highest demand on cleanliness, which led to a lower demand of cleanliness of the entire room, in order to fulfill the demands. In practice, this meant that all the other work stations in that room had a much higher level of cleanliness. This resulted in a higher cost, much more and heavier coverage of clean room garments, a higher frequency in cleaning, etc.

In order to minimize this suboptimal situation of having one room only, the principle of a room in a room was created, that is, clean rooms having a higher cleanliness were built inside a less clean clean room. One limitation of this system is that each clean room in another clean room needs airlocks for the personnel to prepare for entering the clean room. At that time, a lot of effort was put into the development of local zones by having a higher level of cleanliness as compared to the clean room itself. This is how the concept of clean zones started. In the beginning, two systems were developed, one to be used for product protection and one for the protection of the personnel. The first type of clean zone was developed for product protection, which was originally called an open bench or a laminar air flow (LAF) bench. The other clean zone used for the protection of personnel was called a safety bench, and only offered protection for the personnel working with materials that could have an adverse influence on them.

1.7.2 Clean zones today

Today, the concept of clean zones has evolved enormously. It is now possible to protect nearly every aspect of hazardous work, that is, protect the product and process, personnel; double protection, namely, protection of both product/process and personnel; and furthermore, it is also possible to create a totally enclosed environment, such as an isolated zone.

Clean zones can be divided into subparts:

- Product protection
- Personnel protection

There are many names for product protection zones:

- Opened benches
- LAF benches
- Unidirectional flow (UDF) benches
- Unidirectional air flow (UDAF) benches
- Clean air benches

Normally these clean zones are called LAF or UDF benches. These are found in two versions depending on the flow pattern of air through the working chamber of the bench:

- Horizontal
- Vertical

The horizontal benches were the first to be used, but unfortunately it was shown that the personnel and the work that was undertaken on the bench had a negative influence on the air flow, which led to a protection that was not as good as desired. The vertical bench was then developed and shown to lack many of the negative aspects of the horizontal one.

The horizontal LAF/UDF bench, as shown in Figure 1.4, has an internal fan that draws the air from the surrounding environment, normally a clean room, into the bench. The air is directed to a plenum situated at the back of the equipment and then forced through a HEPA-filter and is allowed to flow in a UDF flow through the work area, passing the product. The air in the work bench is then let out into the room in which the bench is placed. This type of equipment only gives protection to the product and the process performed inside the clean zone. There is no protection whatsoever for the operator or the personnel situated inside the room.

The vertical bench has a similar function, as shown in Figure 1.5. The fan placed inside the bench is drawing air from inside the room and allowing it to pass through a HEPA-filter situated at the top of the work zone. The air is flushed into the work area and finally leaves the bench into the room in which it is placed. There is no personal protection, only protection of product and process.

Even though the vertical product-protecting bench offers a better solution than the horizontal one, it cannot be used when dealing with processes requiring heat. This includes work that requires hot surfaces, Bunsen burners, and sealing equipment for plastic bags, to name a few. The upward thermal air from the heat source will meet the downward clean air and turbulence is created, which will lead to a suboptimal environment and loss of desired air quality.

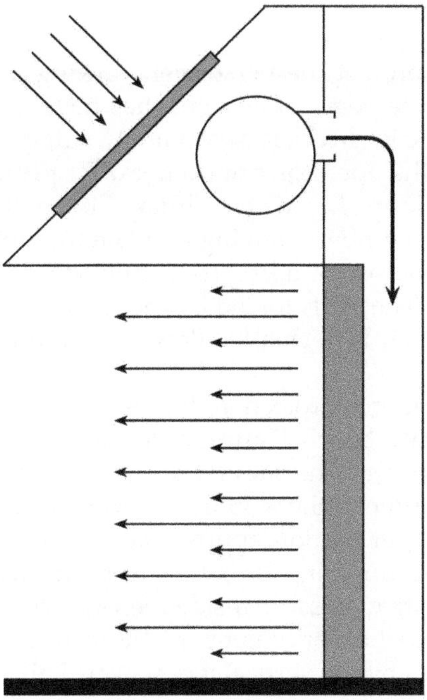

Figure 1.4 Schematic illustration of a horizontal LAF (UDF) unit. This unit is used for product protection only.

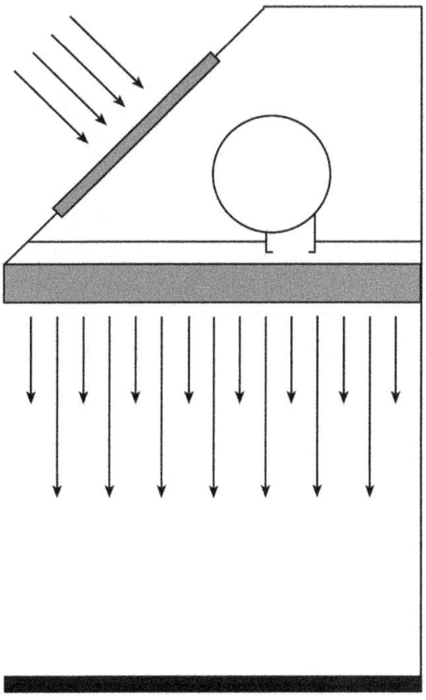

Figure 1.5 Schematic illustration of a vertical LAF (UDF) unit. This unit is used for product protection only.

1.7.3 Safety benches

Safety benches are used to protect the personnel working in the clean zone and in the vicinity of the bench. Over the years, safety benches have gone through many developments and today are available in three classes, namely, safety bench class I, II, and III.

Class I benches protect the operator, but do not offer protection to the items handled in the bench. As shown in Figure 1.6, the fan situated inside the bench creates a negative pressure inside the working chamber, drawing air from the surrounding room into it. This air has the same quality as the surrounding room and will therefore not give any protection to the product handled. The air is forced by the fan through a HEPA-filter situated at the top of the bench, and the air is normally allowed to continue out of the room through a separate ventilation outlet.

Class II benches supply double protection, that is, they protect both personnel and the product being handled inside the bench. Figure 1.7 depicts a schematic illustration of a class II bench. It is equipped with two fans. The one on the top left is used to evacuate a portion, normally one-third, of the air volume in the working chamber through a HEPA-filter. The other fan takes care of the remaining air portion, approximately two-thirds of the total volume, and forces it through a HEPA-filter, directing it downward to the bench surface. The air that has been evacuated creates a negative pressure inside the work chamber, which is compensated by outside air that is drawn into the work chamber. This incoming air is not "clean," but it protects the operator and is forced by the vertically downward airflow to enter perforated holes in the front of the bench. This incoming outside air circulates in a hollow part of the bench. Class II safety benches have a vertically downward flow of clean air, exactly as the vertical LAF bench, and thus cannot be used in connection with processes requiring heat.

The class III bench is a totally or semi-totally enclosed workspace, normally called an isolator or restricted area barrier system (RABS). This type of safety bench supplies

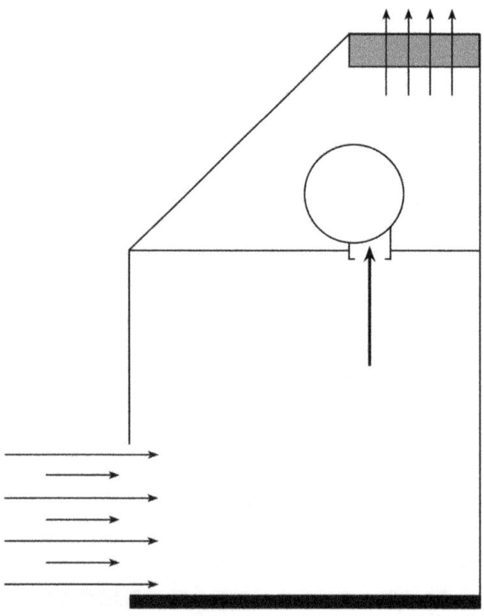

Figure 1.6 Schematic illustration of a class I safety cabinet. This unit is solely used for the protection of the operator and will not protect the product handled.

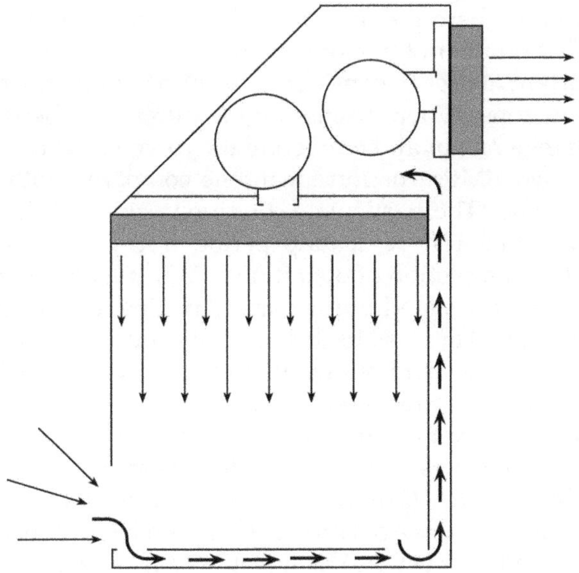

Figure 1.7 Schematic illustration of a class II safety cabinet. This unit will, if used correctly, give protection to the product handled as well as the operator performing the work in the cabinet.

protection for both product and personnel. In the beginning, isolators were developed for handling extremely dangerous chemical substances or microorganisms, but over the years they have been used more and more in microbiological laboratories, for example, sterility testing. In the future, isolators or better-developed class II safety benches are likely to be more common both in industry as well as hospitals. This is due to the fact that they supply a higher security and require lower background cleanliness. At least grade D background air environment is needed for this type of safety bench.

Even though clean zones can be used in fully uncontrolled environments in order to achieve better cleanliness standards, total cleanliness should be the ultimate goal of all processes that take place inside such benches. Total cleanliness depends on the surroundings where the bench is placed. This means that the cleaner the background environment, the higher the safety for the things being handled. In some clean room applications, for example, IVF laboratories, there is a need to use larger equipment inside the clean zones. These items have an enormous impact on the flow or air inside such a zone, and will therefore also create a higher risk for contamination of the cells handled.

1.7.4 How clean rooms and clean zones are described

When describing a clean room and a clean zone, it is not only important to state the cleanliness class or grade. There are two more important aspects to consider. One is to define what operation state the clean room is in because there are three different operation states, namely, (1) as built, (2) at rest, and (3) operational.[4]

"As built" is defined as "the condition where the installation is functioning in the defined operating mode without equipment and personnel." "At rest" is defined as "the condition where the installation is installed and operating, complete with production equipment but with no operating personnel present." Lastly, the "operational state" is defined as "the condition where the installation is functioning in the defined operating mode with the specified number of personnel working."

The second important aspect to consider is to specify how much air is introduced in the room and the clean zone. When discussing the differences between various types of clean rooms, the exchange rate of air supplied to the room should be noted. There are differences between the two GMPs, the European one compared with the U.S. FDA cGMP. The European GMP states, "The particulate conditions given in the table for the 'at rest' state should be achieved after a short 'cleanup' period of 15–20 minutes (guidance value) in an unmanned state after completion of operations." When looking at the U.S. FDA cGMP, it states what nearly all GMPs stated in the past: "An adequate air change rate should be established for a clean room. For class 100,000 (ISO 8) supporting rooms, airflow sufficient to achieve at least 20 air changes per hour would be typically acceptable. For areas of higher air cleanliness, higher air change rates will provide an increased level of air purification."

When it comes to significant clean zones, there is also a difference between the two GMPs. The European GMP states, "Laminar air flow systems should provide a homogeneous air speed of 0.36–0.54 m/s (guidance value) at the working position in open clean room applications. The maintenance of laminarity should be demonstrated and validated."

When it comes to the U.S. FDA cGMP, it states, "Air in critical areas should be supplied at the point of use as HEPA-filtered laminar flow air at a velocity sufficient to sweep particles away from the filling/closing area and maintain unidirectional airflow during operation. The velocity parameters established for each processing line should be justified and appropriate to maintain unidirectional airflow and air quality under dynamic conditions within a defined space."

1.8 Particle generation in clean rooms

As stated before, a clean room is a room that is constructed and used in such a way as to minimize the introduction, generation, and retention of particles. We have thus far discussed how to minimize the introduction, which in short is done by using airlocks and positive pressure inside the clean room. We have also discussed how to minimize the retention of particles in a clean room, which is obtained by using a highly effective ventilation system that is capable of diluting and drawing particles out of the room and the clean zone.

We will now discuss how to minimize the generation of particles inside a clean room.

There are two major sources of particles with a huge impact on the cleanliness of a clean room, namely, people present inside the room and the activities performed.[8–10]

Let's start with the personnel. It has long been known that humans generate and disperse heavy amounts of particles, such as skin parts, microorganisms, small bits of hair, etc. During the space race, NASA in the United States in particular conducted many tests and their results are still used today. A human being sitting totally still without talking is said to disperse approximately 100,000 particles of a size ≥0.3 μm per minute. When the person becomes more physically active, the numbers increase, as shown in Table 1.6. Even though we generate and disperse a lot of particles, including microorganisms, we can enter and perform work properly in a clean environment such as a clean room. For this, three key aspects have to be followed:

1. Use of correct garment
2. Correct number of personnel
3. Correct personnel behavior

Table 1.6 Number of particles emitted by a person at different degrees of activity

Personnel activity	Particle emission per minute (equal to and larger than 0.3 µm)
No movement, sitting, or standing	100,000
Light movement	500,000
Heavy movement	1,000,000
Change position	2,500,000
Slow walk 2.0 mph (0.9 m/s)	5,000,000
Normal walk 3.5 mph (1.6 m/s)	7,500,000
Fast walk 5.0 mph (2.2 m/s)	10,000,000

The garment used in clean rooms positively impacts cleanliness in three ways. It is clean enough, it acts as a filter in order to collect particles generated by the person, and finally, it minimizes the need to use private clothing in clean rooms. The better the personnel gowning, the better the filtration efficiency. This is why the various clean room grades need different garments. If we take a closer look at what is recommended in the European EU GMP, Appendix 1 of Volume 4, the following is stated for each clean room grade[6]:

- Grade D: "Hair, and whenever relevant, beard should be covered. A general protective suit and appropriate shoes or overshoes should be worn. Appropriate measures should be taken to avoid any contamination coming from outside the clean area."
- Grade C: "Hair, and whenever relevant, beard and moustache should be covered. A single or two-piece trouser suit, gathered at the wrists and with high neck and appropriate shoes or overshoes, should be worn. They should shed virtually no fibers or particulate matter."
- Grade A/B: "Headgear should totally enclose hair and, where relevant, beard and moustache; it should be tucked into the neck of the suit; a face mask should be worn to prevent the shedding of droplets. Appropriate sterilized, non-powdered rubber or plastic gloves and sterilized or disinfected footwear should be worn. Trouser-legs should be tucked into the footwear and garment sleeves into the gloves. The protective clothing should shed virtually no fibers or particulate matter and retain particles shed by the body."

It further states, "Outdoor clothing should not be brought into changing rooms leading to grade B and C rooms. For every worker in a grade A/B area, clean sterile (sterilized or adequately sanitized) protective garments should be provided at each work session. Gloves should be regularly disinfected during operations. Masks and gloves should be changed at least for every working session."

The number of people in a clean room also has a huge impact on the total cleanliness. It is easy to understand that if a clean room works well and is clean enough for four people, and that this number increased to six people, there is a risk that the number of particles released inside the room would not be taken care of by the ventilation system. Lastly, concerning behavior in the clean room, every operation has its own rules and instructions concerning what you are allowed as well as not allowed to do. The general view on the behaviors of personnel in a clean room covers the following[8]:

1. Personal hygiene
2. What is allowed to be brought into the clean room
3. Movement pattern

Personal hygiene is of significant importance. Good personal hygiene is often comprised of:

- A full body wash on a daily basis.
- Wash your hair on a regular basis.
- Clean and well groomed nails.
- All clothing shall be clean, including underwear.
- All hair should be covered by a hair protection.
- Men should be clean shaved; alternatively use a beard cover.

A central part within the personal hygiene is hand hygiene, as follows:

- You should frequently wash your hands.
- You should dry your hands thoroughly.
- In some cases you should also disinfect your hands.

Hand washing rules are often tied to the operation and also apply if you wear gloves in the clean room. The operator should wash hands:

- Before leaving/exiting the room
- After a break for eating, drinking, resting, etc.
- After using the toilet
- After coughing or sneezing
- After handling something that is contaminated

References

1. Lister J. On the antiseptic principle in the practice of surgery, *Brit Med Assoc J* 1867; 2: 246.
2. Anon. Clean room and work station requirements. Federal Standard 209, Federal Drug Administration, Washington DC.
3. Anon. Milestones in U.S. food and drug lay history, FDA backgrounder: Current and useful information from Food and Drug Administration. Food and Drug Administration, Rockville, MD, 1995.
4. Clean rooms and Associated Controlled Environments—Part 1: Classification of Air Cleanliness, ISO 14644-1. International Organization for Standardization (ISO), Geneva, Switzerland, 1999.
5. Ramstorp M. Microbial contamination control in pharmaceutical manufacture. In: *Microbiology and Sterility Assurance in Pharmaceuticals and Medical Devices*, Saghee M.R., Sandle T., and Tidswell E.C. (Eds.), Business Horizons, New Delhi, India, 2010, pp. 615–700.
6. The Rules Governing Medical Products for Human and Veterinary Use, Volume 4, Annex 1 "Manufacture of Sterile Medicinal Products," The European Commission, Brussels, 2008.
7. Commission of the European Parliament, 2004. Directive 2004/23/EC of the European Parliament and of the Council of March 31, 2004 on setting standards of quality and safety for the donation, procurement, testing, processing, preservation, storage and distribution of human tissues and cells. http://eur-lex.europa.eu/LexUriServ/LexUriServ.do?uri=CELEX:32004L0023:EN:NOT (accessed March 15, 2015).
8. Austin PR. *Encyclopedia of Cleanrooms, Biocleanrooms and Aseptic Areas*, Contamination Control Seminars, Livonia, MI.
9. Ramstorp M. *Introduction to Contamination Control and Cleanroom Technology*. Wiley VCH Verlag GmbH, Weinheim, Germany, 2000.
10. Ramstorp M, Gustavsson M, and Gudmundsson A. Particles generated from humans—A method for experimental studies in cleanroom technology. *J Indoor Air* 2005; 15 (suppl. 11): 1572–6.

chapter two

Clean room technology

An overview of clean room classification standards

Raul A. Sadir, Adriano Villarmosa, and Luciano Figueiredo

Contents

Abstract

Clean rooms and controlled environments provide different air cleanliness levels, which are essential to many manufacturing, health, and pharmaceutical sectors that require control of environmental pollutants. The steps involved in the implementation of a clean room or controlled environment comprise: (1) needs assessment with regard to the operation and/or process; (2) risk analysis; (3) design; (4) installation; (5) balancing the air system; (6) testing; (7) operation; and (8) monitoring and maintenance. This chapter is dedicated to explaining the key variables in clean room implementation and air cleanliness classification according to the International Standardization Organization (ISO) 14644 standard.

2.1 Clean room implementation: An overview

The user specification requirements will define the clean room's intended use. In the human in vitro fertilization sector, the control of environmental pollutants should include removal of both particulate matter, which may carry microbials, and volatile organic compounds (VOC), which have been associated with poor embryo development.[1,2] In this sense, the most suitable layout for the specific procedures, routines, and work demands are determined. A set of standards and regulations will guide design and fabrication.[3]

The proper material for fabrication is selected, which should take into consideration the ultimate application of the clean room and the chemical products to be utilized for aseptic cleaning. The design must consider "how" and "what" services should be provided to the clean room, such as water supply, air, and specialty gases.

On completion of fabrication and installation, a validation process is carried out. At this stage, the clean room must be tested to make sure it is operating as per the design specifications. Usually, fine-tuning adjustments are done to ensure proper balancing of the airflow and adjustment of the pressure differential between different rooms. After validation at both rest and operational states, periodic tests must be conducted to monitor the clean room's performance and to ensure it keeps operating in accordance with optimal design conditions. Briefly, the following tests are carried out after the system has been balanced and the room thoroughly cleaned: downstream airflow rate, particle counting, room pressure differential measurement, air temperature and humidity, and noise level assessment.[4] These issues will be considered elsewhere within this book.

The proper operation of the clean room environment is mandatory to prevent contamination during specific procedures or manufacturing processes. To achieve such a level of operational accuracy, periodic air monitoring tests must be carried out at the appropriate times. Additionally, there must be strict procedures for controlling personnel, equipment, and materials accessing the clean room. Personal hygiene and proper attire should be used in accordance with the personal protective equipment (PPE) and collective protective equipment (CPE) standards adequate for each specific application, including lab coats, coveralls, gloves, masks, head caps, shoe covers, biosafety cabinets, etc.

2.2 International standards for clean room classification

The international standardization organization (ISO) 14644 is the main standard on clean rooms and controlled environments.[5] The norm is divided into 10 parts, which cover the following topics:

- Part 1: Classification of air cleanliness

  This section defines ISO classes to be used in determining air cleanliness of the clean rooms and associated controlled environments. This standard also describes the standard method for testing, as well as the procedure for determining the concentration of airborne particles.
- Part 2: Testing and monitoring specifications for attesting continuous compliance with ISO 14644-1

  This section provides information, including necessary intervals, for clean room testing to confirm its compliance with the ISO 14644-1 standard.
- Part 3: Test methods

  It presents a description of methods that can be used for testing a clean room and ensuring it is indeed operating properly.

- Part 4: Design, fabrication, and start-up
  This section provides guidelines on how to design, build, and prepare a clean room for customer delivery.
- Part 5: Operations
  The basic requirements for operating a clean room or controlled environment are presented.
- Part 6: Terminology
  This section compiles all the definitions of words listed in the individual parts of the ISO related to clean rooms and associated controlled environments.
- Part 7: Separation/partition devices (clean air partitions, isolators, mini-environments)
  This part provides information on advanced technology clean air devices, such as isolators and mini-environments.
- Part 8: Classification of molecular airborne contamination
  The means to classify the concentrations of specific chemical substances suspended in the air, and test methods are indicated.
- Part 9: Classification of particles cleanliness in surfaces
  This section provides means to classify, and includes additional information about particle contamination in surfaces.
- Part 10: Classification of chemical substances cleanliness in surfaces
  This part provides guidelines to classify and includes additional information on surface contamination by chemical substances.

The former U.S. Federal Standard 209 was the first to establish how classification of clean rooms was to be made.[6] Despite being withdrawn in 2001, the U.S. Federal Standard 209 is still widely used. Moreover, this standard served as a basis for the current ISO 14644-1:1999—Clean Rooms and Associated Controlled Environments—Part 1: Classification of Air Cleanliness.[7] Table 2.1 provides classes of air cleanliness for airborne particles in clean rooms and clean areas according to ISO 14644-1:1999.

The ISO classification shown in Table 2.1 is based on the following equation:

$$C_n = 10^N \times \left[\frac{0.1}{D}\right]^{2.08}$$

where:

C_n is the maximum concentration allowed (in particles/m³ of air) of airborne particles in the air that are equal to, or greater than, the size considered for the particle. C_n is rounded up, using at least three significant figures.

N is the number of ISO classification, which cannot be greater than 9. Numbers of intermediary classifications can be specified, using 0.1 as the smallest increment allowed for N.

D is the size considered for the particle in μm.

0.1 is a constant with a dimension of μm.

The former Federal Standard 209 takes into consideration the number of particles per cubic feet of air for clean room classification. In contrast, classes of cleanliness are based on the number of particles per cubic meter of air according to ISO 14644-1 (Table 2.2).

Table 2.1 Classes of air cleanliness for airborne particles in clean rooms and clean areas according to ISO 14644-1:1999

ISO classification	Maximum concentration limits (particles/m^3 of air) for particles equal to and larger than the sizes shown below					
	≥0.1 μm	≥0.2 μm	≥0.3 μm	≥0.5 μm	≥1.0 μm	≥5.0 μm
ISO Class 1	10	2				
ISO Class 2	100	24	10	4		
ISO Class 3	1000	237	102	35	8	
ISO Class 4	10,000	2370	1020	352	83	
ISO Class 5	100,000	23,700	10,200	3520	832	29
ISO Class 6	1,000,000	237,000	102,000	35,200	8320	293
ISO Class 7				352,000	83,200	2930
ISO Class 8				3,520,000	832,000	29,300
ISO Class 9				35,200,000	8,320,000	293,000

Table 2.2 Comparison between cleanliness classes in accordance to the former standard FS 209 and the current ISO 14644-1:1999

Norm	Cleanliness class					
ISO 14644-1	3	4	5	6	7	8
FS 209	1	10	100	1000	10,000	100,000

According to ISO standard 14644-1:1999, there are three different occupancy situations for clean room classification, as follows:

As built: defines a clean room in which installation is complete and the room is fully operational, but equipment and personnel are nonexistent.

At rest: the installation is complete with the air system installed and operational as per customer and supplier specifications. Equipment is included, but no personnel are actually working within the facility.

In operation: in this situation, the installation is fully operational as per design specifications, including equipment and personnel.

ISO 14644-1:1999 also includes a clean room classification method for particle sizes outside those specified in Table 2.1. Smaller particles (e.g., ≤0.1 μm), for instance, known as ultrafine particles, should be controlled in semiconductor industries, while large particles (≥5.0 μm), know as macro particles, are important for automotive industry (painting process) and hospitals.

2.3 *Design and fabrication*

Nowadays, technology advances with regard to construction materials and accessories have made it possible to build clean rooms and controlled environments for most user requirement specifications. Some key features of clean room construction include:

- Walls and ceilings hermetically sealed.

- Internal surfaces must be smooth, easy to clean and impact resistant, as well as being able to withstand attack and penetration of chemical process, cleaning supplies, disinfecting products, and water.
- Some clean room applications require fabrication with antistatic materials or low VOC emission materials.

Clean room design must comply with the following characteristics:[3]

1. Airflow obstruction should be avoided. Columns and wall protrusions/indents should be kept at a minimum; rectangular- or square-shaped rooms are preferable. The design should minimize airflow turbulence, making it easier to drag and remove airborne particles.
2. The construction material should be selected among those with low particle generation and retention. Surfaces should be coated with the most appropriate paint. Wood and non-sealed light fixtures that may require constant cleaning are not recommended. Likewise, knurls or grooves in window sills and door frames should be avoided. Porous flooring with grout, wood lockers, electrical motors, foot rests in work benches, fibrous cabling insulation, and electrical wall switches are to be avoided as well.

   On the contrary, round corners between floor and wall, and wall and ceiling are recommended to minimize particle retention. Epoxy base coatings for painting walls and ceilings, or stainless steel and laminated panels suitable for clean rooms are preferable. Sealed light fixtures embedded in the ceiling are also recommended. Doors with embedded hinges should be made of stainless steel, glass, or plastic suitable for clean rooms. Auxiliary systems such as compressed air, vacuum, ductwork, electrical network, etc., must be properly fitted to walls, ceilings, and floors.

2.4 Air filter properties and classification

Air filters are classified according to the European standards EN-779 (coarse/pre-filters, medium, and fine filters) and EN-1822 (EPA, HEPA, and ULPA filters) (Tables 2.3 and 2.4).[8,9]

Pre-filters (or coarse filters) are used for filtering particles greater than 10.0 μm. Such filters are rated according to their gravimetric efficiency as G1, G2, G3, and G4 (Table 2.3). Gravimetric efficiency is used to measure efficiency by comparing the relative weight of the particles retained by the filter against the total weight of particles emitted.

Fine and medium filters are used for filtering particles greater than 1.0 μm. Filter rating, namely, M5, M6, F7, F8, and F9, is in accordance with their spectral efficiency. Spectral efficiency is measured by counting downstream particles after filter challenge with diethylhexyl sebacate (DEHS) aerosol and a reference particle size of 0.4 μm.

Table 2.3 Coarse filter grading system as per the European Standard EN 779:2012

Coarse filters	
Grade	Gravimetric efficiency
G1	$50 \leq Am < 65\%$
G2	$65 \leq Am < 80\%$
G3	$80 \leq Am < 90\%$
G4	$Am \leq 90\%$

Note: Am: "Arrestance Moyenne" (average retention).

Table 2.4 Medium and fine filter grading system as per the European Standard EN 779:2012

Medium and fine filters	
Grade	**Spectral efficiency DEHS 0.4 μm**
M5	40 ≤ Em < 60%
M6	60 ≤ Em < 80%
F7	80 ≤ Em < 90%
F8	90 ≤ Em < 95%
F9	Em ≤ 95%

Note: Em: "Efficacité Moyenne" (average efficiency).

EPA and HEPA filters, rated as E10, E11, E12, H13, and H14 according to their efficiency grade, are used for filtering particles greater than 0.3 μm. In contrast, ULPA filters are used for filtering particles greater than 0.12 μm. The latter are rated as U15, U16, and U17 according to their efficiency grade. EPA, HEPA, and ULPA filter efficiency is determined by the most penetrating particle size (MPPS) method. The method is based on the filter efficiency, determined by laser measurement, to retain the most penetrating particles (normally between 0.1 and 0.2 μm) (Table 2.5).

Activated carbon filters are used for filtering gases such as CO_2, alcohols, aldehydes, refrigerating gases, acetone, styrene, benzene, and toluene. Activated carbon is best for removing compounds with high molecular weight, such as benzene, toluene, and xylene. Polar molecules, like aldehydes, will adsorb with weak bonds. Hence, oxidizing media may be necessary for situations involving high aldehyde concentrations. The usual carrier medium is alumina, which is made by treating aluminum ore to make it porous and highly adsorptive. Alumina is usually impregnated with potassium permanganate to create a powerful oxidizing media. These media bind gases, which are then chemically broken down by oxidation.

The importance of VOC air filtration to assisted reproductive technology (ART) relies on the fact that materials used inside the laboratories release variable amounts of VOCs, which have been associated with embryo toxicity. Installation of VOC filters is therefore

Table 2.5 EPA, HEPA, and ULPA filter grading system as per the European Standard EN 1822:2009

EPA, HEPA, and ULPA filters				
	Integral value MPPS		Local value MPPS	
Grade	Efficiency	Penetration	Efficiency	Penetration
E10	≥85%	15%	–	–
E11	≥95%	5%	–	–
E12	≥99.5%	0.5%	–	–
H13	≥99.95%	0.05%	99.75%	0.25%
H14	≥99.995%	0.005%	99.975%	0.025%
U15	≥99.9995%	0.0005%	99.9975%	0.0025%
U16	≥99.99995%	0.00005%	99.99975%	0.00025%
U17	≥99.999995%	0.000005%	99.9999%	0.0001%

Note: EPA: efficiency particulate air filters; HEPA: high efficiency particulate air filters; MPPS: most penetrating particle size; ULPA: ultra low penetration air filters.

recommended in the extraction points for return air that will be recirculated in the clean room or controlled environment.[1,2]

In a basic three-stage air filtration system for airborne particulate matter, incoming air first goes through the coarse/pre-filters stage, which is responsible for filtering larger particles. These inexpensive filters will provide initial contamination control, and have to be replaced often. In daily operations, the method used to determine whether pre-filters need to be replaced (when saturation level is reached) is visual; the darker the filter, the dirtier it is, which means that the filtration media is saturated. The second-stage filtration utilizes fine-dust filters to remove fine particles. The combination of second- and first-stage filtration allows filtered air to reach the HEPA filters at an optimal cleanliness grade. The method used for assessing the saturation level of fine-dust filters is by means of assessing the air pressure drop (ΔP). In some controlled environments, the second-stage filtration is enough to provide adequate contamination control. Last, the third-stage filtration comprises HEPA filters that are responsible for filtering smaller particles. HEPA filters are essential for clean room classification. Like fine filters, the method used for assessing saturation level is by means of reading the pressure drop (ΔP).

In some specific cases, for instance, clean rooms or controlled environments related to ART facilities, VOC air filtration should be incorporated to the air particulate filtration system. Replacement of VOC filters should be done at six-month intervals.

2.5 Air filtration systems

A properly designed and implemented air filtration system will provide adequate contamination control for both particles and VOCs, thus allowing activities sensitive to contamination to be performed safely. As mentioned earlier, filtration systems for particulate matter in clean room or controlled environments basically consist of two- or three-stage air filtration. In some specific cases, such as an IVF laboratory, additional filtration to toxic gases is recommended.

2.5.1 Centralized heating, ventilation, and air conditioning (HVAC) filtration systems

Centralized HVAC filtration units combine adequate supplies of pressurized air flow with temperature and humidity control (Figure 2.1). In such systems, pre-filters are installed at the inlet of outside air. A bank of pre-filters and fine filters is assembled in a filtration box installed in the main ductwork. To complete the set, air diffusers are assembled with terminal HEPA filter units at the end of every ductwork outlet. Optionally, VOC filters are installed just after the pre-filters and also in the return air intake (Figure 2.1). In addition to the central HVAC unit, such systems rely on accessories to control airflow, including dampers, valves, diffusers, and frequency inverters. These components are essential for balancing the air system and allow for adjustments of the pressure differential between rooms.

In some situations, where space constraints do not allow for the installation of terminal HEPA filter units, it is possible to assemble a filtration box with HEPA filters installed immediately after the fine filters (Figure 2.2). This type of system can be also configured as a "bag-in-bag-out" filtration box. The main difference lies in the fact that "bag-in-bag-out" filtration boxes can be wrapped in plastic bags, ready for disposal, whenever filter replacement is needed. This model prevents direct contact of maintenance personnel with filters that may be impregnated with contaminants. "Bag-in-bag-out" filtration boxes are

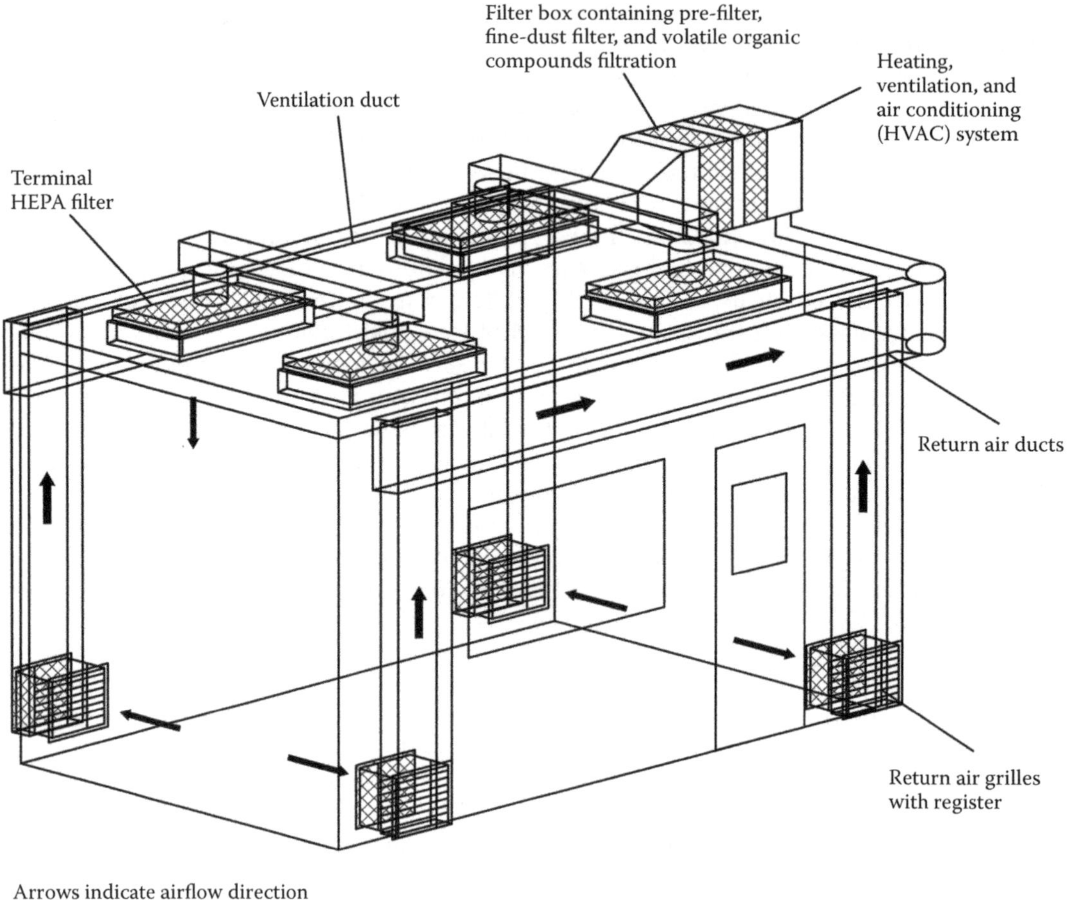

Figure 2.1 Illustration depicting a classic example of centralized air filtration system.

normally used in pharmaceutical industries, in which manufacturing processes release contaminants that may impregnate into the filters.

2.5.2 Compact filtration systems

For small areas and/or low budget facilities, compact air filtration systems are available (Figures 2.2 and 2.3). These systems have been particularly adopted in facilities where an existing structure has to be adapted but space constraints exist. Nowadays, several manufacturers offer compact air filtration systems. Depending on the user specification requirements, such systems may provide effective air filtration at low cost.

Compact air filtration systems normally use individual equipment for supplying filtered air to up to two rooms or environments with a maximum area of 20 m^2 (215 ft^2). Such systems are equipped with pre-filters, HEPA filters, and even activated carbon filters, and operation involves high airflow and high air renewal rates by taking in outside air. In addition to air filtration, temperature and humidity control, as well as positive pressurization to allow maintenance of pressure differential between rooms are provided by compact systems.

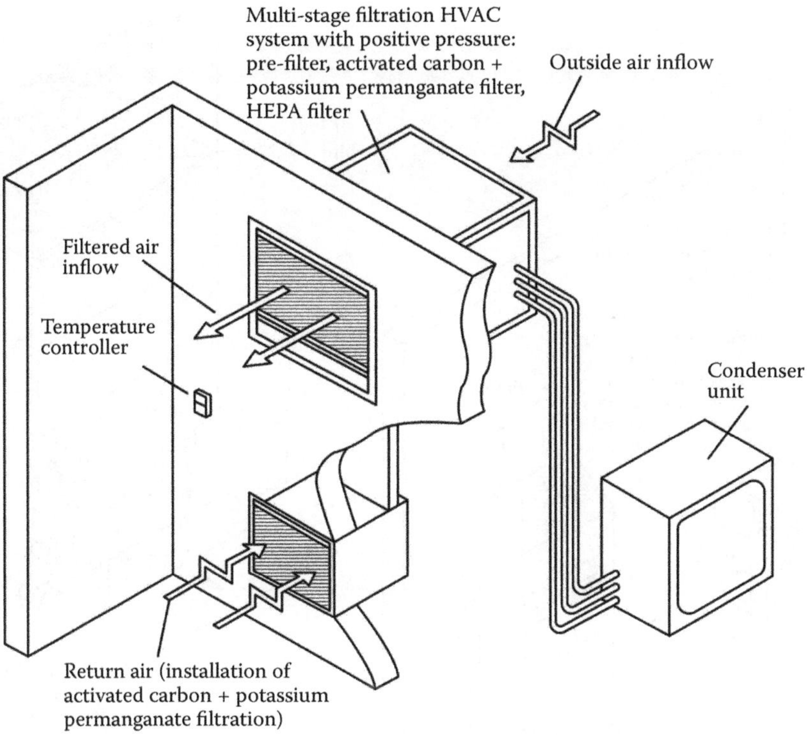

Figure 2.2 Illustration depicting a compact air filtration system. The filtration unit is placed outside the clean room or controlled environment on an adjoining wall.

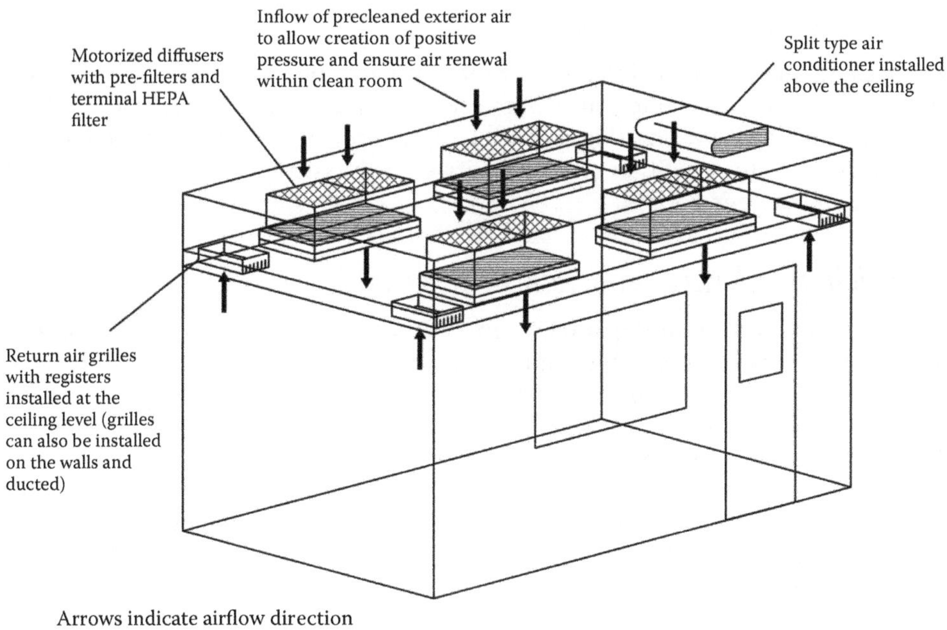

Figure 2.3 Illustration depicting a compact air filtration system using fan units.

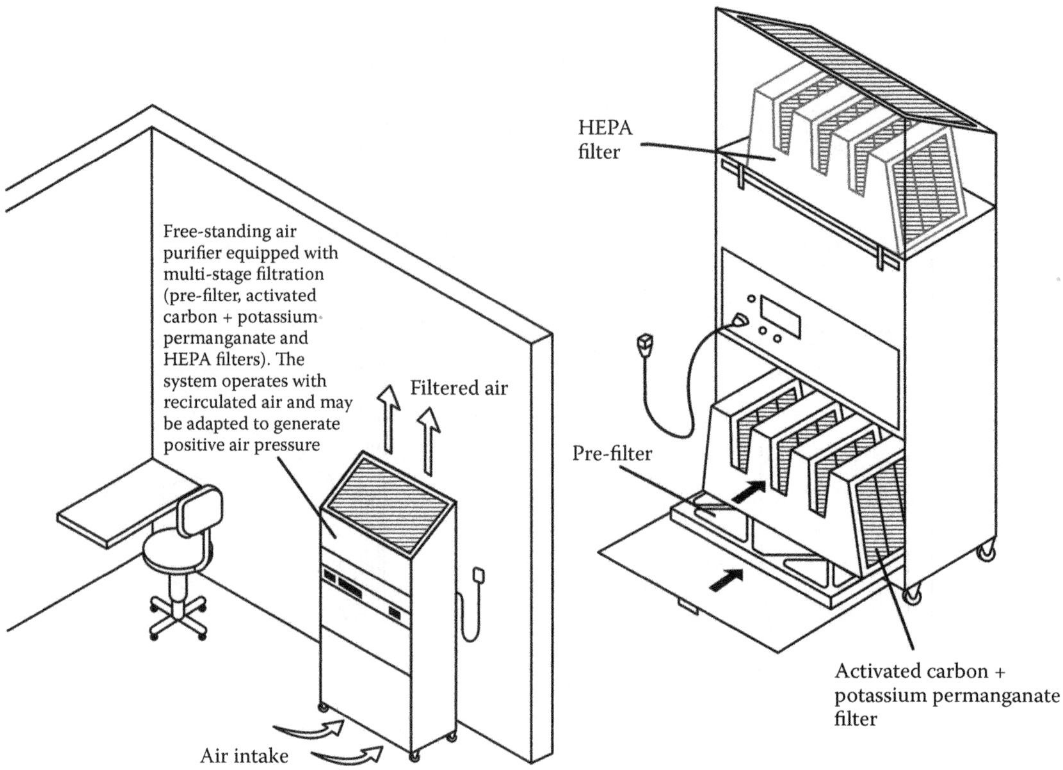

Figure 2.4 Illustration depicting a portable four-stage free-standing air filtration system.

2.5.3 Portable filtration systems

Portable systems are installed inside the room or controlled environment. Such systems comprise a three-stage (pre-filter, fine filter, and HEPA) or four-stage (pre-filter, fine filter, VOC filter, and HEPA) filtration (Figure 2.4). Unlike centralized HVAC and compact units, portable filtration systems neither supply positive air pressurization nor allow for air pressure differential between rooms.

2.6 Which air filtration system to choose?

The most suitable air system depends on three main factors: (1) the air cleanliness class to be achieved; (2) the main purpose of the controlled environment; and (3) the risks that the product and/or process will involve. On completing this preliminary risk assessment, the structural conditions are also analyzed taking into consideration if it is an existing or new facility. Also important is to define what type of air is to be filtered, that is, how polluted the air is where the facility is located. This analysis should include concentration levels of particulate matter and toxic gases. Equally important is to define the budget to be invested in air filtration and whether specific regulatory requirements are to be followed. This assessment will provide information for the engineering and design teams to recommend the best cost-effective system to the installed.

Industrial applications such as aerospace, micro-electronics, automotive painting, pharmaceutical, medical appliances, food, and healthcare are among the products and/or processes that can benefit from air filtration and contamination control. All of the above have, at some point, one or more critical stages that require some level of air contamination control.

2.7 Care of air filtration system and maintenance schedule

Filter replacement should follow design specifications. Periodic maintenance schedules vary according to the types of particulates and chemicals being filtered and the relative contamination, both outside and inside the location where the system is installed. Maintenance periodicity is a very common query by final users, and manufacturers usually argue against specific time frames for filter replacement. It is better to first recording a log history of testing results to better determine filter changes according to each application. In new installations, it is recommended that testing be carried out in short intervals to monitor the actual condition of each filtration stage. Hence, filter changes are done according to the need of each filtration stage. Usually it takes about two years of operation to collect enough data; the customer and maintenance service will then have enough information about the actual conditions of the system.

It is worth mentioning that when a given filtration stage is saturated, all filters within that particular filtration stage must be replaced. Otherwise, the system will be unbalanced and will not operate as per the design specifications.

Replacing pre-filters or medium filters in the right time will extend the life of the fine filters. The same concept applies for replacing fine filters to protect and extend the life of the HEPA filters. A well-established and evidence-based replacement schedule, in addition to keeping the system running as per design specifications, reduces maintenance costs.

2.8 Air quality requirements according to the Brazilian Cell and Tissue Directive (BCTD)

In Brazil, units conducting in vitro manipulation of human gametes and embryos, including in vitro fertilization (IVF) treatments, are obliged to comply with specific regulatory requirements, including air filtration in critical areas where gamete and embryo manipulation take place. Such regulation was made effective by the Brazilian Health Surveillance Agency (ANVISA) in 2006 and subsequently revised in 2011.[10] A detailed description and critical analysis of the BCTD is provided elsewhere within this book (Chapter 18).

Briefly, clean room or controlled environments should be provided to operating theaters where oocyte collection and sperm retrieval are carried out, and reproductive laboratories. Compliance with the BCTD requires a separate changing room and a physical barrier preventing access to the aforesaid critical areas. A scrubbing area for hand hygiene is mandatory and it should be located between the changing room and the operating theater.

As far as air filtration is concerned, the minimum requirements are as follows:

2.8.1 Oocyte, ovarian, and testicular tissue harvesting room

The room should have a positive air pressure differential in relation to the adjoining areas. The ambient temperature and relative humidity should be controlled and kept between 23°C and 27°C (73.4°F and 80.6°F) and 40% and 70%, respectively. The total airflow rate of at least 18 $(m^3/h)/m^2$ (1 cubic feet per minute [cfm]/ft^2) should be supplied to the room, and incoming air must be filtered by at least G4 filters. At least 6 $(m^3/h)/m^2$ $(0.33\ cfm/ft^2)$ airflow should be supplied by outside air.

2.8.2 *Sperm processing room*

In situations where sperm processing is carried out outside the IVF laboratory, the minimum requirements are as follows: Ambient temperature and relative humidity should be controlled and kept between 21°C and 27°C (70.8°F and 80.6°F) and 40% and 70%, respectively. Air supplied to the room should be filtered using at least G3 grade filtration. Such rooms should be equipped with biosafety cabinets (Class II Type A1) with its work area classified as ISO class 5, and processing of specimens should be carried out within such controlled environments.

2.8.3 *IVF laboratory*

The room should have a positive air pressure differential in relation to the adjoining areas. The ambient temperature and relative humidity should be controlled and kept between 23°C and 27°C (73.4°F and 80.6°F) and 40% and 70%, respectively. A total airflow rate of at least 45 $(m^3/h)/m^2$ $(2.46\ cfm/ft^2)$ should be supplied to the room, and incoming air must be filtered with at least G3 filters in association with carbon activated filters and F8 filters. At least 15 $(m^3/h)/m^2$ $(0.82\ cfm/ft^2)$ airflow should be supplied by outside air. Handling of biological material, including cells, embryos, and reproductive tissue, and culture media should be carried out within biosafety cabinets (Class II, Type A1) or unidirectional air flow equipment with their respective working areas classified as ISO class 5. Alternatively, handling of biological material can be carried out in ISO class 5 clean rooms according to ISO 14644-1:1999 standards.[7]

Water sanitation stations, such as sinks, drains, or lavatories, are not allowed inside the IVF lab.

2.8.4 *Storage room for cryopreserved biological material*

Should cells or tissues storage be done in liquid nitrogen tanks or with a safety system using liquid nitrogen for freezing with temperatures of –135°C (–211°F) or below, the room must be equipped with the following: (1) a door with a glass panel; (2) a dedicated exhaust system with a minimum total airflow of 75 $(m^3/h)/m^2$ $(4.1\ cfm/ft^2)$; (3) an air supply with at least G1 grade filtration; and (4) an ambient oxygen level sensor with sound and visual alarms. Exhaust grilles must be installed at the floor level, and exhaust air discharged directly to the outside of the building.

References

1. Esteves SC, and Bento FC. Implementation of air quality control in reproductive laboratories in full compliance with the Brazilian Cells and Germinative Tissue Directive. *Reprod Biomed Online.* 2013; 26: 9–21.
2. Esteves SC, and Bento FC. Air quality control in the ART laboratory is a major determinant of IVF success. *Asian J Androl.* 2015 Nov 10. doi: 10.4103/1008-682X.166433. [Epub ahead of print]
3. White W. (ed.). *Cleanroom Technology: Fundamentals of Design, Testing and Operation,* 2nd ed., Wiley, 2010.

4. International Organization for Standardization, 2000. ISO NBR 14644-2:2006 on cleanrooms and associated controlled environments—Part 2: Specifications for testing and monitoring to prove continued compliance with ISO 14644-1. Associação Brasileira de Normas Técnicas (ABNT), Brasilia, DF, Brasil.
5. International Organization for Standardization, 1999. ISO NBR 14644:2005 on cleanrooms and associated controlled environments. Associação Brasileira de Normas Técnicas (ABNT), Brasilia, DF, Brasil.
6. Federal Standard 209E. https://set3.com/papers/209e.pdf (accessed 2/12/2015).
7. International Organization for Standardization, 1999. ISO NBR 14644-1:2005 on cleanrooms and associated controlled environments—Part 1: Classification of Air Cleanliness. Associação Brasileira de Normas Técnicas (ABNT), Brasilia, DF, Brasil.
8. EN-779:2012. Particulate air filters for general ventilation. http://www.freudenberg-filter.com/fileadmin/templates/EN_downloads/CI/EN779_CI_02_IN_126_October_2012_EN_low.pdf (accessed 2/12/2015).
9. EN 1822:2010. High efficiency particulate air filters (HEPA and ULPA). http://www.tripleair-technology.com/downloads/The-new-series-of-BS-EN-1822.pdf (accessed 2/12/2015).
10. ANVISA. Brazilian National Agency for Sanitary Surveillance, 2006. Resolução no. 33 da Diretoria colegiada da Agência Nacional de Vigilância Sanitária (amended by RDC23 of 27 May 2011 on setting standards of quality and safety for the donation, procurement, testing, processing, preservation, storage and distribution of human tissues and cells). http://bvsms.saude.gov.br/bvs/saudelegis/anvisa/2011/res0023_27_05_2011.html (accessed 8/11/2015).

chapter three

The critical role of air quality

Novel air purification technologies to achieve and maintain the optimal in vitro *culture environment for IVF*

Kathryn C. Worrilow

Contents

Abstract

Successful preimplantation embryogenesis and the reproductive potential of the human embryo are critically dependent on a number of variables including the changing organic chemistry of the ambient air within the *in vitro* fertilization (IVF) laboratory. New data has indicated that a significant yet delicate balance exists between the dynamic and changing nature of the laboratory ambient air and the effects it may exert on successful embryogenesis. The continual advancement of assisted reproductive technologies (ARTs), such as the extended culture of the genomically active human embryo and the return of a single embryo to the patient, demand a more critical environment. The origin of the ambient air serving an IVF laboratory is often a combination of outside fresh or source air and the air recirculated from the IVF laboratory and clinical procedure rooms. Each source of ambient air is perpetually dynamic in its contribution of airborne chemical and biological pathogens to the *in vitro* culture environment. Activities occurring outside the IVF laboratory cannot be controlled by the IVF program and contribute a significant level of embryotoxic chemical and biological contaminants to the laboratory environment. This chapter will discuss the most prevalent embryotoxic constituents within outside source and recirculated air, the role of volatile organic compounds (VOCs), viable and nonviable particulates in preimplantation toxicology, and finally, novel mechanisms by which the variable of air can be comprehensively controlled and eliminated, thereby providing the opportunity to maximize clinical outcomes and the level of patient care offered.

3.1 Introduction

Human conception involves the coordination of a complex cascade of biochemical and molecular intracellular signaling events between human gametes, resulting in the production of viable embryos capable of implantation and the establishment of a viable pregnancy. The physiological continuum involved in the *in vitro* culture of the human embryo constitutes one of the most challenging applications of cell culture technology. Successful preimplantation embryogenesis is critically dependent on the culture environment provided by the IVF laboratory. With the exception of the pioneering work of Cohen, Hall, Gilligan, and Boone, there have been few studies focusing on a significant source of environmental influence, the laboratory ambient air.[1–6] Human embryos are largely unprotected as they lack physical barriers typically provided by epithelial surfaces, immunological defense mechanisms, and detoxifying mechanisms provided by a functioning liver. It is highly likely that gametes and embryos grown *in vitro* are more sensitive to environmental influences than are complex organisms with more developed mechanisms for protection. Many incubators utilized in the *in vitro* culture of human embryos consist of 90–95% ambient air. Although the use of tabletop incubators, time-lapse digital imaging, and other such protocols offer a slight reduction in the level of exposure to ambient air, these chambers are not air-tight and many of the supporting processes still necessary in IVF allow direct exposure of the tissue culture media and oil to the constituents of the ambient air. New and significant data have demonstrated a critical association between levels of chemical and biological pathogens in the laboratory ambient air, their influence on epigenetic processes, and the role they play in preimplantation toxicology toward successful embryogenesis, implantation, and conception.[7–9]

Most IVF programs incorporate varying mechanisms of air filtration towards the protection of their *in vitro* culture environment. It is most common to use a combination of adsorbing activated carbon, oxidizing potassium permanganate ($KMnO_4$), and high efficiency particulate air (HEPA) filtration with positive pressure, and an adequate number of air changes per hour within the laboratory and clinical space. Recent data has indicated that the use of carbon, $KMnO_4$, and HEPA filtration, alone or in combination, is inadequate in remediating VOCs, viable particulates, and nonviable particulates to the levels necessary for an optimal *in vitro* culture environment.[6,7,9,10] These systems are also challenged and often overwhelmed by the large number of sources of airborne contaminants common to most IVF programs. Filters and filter media are not absolute. They are dynamic in that they are influenced by the environment to which they are exposed. It has been demonstrated that HEPA filtered laboratory air can carry far greater levels of VOCs and threatening contaminants than unfiltered outside air.[2] Equipment, instrumentation, and personnel activities within the IVF laboratory are significant sources of off-gassing and therefore can emit high levels of VOCs into the air environment.[1–3,11,12]

Laboratory personnel, alone, constitute one of the greatest sources of bioburden, adding bacteria, viruses, and mold spores to the culture environment.[12] The design of the IVF laboratory, heating, ventilation, and air conditioning (HVAC) and air purification systems are therefore critical in determining the future success of human embryogenesis and clinical outcomes.

The necessity of exceptional air quality and an independent air handling system is also influenced by the progressive development of ARTs. One such technological advancement involves the return of a single embryo or blastocyst to the patient. The blastocyst must be supported and maintained outside of the female reproductive tract for five to six days versus the more typical two to three days employed in standard IVF protocols. The transfer of a single blastocyst increases the likelihood of a singleton pregnancy, reduced obstetrical complications, and reduced likelihood of neonatal intensive care for the infant. The goal of many providers within the ART community is to transfer only one embryo to each patient to better assure a healthier outcome for both the mother and the infant. Extended periods of embryo culture dictate enhanced culture environments including but not limited to the laboratory and incubator ambient air and the supporting media and tissue culture oil. A suboptimal laboratory or culture environment will compromise preimplantation embryogenesis, the production of viable blastocysts and, therefore, successful implantation and conception.

3.2 Constituents of ambient air: Outside source and recirculated air

The outside source or fresh air component of the ambient air serving the IVF laboratory and clinical procedure rooms is influenced by a number of activities both common to and outside of the control of the IVF program. Common occurrences include but are not limited to road and rooftop resurfacing, construction, vehicle traffic and exhaust, industrial emissions, waste management, restaurant exhaust, accidents, generator exhaust, and seasonal pollutants. Construction incidents generate numerous embryotoxic VOCs, including ketones, aldehydes, benzenes, alkenes, formaldehyde, acetone, toluene, and styrene.[12–14] The placement of new asphalt on a road, parking lot, or onto a medevac landing pad releases significant levels of the embryotoxic VOCs, acrolein and toluene.[12] Vehicle exhaust contains multiple classes of VOCs including sulfur dioxide, formaldehyde, and nitrogen oxides.[1,15] A large number of embryotoxic VOCs are also of biogenic sources such as trees, shrubs, and vegetation. Biogenic sources of VOCs can be both significant and seasonal in their impact. In addition to the overwhelming contribution of VOCs, these common activities are also a source of significant viable and nonviable particulates.

Within the IVF laboratory, there are a number of common sources of VOCs, viable and nonviable particulates.[12] Sterile tissue cultureware emit embryotoxic styrene, ethylbenzene, and benzaldehyde; compressed gases contain embryotoxic levels of freon, benzene, and xylene; refrigerants contain chloroethane and dichlorodifluoromethane; and common cleaning and fixation materials contain isopropyl alcohol and acetone.[1,3,11,16,17] The IVF laboratory and clinical staff are also a common source of high levels of VOCs, viable and nonviable particulates.[12,18] New equipment as well as construction materials used in the building of the laboratory and clinical areas may offer sources of airborne pathogens. Gasketing, caulking, paint, floor and ceiling materials, pressed particle board, adhesives, and bonding materials can each contribute to the VOC burden within the IVF laboratory and clinical spaces.[13,14,19–21] These sources can also require a lengthy period of time to fully and properly off-gas. While there are additional sources of airborne pathogens beyond those discussed, many are unavoidable as they are present in protocols and materials necessary to perform the various processes involved in IVF.

3.3 *Airborne pathogens: Volatile organic compounds*

3.3.1 *The role of volatile organic compounds (VOCs) in preimplantation toxicology*

A number of studies have evaluated the impact of ambient air quality on specific measures of human embryogenesis and clinical outcomes. Pioneering work led by Cohen, Hall, Gilligans, and Boone, and others have clearly linked the presence of VOCs and biologicals or viable particulates with compromised embryo development and clinical outcomes.[1–6] Numerous studies have demonstrated that low levels of VOCs within the IVF laboratory compromised clinical outcomes.[1–3,5,6] VOCs encompass those contaminants specific to chemically active compounds and can be highly embryotoxic. Studies exploring the mechanisms of action of VOCs have demonstrated that VOCs can attach directly to DNA during embryonic growth and development.[22,23] Furthermore, increased DNA fragmentation has been linked to increased levels of episodic air pollution and VOCs.[24] Hall and his colleagues identified an inverse relationship between mouse embryo development and varying acrolein concentration.[2] Acrolein is highly embryotoxic as it is both water soluble and carries the ability to impact the molecular mechanisms associated with cell replication.[13,18,25,26] The rate of entry of VOCs into growth media and tissue culture oil is dictated, in part, by the vapor pressure and coefficient partition associated with the molecular structure of the VOC.[27] For example, the embryotoxic VOCs ethanol, acetone, and formaldehyde are water soluble and thus capable of partitioning into the tissue culture media whereas benzene, isobutylene, and styrene are primarily oil soluble, allowing them to remain harbored in the oil overlay of a culture dish. There are also VOCs which are considered biphasic and carry the capacity to partition into both water (media) and oil.[27] Studies have demonstrated that specific organic compounds can be absorbed by an oil overlay and shared with individual droplets of media, thus altering the composition of the culture media.[28] It has also been demonstrated that concomitant with the *in vitro* culture of human embryos in an environment containing strict control of air quality is an increase in specific measures of embryo development and clinical outcomes.[9,29–32]

A more recent study by the author and her colleagues, encompassing eight years of clinical outcomes, evaluated the dynamic levels of VOCs, and viable and nonviable particulates within the ambient air of the IVF laboratory, measures of preimplantation embryogenesis, and clinical outcomes. The study evaluated the clinical data of 950 IVF couples collected over 48 testing quarters. Qualitative and quantitative levels of airborne VOCs, and viable and nonviable particulates were evaluated during clinical operation throughout the study. Airborne VOCs and aldehydes were identified and quantitated using multiple TO-11 and TO-15 assays. Samples were collected over time in both the source air, between each stage of air filtration within the HVAC system, and during operation within the IVF laboratory. Microbial bioaerosol assays evaluated multiple samples of 150 liters of air collected over time. The assays included the use of spore trap samples and cultureable air samples. To better understand the potential impact of each stage of air filtration on clinical outcomes, the study also examined

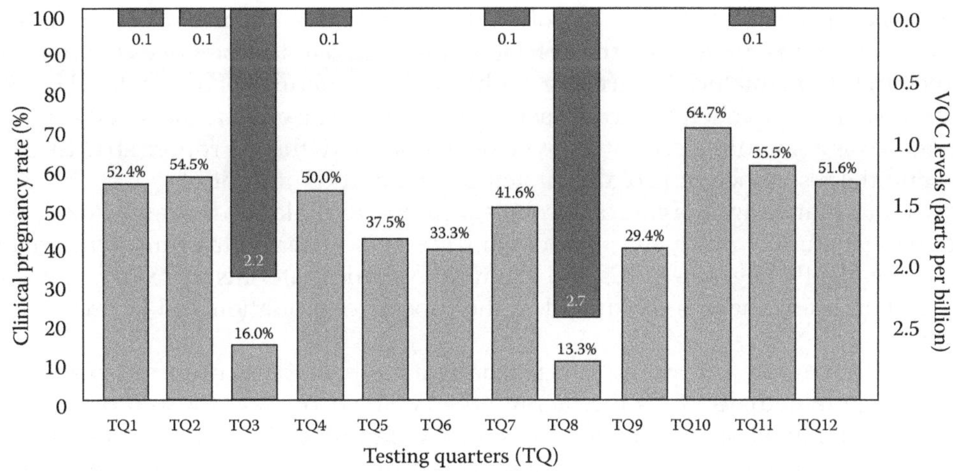

Figure 3.1 Relationship between clinical pregnancy rates (CPR) and the presence of low levels (parts per billion; ppb) of volatile organic compounds (VOCs) and chemically active compounds (CACs). The entire study evaluated 950 IVF couples and data were collected over 48 testing quarters.

the time period in which particulate, gas phase filters, and UV lamps were replaced relative to markers of preimplantation embryogenesis and clinical pregnancy rates. Using the time period in which each air purification component was changed as the dependent variable, and fertilization rates, embryo morphology, +beta hCG, and clinical pregnancy rate as the independent variables, the data were subjected to a time series analysis.

There were no statistically significant differences observed in the fertilization rates, zygote, embryo, and blastocyst morphologies associated with increased levels of VOCs. In contrast, increased levels of VOCs (Figure 3.1) were associated with a statistically significant decrease in clinical pregnancy rates.[5,6,9,10] Although criteria have not been well defined in the past, it has been generally recommended that IVF laboratories and associated clinical spaces maintain VOC levels below 300 ug/m^3. The eight-year study demonstrated that levels of VOCs far less than previously recommended could compromise clinical outcomes.[10]

3.3.2 *Mechanisms for remediation of VOCs*

There are multiple classes of VOCs. Each biochemical classification of VOCs varies in its molecular weight, size, and polarity, and thus responsiveness to agents of removal. The mechanisms of removal specific to each molecular and biochemical classification vary considerably. VOCs are not captured by HEPA filtration, as their physical size is 100 to 1000 times smaller than the effective capture rate.[16] Although additional mechanisms are necessary for the successful mitigation of a broad range of VOCs, two commonly used mechanisms involve the use of activated carbon and potassium permanganate in the protection of an IVF laboratory environment.

Activated carbon will adsorb the higher molecular weight hydrocarbon within the ambient air. Carbon contains pores of varying size, allowing materials to diffuse within its matrix. The surfaces of the pores provide a field of molecular attraction capturing and holding large flat electron-rich molecules.[33] Benzene and toluene are strong examples of such chemical species.[34] Although it is often the main line of defense in reducing overall VOC loads within the air serving the IVF laboratory, activated carbon does not hold small molecules tightly or materials carrying highly polar structures. Low molecular weight organics are not effectively removed by activated carbon. The effectiveness of the activated carbon matrix is also influenced by the type of carbon used, the micropore structure of the matrix, and the resonance time of the air, temperature, and humidity.[31]

Low molecular weight organics, alcohols, ketones, and aldehydes can be oxidized by the permanganate ion producing carbon dioxide and water. Potassium permanganate serves to chemically degrade VOCs and chemical organic materials by oxidizing the molecules. The permanganate is consumed in the process of oxidation and is irreversible in application.

Both active carbon and potassium permanganate have been used in isolation or in combination to remediate VOCs threatening the IVF environment for well over 20 years. Although each remediate particular biochemical families of VOCs, activated carbon and potassium permanganate are not able to capture or remediate all known VOCs.[27] Photocatalytic oxidation (PCO) technologies offer another commonly used means of VOC remediation. PCO technology has been used successfully for years and the details underlying the technology are discussed further in Chapter 11. Engineered molecular media have been developed specific to the protection of the human embryo and use of such media will comprehensively remediate all known biochemical families of VOCs. The use of engineered media in newer, more aggressive air purification technology and the associated clinical outcomes are discussed in greater detail in Section 3.5 of the chapter.

3.4 Airborne pathogens: Viable particulates

3.4.1 The role of viable particulates in preimplantation toxicology

In addition to the role of embryotoxic VOCs in preimplantation toxicology, data from the 8-year study also demonstrated that viable particulates or biologicals such as bacteria, viruses, and mold spores play a critical role in successful human embryogenesis.[7,10] Although significant differences were not observed in measures of preimplantation embryogenesis, there was a statistically significant relationship between the UV lamp intensity, increased levels of viable particulates, and clinical outcomes. Decreased lamp intensity was concomitant with an increased level of viable particulates and a statistically significant decrease in clinical pregnancy rates. Immediately following 9 of the 12 UV lamp change-out or replacement periods and thus an increase in lamp intensity and decrease in viable particulates, the +beta hCG and clinical pregnancy rates demonstrated statistically significant increases (Figure 3.2). The proliferation of mold within the HVAC system, ductwork, and final filters serving the IVF laboratory is common as the IVF laboratory provides the ideal temperature and humidity for such growth. Fewer than 100 fungal spores can produce multiple embryotoxic mycotoxins and fungal VOCs. Viable particulates often use nonviable particulates or microscopic dust particles as vehicles of transport. Such attachment allows a clustering of airborne biologicals within specific areas of the laboratory and clinical procedure rooms. The study conducted by the author and her colleagues demonstrated a statistically significant relationship between the presence of low levels of viable particulates and decreased clinical pregnancy rates. Recommendations specific to IVF—appropriate levels of viable particulates are not well defined. Critical to the success of an IVF program is the direct and comprehensive remediation of all viable particulates. Although playing a lesser role in preimplantation toxicology, levels of nonviable particulates should also be maintained and

UVC change-out	Post UVC change-out delta change in β hCG	Post UVC change-out delta change in CPR
UVC Δ #1	↑ 34%	↑ 29.5%
UVC Δ #2	↑ 8.3%	↑ 12.4%
UVC Δ #3	↑ 35.3%	↑ 29.4%
UVC Δ #4	↑ 11.0%	↑ 2.3%
UVC Δ #5	↑ 10.5%	↑ 24.8%
UVC Δ #6	↓ 1.1%	↑ 1.5%
UVC Δ #7	↓ 10.4%	↓ 32.9%
UVC Δ #8	↑ 10.0%	↑ 3.3%
UVC Δ #9	↑ 12.5%	↑ 25.0%
UVC Δ #10	↑ 11.7%	↑ 23.6%
UVC Δ #11	↓ 5.6%	↑ 11.1%
UVC Δ #12	↑ 41.8%	↑ 35.9%

Figure 3.2 The impact of UVC intensity on viable particulate loading and clinical outcomes (eight-year evaluation). A statistically significant relationship was demonstrated between the change-out of UVC lights, varying levels of viable particulate loading, + β hCG, and the clinical pregnancy rates. The relationship highlighted the significance of UVC intensity and longevity, and its effectiveness on ambient air bioburden levels and clinical outcomes.

controlled. Ongoing studies are exploring the mechanisms of action of viable particulates on preimplantation embryogenesis and their role in toxicology.

3.4.2 Mechanisms for remediation of viable particulates

A common mechanism of remediation for viable particulates is that of HEPA filtration. HEPA filtration is classified as achieving 99.97–99.99% effectiveness in removing particles greater than 0.3 μm in size. The efficiency of the HEPA filter can decrease to 99.94–99.95% for numerous reasons. Air bypass around the HEPA filter, the presence of a breach in integrity, or a "pin-hole" leak in the filter matrix and/or improper maintenance will allow a decrease in efficiency. Such a decrease in efficiency can allow approximately 7.2 million particles to penetrate the filter and enter the laboratory and clinical spaces.[35] Assuming that there is no bypass or breach in filter media integrity, viable particulates greater than 0.3 μm in size will be captured by HEPA filtration. Those biologicals captured on the HEPA matrix will then have the opportunity to continue to proliferate, remain viable, and enter the laboratory and clinical spaces.

Another means of remediation of viable particulates involves the use of ultraviolet light (UV). UV light serves to perturb the bacterial, fungal, and viral cell wall and destroy the DNA and RNA of the organism.[36] Vegetative bacteria are the most susceptible to UV irradiation while bacterial and fungal spores are the most resilient.[35] One, however, must be exceptionally careful as the use of the wrong wavelength, intensity, and positioning of the UV source can produce a highly toxic environment for the human embryo. Use of UV light of the C wavelength, or UVC, is the most appropriate but one must carefully evaluate the intensity, positioning, and potential byproducts generated. Some forms of UV, in combination with other media, can produce ozone and, in reaction with particular VOCs, create toxic intermediary molecules.

3.5 *Novel air purification technology and clinical outcome data*

Both recent and significant clinical outcome data (Figures 3.3 and 3.4) have demonstrated that strict adherence to the recommended levels of airborne pathogens, VOCs, viable particulates, and nonviable particulates will support an IVF laboratory capable of offering a continuum of excellence from oocyte collection through blastocyst development and, ultimately, to a viable pregnancy. Removal of airborne pathogens in the ambient air and comprehensive control of the ambient air serving the *in vitro* culture environment is critical to successful preimplantation embryogenesis. Each category of airborne pathogens demands targeted and effective mechanisms of remediation. Years of research by the author and her colleagues have allowed the development of a proprietary and targeted engineered molecular media which uses specific combinations of chemical and physical constituents to remediate all known biochemical families of VOCs. Viable particulates are inactivated and destroyed using genomically modeled inactivation and nonviable particulates are

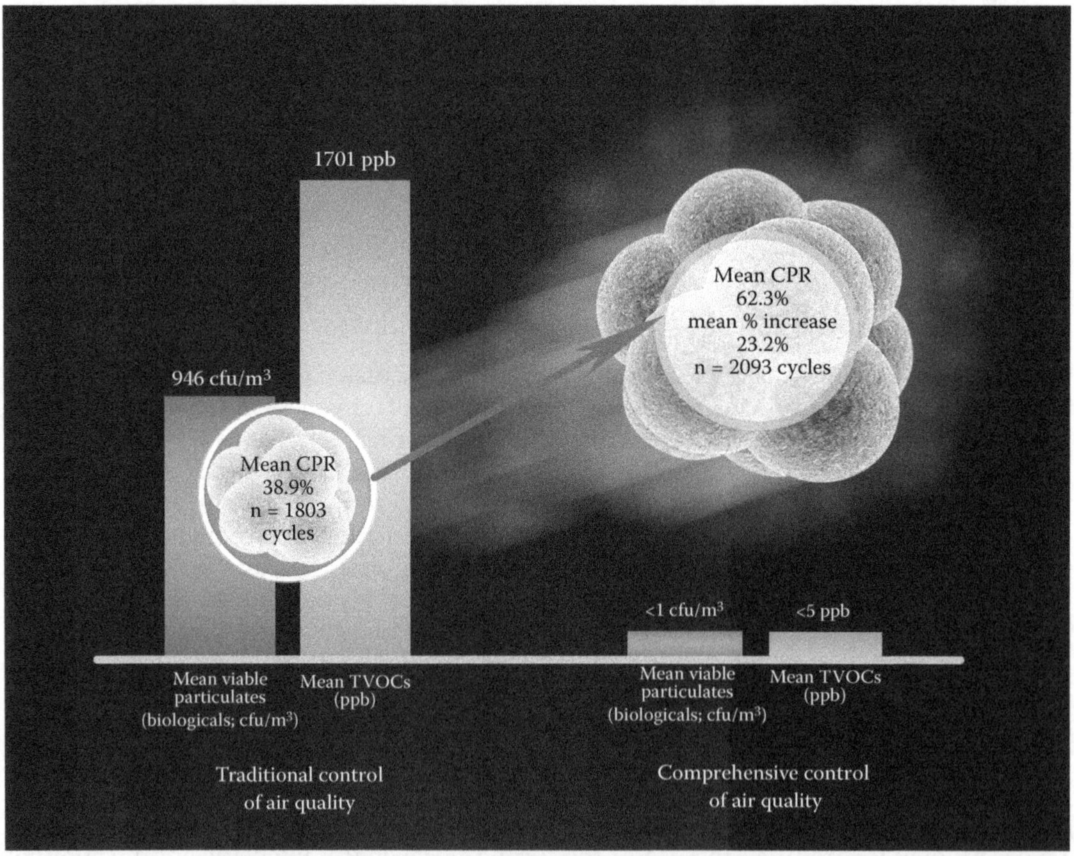

Figure 3.3 **(See color insert.)** Statistically significant increase in clinical pregnancy rates (CPR) concomitant with comprehensive control of ambient air quality; viable particulates and total volatile organic compounds (TVOCs).

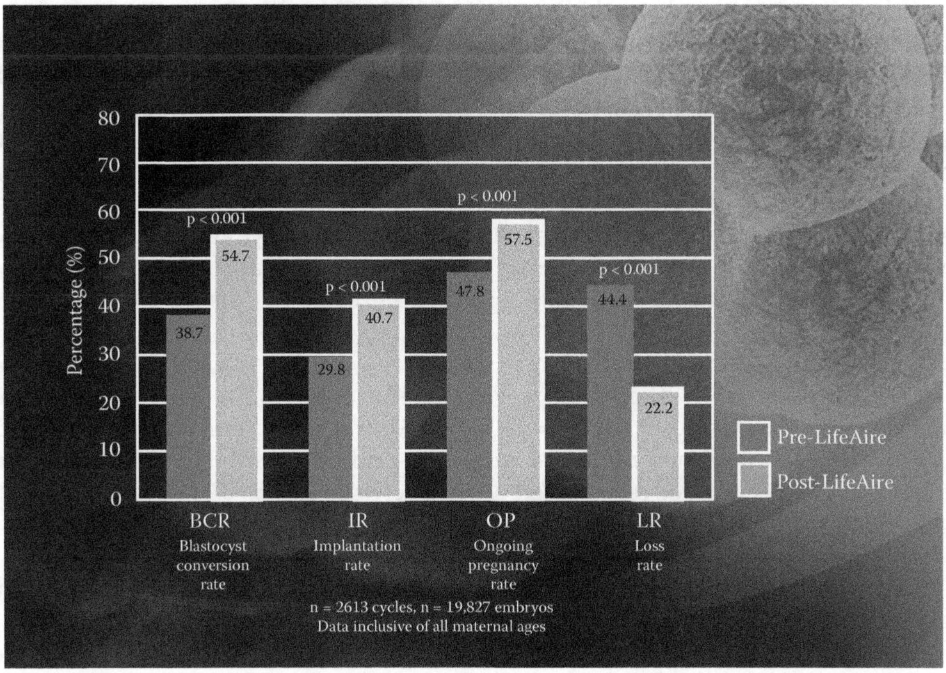

Figure 3.4 **(See color insert.)** Statistically significant increase in BCR, IR, and OP rates and statistically significant decrease in LR with comprehensive control of ambient air quality—a multi-site study including 2613 non-donor patient cycles and 19,827 embryos. The data are inclusive of all maternal ages.

captured via final filtration. The proprietary combination of media is placed within the ductwork serving and protecting the IVF laboratory and clinical space. An in-duct system was designed, as space is a premium within the IVF laboratory and clinical areas. The in-duct system targets all airborne pathogens contributed by the outside source air as well as those generated within the laboratory. An in-room air filtration system will only remove airborne pathogens once present in the space. VOCs and viable particulates can exert their negative impact on mechanisms of replication, influence epigenetic variations and embryo development in a very short time frame. Over 15 years of research has defined the ambient air criteria necessary to support the optimal *in vitro* culture environment.[9,10] Data have indicated that strict maintenance of these criteria should be maintained so as to maximize clinical outcomes.[9]

Recently launched to colleagues, the design of the dedicated air purification system has been successful in providing the optimal air to the laboratory and clinical spaces—air that meets the ambient air criteria defined for successful human embryogenesis. The technology has allowed the successful operation of IVF processes in complete isolation of the environmental influences provided by the dynamic outside and laboratory environments. Use of the novel air purification system will support an IVF laboratory environment capable of offering a continuum of excellence from oocyte collection through embryonic genome activation, blastocyst development, and embryo transfer.

A multi-center analysis of numerous IVF programs using the novel air purification technology (Aire~IVF®, LifeAire Systems) examined the impact of comprehensive control of airborne pathogens on measures of embryogenesis and patient outcomes. Clinical outcome data from all non-donor IVF patients (n = 2613) cycling through seven independent IVF programs were evaluated over a 24–36 month period. Data was collected for 1274 patients cycling in an environment protected by pre-existing mechanisms of air filtration and 1339 patients after the installation of the LifeAire Systems technology. The blastocyst conversion rate was defined by zygotes reaching the blastocyst stage by Day 5, implantation rate by positive fetal cardiac activity per transferred embryo, ongoing pregnancy by positive fetal cardiac activity, and loss rate as an intrauterine gestational sac without subsequent fetal cardiac activity. Multivariate analyses evaluated differences in patient demographics, etiology, and pre- and post-installation variables. Statistical analyses included odds ratios calculated with 95% confidence intervals and $\alpha = 0.05$ using MedCalc Software 13.1.2, Ostend, Belgium.

Embryos cultured after installation of the Aire~IVF system demonstrated a statistically significant increase in the blastocyst conversion rate (38.7% vs. 54.7% [$p = 0.001$]), implantation rate (29.8% vs. 40.7%, [$p = 0.001$]), and ongoing pregnancy (47.8% vs. 57.5% [$p = 0.001$]) from all combined maternal ages, pre- and post-Aire~IVF rates, respectively. The mean number of embryos transferred decreased from 2.38 to 2.04 ($p = 0.051$) and those embryos cultured in an Aire~IVF environment demonstrated a statistically significant decrease in loss rate (44.4% vs. 22.2% [$p = 0.001$]) (Figure 3.4).

Embryotoxic VOCs and viable particulates play a critical role in preimplantation toxicology and in the influence of ambient air on epigenetic processes. Concomitant with comprehensive removal and control of airborne pathogens within the *in vitro* culture environment was a statistically significant increase in blastocyst conversion rate, implantation rate, ongoing pregnancy, and a decrease in loss rate. Comprehensive control of the ambient air is critical to successful preimplantation embryogenesis. Ongoing studies are examining the relationship and mechanisms of action of varying biochemical families of VOCs, viable, and nonviable particulates on the regulation of early preimplantation embryo development and implantation.

References

1. Cohen J, Gilligan A, Esposito W, Schimmel T, and Dale, B. Ambient air and its potential effects on conception in vitro. *Hum Reprod* 1997; 12(8): 1742–9.
2. Hall J, Gilligan A, Schimmel T, Cecchi M, and Cohen J. The origin, effects and control of air pollution in laboratories used for human embryo culture. *Hum Reprod* 1998; 13: 146–55.
3. Cohen J, Gilligan A, and Willadsen S. Culture and quality control of embryos. *Hum Reprod* 1998; 13: 137–44.
4. Boone WR, Johnson JE, Locke A-J, Crane IV M, and Price TM. Control of air quality in an assisted reproductive technology (ART) laboratory. *Fertil Steril* 1999; 71: 150–4.
5. Worrilow KC, Huynh HT, Gwozdziewicz JB, Schillings W, and Peters AJ. A retrospective analysis: The examination of a potential relationship between particulate (P) and volatile organic compound (VOC) levels in a class 100 IVF laboratory cleanroom (CR) and specific parameters of embryogenesis and rates of implantation (IR). *Fertil Steril* 2001; 76: S15–6.
6. Worrilow KC, Huynh HT, Bower JB, Schillings W, and Peters AJ. A retrospective analysis: Seasonal decline in implantation rates (IR) and its correlation with increased levels of volatile organic compounds. *Fertil Steril* 2002; 78: S39.
7. Worrilow KC. The impact of UVC irradiation on clinical pregnancy rates in an ISO 5 cleanroom in vitro fertilization laboratory. *ASHRAE IAQ* 2009; 4–6.
8. Munch EM, Sparks AE, Van Voorhis BJ, and Duran EH. Poor air quality and its impact on early embryo development. *Fertil Steril* 2014; 101(2): S18.

9. Forman M, Sparks A, Degelos S, Koulianos G, and Worrilow KC. Statistically significant improvements in clinical outcomes using engineered molecular media and genomically modeled ultraviolet light for comprehensive control of ambient air (AA) quality. *Fertil Steril* 2014; 102(3): e91.
10. Doshi A, Karunakaran S, Worrilow KC, Varghese A. (2013). What makes an IVF lab successful? In: Varghese AC, Sjoblom P, and Jayaprakasan K (eds.). *A Practical Guide To Setting Up An IVF Laboratory*, Jaypee Brothers Medical Publishers, Ltd., London, March 2013, pp. 13–23.
11. Gilligan A, Schimmel T, Esposito Jr B, and Cohen J. Release of volatile organic compounds such as styrene by sterile Petri dishes and flasks used for in-vitro fertilization. *Fertil Steril* 1997; 68(Suppl 1): S52–3.
12. Lawrence C, Mortimer S, and Mortimer D. VOC levels in a new IVF laboratory with both central and in-laboratory photocatalytic air purification units. *Alpha Scientists in Reproductive Medicine* 2007; 36. http://alphascientists.com.
13. Brown SK. Chamber assessment of formaldehyde and VOC emissions from wood-based panels. *Indoor Air* 1999; 9: 209–15.
14. De Bortoli M, Kephalopoulos S, Kirchner S, Schauenburg H, and Vissers H. State-of-the-art in the measurement of volatile organic compounds emitted from building products: Results of European interlaboratory comparison. *Indoor Air* 1999; 9: 103–16.
15. Vrashney CK, Padhy PK. Total volatile organic compounds in the urban environment of Delhi. *J. Air Waste Manag Assoc* 1998; 48: 448–53.
16. Esteves SC, Gomes AP, and Verza Jr S. Control of air pollution in assisted reproductive technology laboratory and adjacent areas improves embryo formation, cleavage and pregnancy rates and decreases abortion rate: Comparison between a class 100 (ISO 5) and a class 1000 (ISO6) cleanroom for micromanipulation and embryo culture. *Fertil Steril* 2004; 82: S259–60.
17. Hyslop L, Prathalingam N, Nowak L, Fenwick J, Harbottle S, Byerley S et al. A novel isolator-based system promotes viability of human embryos during laboratory processing. *PLos ONE* 2012; 7(2): 1–11.
18. Johnson JE, Boone WR, and Bernard RS. The effects of volatile compounds (VC) on the outcome of in vitro mouse embryo culture. *Fertil Steril* 1993; 60(Suppl 1): S98–9.
19. Lundgren B, Jonsson B, and Ek-Olausson B. Materials emission of chemicals—PVC flooring materials. *Indoor Air* 1999; 9: 202–8.
20. Sparks LE, Guo Z, Chang JC, and Tichenor BA. Volatile organic compound emissions from latex paint—Part 1–chamber experiment and source, model development. *Indoor Air* 1999; 9: 10–17.
21. Chang JC, Fortman R, Roache N, and Lao HC. Evaluation of low VOC latex paints. *Indoor Air* 1999; 9: 253–8.
22. Dadvand P, Rankin J, Rushton S, and Pless-Mulloli T. Association between maternal exposure to ambient air pollution and congenital heart disease: A register-based spatiotemporal analysis. *Am J Epidemiol* 2011; 173(2): 171–82.
23. Meng Z and Zhang LZ. Chromosomal aberrations and sister-chromatid exchanges in lymphocytes of workers exposed to sulfur dioxide. *Mutat Res* 1990; 241(1): 15–20.
24. Rubes J, Selevan SG, Evenson DP, Zudova D, Vozdova M, Zudova Z et al. Episodic air pollution is associated with increased DNA fragmentation in human sperm without other changes in semen quality. *Hum Reprod* 2005; 20(10): 2776–83.
25. Little SA and Mirkes PE. Relationship of DNA damage and embryotoxicity induced by 4-hydroperoxydechosphamine in postimplantation rat embryos. *Teratology* 1990; 41: 223–31.
26. Zitting A and Heinonen T. Decrease of reduced glutathione in isolated rat hepatocytes caused by acrolein acrylonitrile, and the thermal degradation products of styrene copolymers. *Toxicology* 1980; 17: 333–51.
27. Lillo-Rodenas MA, Cazorla-Amoros D, and Linares-Solano A. Behaviour of activated carbons with different pore size distributions and surface oxygen groups for benzene and toluene adsorption at low concentrations. *Carbon* 2005; 43(8): 1758–67.
28. Miller KF and Pursel VG. Absorption of compounds in medium by the oil covering microdrops cultures. *Gam Res* 1987; 17: 57–61.

29. Esteves S, Verza Jr S, and Gomes AP. Comparison between International Standard Organization (ISO) type 5 and type 6 cleanrooms combined with volatile organic compounds filtration system for micromanipulation and embryo culture in severe male factor infertility. *Fertil Steril* 2006; 86: S353–4.
30. Knaggs P, Birch D, Drury S, Morgan M, Kumari S, Sriskandakumar R, and Avery S. Full compliance with the EU directive air quality standards does not compromise IVF outcome. *Hum Reprod* 2007; 22: i164–65.
31. Boone WR and Higdon III HL. Quality control management. In: Nagy ZP, Varghes AC, Agarwal A (eds.). *Practical Manual of In Vitro Fertilization: Advanced Methods and Novel Devices,* Springer, New York, 2012, pp. 33–39.
32. Esteves SC and Bento FC. Implementation of air quality control in reproductive laboratories in full compliance with the Brazilian Cells and Germinative Tissue Directive. *Reprod Biomed Online.* 2013; 26(1): 9–21.
33. Chiang YC, Chiang PC, and Huang CP. Effects of pore structure and temperature on VOC adsorption on activated carbon. *Carbon* 2001; 39: 523–34.
34. Cooper DC and Alley FC. *Air Pollution Control: A Design Approach.* 4th ed. Waveland Press, Inc., Long Grove, IL, 2011.
35. Schwarzenbach RP, Gschwend PM, and Imboden DM. *Environmental Organic Chemistry,* 2nd ed., John Wiley & Sons, Hoboken, NJ, 2003.
36. Kowalski W. *Ultraviolet Germicidal Irradiation Handbook.* Springer-Verlag, Berlin, 2009.

section two

Design and construction

chapter four

Building an environmentally clean and highly productive IVF laboratory suite

Antonia V. Gilligan

Contents

Abstract

The term IVF laboratory suite refers to the set of rooms used for the medical requirements of egg retrieval, plus the laboratory requirements for cryopreservation, embryo culture, and entry anterooms. These will be located in a specifically designed and constructed portion of the practice. This area will be physically isolated by a series of sealed walls and ceilings, positively pressurized, equipped with its own dedicated ventilation system with particulate and chemical filtration. All materials used in the suite should be vetted for embryotoxic components.

4.1 Introduction

The design, construction, use, and maintenance of a modern assisted reproductive technology (ART) laboratory suite are not simple tasks. Its accomplishment requires a team of architects, mechanical and civil engineers, builders, and mechanical specialists for the installation of ventilation systems. It will also require the input of the future occupants from medical director, doctors, scientific directors, embryologists, andrologists, and nurses. Failure to build with this assortment of skill sets in mind, as well as the practice's specific needs, will result in a poorly functioning facility and added cost for corrections.[1] A full study of the future work flow of the practice is needed. Planning is required to ensure it is kept fully functional throughout its working life of 10–15 years. The group and end users must also be informed of the adverse effects of poor environmental quality in the IVF laboratory suite.[2,3] The intent of this chapter is directed at the attainment of the final product. No brief summary could possibly cover every facet. The goal of this chapter is to provide a brief exploration of the task required.

4.2 Site selection

The IVF laboratory suite will be enclosed in a variety of structures ranging from small, stand-alone arrangements outwardly looking like simple doctors' offices to large spaces in professional office buildings. Often the site is selected for many reasons such as cost and location to a service market or nearby medical institution. Each approach has its own advantages and drawbacks. Ideally, environmental quality should be in the decision matrix.

Sites near significant point sources of contaminants should be avoided or evaluated carefully. Such locations would include fossil fuel power plants, refineries, asphalt plants, printing operations, and dry cleaners. A Phase I review, where these are examined, should be considered. This review is done by environmental firms and includes an onsite inspection, baseline analysis of the prospective location, and a review of public documents from local, state, and federal regulations.

The inspection must include baseline sampling for toxic organics (as listed by the U.S. EPA). The baseline samples should be done by recognized analytical methods (U.S. EPA TO-15 and U.S. EPA TO-11) providing both identity and concentrations at the microgram/cubic meter ($\mu g/m^3$) level by an accredited environmental lab. Measurements at milligram/cubic meter (mg/m^3) are not sufficiently rigorous because of the potentially high detection limits. Avoid handheld analysis by photoionization detectors as the investigation tool.

If the facility is in a mixed use building, determine what is in it now or will be in the near future if at all possible. Fellow occupants can be a problem. Dry cleaners and internal parking garages can complicate ventilation and filtration options. Access to the roof is preferred as the location of the air intake. Elevated air intakes above ground level particulates and chemical emissions including building emissions, street paving, fertilizers, and pesticides are preferred. Site selection should also factor in potential growth of the practice. The site should allow the IVF laboratory suite to grow as the patient load increases.

Last, besides knowing the business plan, the budget for the design, construction, equipment, clinical and lab technology should be known at the start of the project. Funds are limited and the principals should weigh the advantages of various options. Is a designed décor really a key requirement?

4.3 Design process

Many designers and contractors will represent their qualifications including building clean rooms, medical offices, or ART facilities. Do not take these at face value. They may think they know what is needed. Many do not. Ask the current end users of these designs and inspect what they have done. Do not assume that design and construction projects have met the standards of a modern high technology ART IVF laboratory suite. Typical medical standards for operating room (OR) door widths and bathroom facilities should of course be followed,[4] but other typical techniques (Formica-particle board case work, hung ceilings with just washable panels and high hat lighting) are not applicable to the IVF laboratory suites' more rigorous and specific design requirements.

The knowledge of how to build a highly functioning lab requires the architects, designers, etc., and the medical and embryology teams to develop a common understanding of the requirements. Present the design and build team with the literature on environmental needs. Conversely, the team of designers must brief the practice on their unique jargon and candidly tell them what can and cannot be done at the budget level.

The design process should be reiterative. After the knowledge transfer described above and the site evaluation is finished, a first draft of a plan should be developed. This should be reviewed by the practice in depth. Before hiring a general contractor and subcontractors, have them review the early draft designs. Collect their input and initial cost estimates.

The source of fresh air is a huge variable. Taking air from a loading dock or a parking deck is an invitation to poor performance or a far more costly filtration system. The ideal location is the roof, away from sanitary vents or general building exhausts.

Materials to be used in the final design must not have materials off-gassing that are potentially toxic contaminants. These include in particular particle board,[5] wood, linoleum, adhesives, poorly mixed epoxy paints, flooring, and oil-based paints.

Regardless of this effort, a heating, ventilation, and air conditioning (HVAC) plan will require a particulate and chemical filtration system. The extremely small size of chemical pollutants will not be trapped by any high efficiency particulate air (HEPA) or ultra low penetration air (ULPA) filters. And the chemical filtration should not be based on some "universal technology." Simple pleated filters with a section of activated carbon are totally inappropriate, lacking removal capacity and poor residence time. The selected media after testing is commonly a mix of activated carbon and an oxidizing component such as potassium permanganate ($KMnO_4$). However, there are other technologies that have been used. Photochemical oxidation (PCO) and PCO augmented with a smaller sized $KMnO_4$ cartridge have been used. Systems that use ozone should not be used. Finally, there are new and proprietary technologies that provide a very high level of effectiveness (LifeAire Systems).

After gaining these inputs of work flow and environmental concerns, a second design for bid should be produced and used for practice review, cost, schedule, and code approval. It is not unusual for this phase to take time.

4.4 *Bid process*

Until this point, costs have been ascertained considering what is needed. The bid process is the commencement of using "real money." The process will be primarily directed at the future general contractor who will bring in subcontractors as needed. The choice of contractor may not be the sole variable of the practice. It could be dictated by the medical institution such as a professional medical building, building owner, or hospital associated with the practice. It could require using a firm associated with the building owner. Some firms will reply that ART lab building is so difficult it will require a significant cost increase compared to typical medical projects. This is a valid point in that the AHU and filters will add capital costs, but the majority of the unique work requires available materials and diligence. Overseeing the labor in cleaning, sealing, and clean building techniques is not as expensive as some will claim, particularly if done by a non-unionized firm.

Solicitation of three bids by reputable firms is recommended, followed by a negotiation. Previous building of advanced laboratories is part of the "due diligence." Every project has "issues," but some are minor. Some are total game stoppers. Failure to meet design specifications is a "Very Big Deal." There may be a dispute among the parties and often the practice has limited recourse except legal action. This can be very expensive, long, and often ends without a favorable outcome. The remediation of defects is commonly costly and may delay the commencement of medical services.

There is an alternate arrangement that gives the practice leverage. Design the contract requiring the general contractor and subcontractors to meet the clearly defined ART lab specifications in the bid package. Holding 10% of the cost as a guarantee of performance is a powerful motivator to achieve compliance to specifications.

4.5 Construction briefing

The persons doing the work and supervising them usually have little idea of what will be done in the IVF laboratory suite. They need to be motivated to meet fully some of our construction techniques and goals. This requires driving the basic knowledge down to these essential craftsmen. A meeting to educate them on the reasons, the techniques, and the fact that their work will be tested comes as a surprise to many. Tell them the materials used will be audited. If unapproved materials are used, they will be replaced at no cost to the practice. Common violations are using fiberglass batting that will release formaldehyde or case work made of medium density particle board, even if represented as formaldehyde free. Experience has shown that the more they know the better. A small talk by the medical director and scientific director at the briefing about the hopes of the families often strikes a chord. Most people work more conscientiously when they are taught and inspected. A presence by the practice staff on the build site, surprise visits taking photos of the project, and casually replying to questions can pay big dividends.

4.6 Construction techniques

The design prints should call out the unique construction needs of positive pressure, rigorous construction of the walls and ceilings, safe materials, and sealing of all penetrations. Penetrations can be sealed with silicones, Tyvek, plaster mud, and tape. All electrical conduits should be sealed at junction boxes, outlets, and switches. Sealing of large holes with gypsum board, formaldehyde-free fiberglass with a surface coat of silicon sealant followed by a weatherproof gasket works well. A better solution is sealed "intrinsically safe" wiring, which will exceed this standard.

The AHU and ductwork is the circulatory system of the IVF laboratory suite. If this is dirty, the lab will suffer. They must be cleaned to remove soil and also the rust inhibitor that prevents oxidation on the metal components. It can be removed by a thorough and rigorous cleaning with alcohol-moistened lint-free cloths by wiping the inside and then sealing of the ends with 6 mil polyethylene sheeting until installation is completed. Store these pieces in a secure area where they will not be fouled. Assemble in a stepwise fashion so the ends are not left open except when connecting pieces is a requirement of clean construction.

The work site should be "clean." A disorganized collection of uncontrolled materials with construction debris on the floor is a warning sign and needs to be corrected immediately. Take pictures if this occurs. Taking pictures is wise for other reasons. Once the lab is complete, certain components will be buried. The prints will show the intended location, but if these have been moved for building or space reasons, "as built" revisions to the prints should be provided. Any flammable solvents in quantities over a half gallon, welding or brazing materials, and gases should be stored in compliance with local and National Fire Protection Association (NFPA) codes.

Medical gas lines are also a one-time build item. Acceptable materials range from stainless steel to medical grade copper. These must be oil-free with capped ends and meeting ASTM specifications for medical gas work. Tygon line with Teflon has been used for short gas lines if they meet local medical gas codes. The installer should be certified. Do not accept a non-certified installer. An apprentice working under the direct supervision of a certified supervisor can be used. If you see medical gas lines with tape as a seal, demand that all work be removed at the contractor's cost and start anew with the specified materials. Medical line cleanliness, along with the cleanliness of the AHU and ductwork, are items to be done exactly. Do not compromise. A polite and firm attitude is essential. Once these are in, fixing the problems is extremely costly and will delay initiation of clinical operations.

4.7 Pre-commissioning

As the project approaches completion, key items will require inspection and certification. Fire and building code inspections can be anticipated. A licensed/certified air balance firm must test the air distribution system. This is not a minor item. The air supply and distribution to the IVF laboratory suite will need to be verified including ventilation rates and levels of specified positive pressure. A medical gas report must also be essential. The AHU must be cleaned after loading and the particulate and VOC removal technologies are about to enter service. It should be run for at least two weeks to verify full specification compliance and should also be used for burning-in the IVF laboratory suite. What is burning-in? It uses an increase in temperature to 85–93°F for at least two weeks. This will promote the off gassing from the various building materials and will lower the VOC levels in the finished lab before clinical operations are commenced.

An inspection and review of the IVF laboratory suite and HVAC must be done at this point. What is missing, have the gas lines been fully installed, are all penetrations and doors sealed, any flooring and wall defects corrected, lighting working and what is the level of positive pressurization? The participants must include the practice, the architect, the HVAC sub- and general contractor. A final "punch list" should be generated and completed as soon as possible.

The beginning of cleaning should now start. The contractor must not dismiss this as "broom clean." All walls, floors, casework, and diffusers should be HEPA vacuumed. Any debris such as cardboard and gas fittings needs to be removed. At this point, tacky mats should be placed on the entry doors. "Bunny suits" must be worn with shoe covers and hair nets at this point. Ideally, the lab equipment such as laminar flow hoods, incubators, air tables, microscopes/micro manipulators, Dewars, OR/procedure room tables, crash carts, and lighting should be installed now. This process can be time consuming and is messy. A final lab inspection of all of these tasks must be completed. After it is complete, nursing and staff should clean the lab. HEPA vacuuming should be redone. Cleaning surfaces with low VOC detergents should be done, followed by 70% ethanol wipe-down on critical surfaces such as bench tops and laminar flow hoods. Six percent hydrogen peroxide can be a safe alternate disinfectant. All methods should be followed by reagent grade water as a final rinse. A final lab inspection of all of these tasks must be completed.

4.8 Commissioning of the IVF laboratory suite

No lab should be tested until it is complete and meets the criteria that it is ready to immediately start operation, that is, the "conditions of use." Premature testing is a fool's errand and could cause problems in the future. Testing should consist of the following:

1. Pressurization throughout the suite must be quantified by a micro-manometer accurate to 0.001 inches of water. It should be repeated multiple times to ensure it is stable. If pressure monitors are used on the lab's perimeter, their readings should be the same as this commissioning instrumentation.
2. Laser particle counting (209e) can be done, but it should be supplemented by particle characterization (Air-O-Cell). This technique uses a proprietary trap that is open and examined under stereo and bright field microscopy. This technique will reveal possible mold spores, pollen, and fibers.
3. VOCs should be determined by U.S. EPA TO-15 at the chemical filter, the diffusers, and on the IVF lab bench top. Incubator testing of at least one new incubator representative of the set used in the culture is a wise precaution. The level of aldehydes should be done at the same points by U.S. EPATO-11.[6] These tests must follow EPA methods and be at $\mu g/m^3$. Methods at better detection limits should not be considered.[7] Isolation and fresh air ventilation should be determined by tracer gas exchange and infiltration testing.[8]

While the testing is being done, it is wise to train the lab staff on the techniques for sampling for VOCs and aldehydes. Training on sampling the lab and chemical filter may be wise depending on the technology.

4.9 Commissioning report and supporting documents

A written report of the results of testing should be prepared. It should list the personnel and their contact information, and who designed, built, and did any required certifications. An executive summary followed by recommendations should be included. A section on methods used including equipment calibrations and QC/QA is essential. The chemical data and comparison to levels in highly productive IVF laboratory suites is also a must. A discussion section of the data is obviously required.[9]

A plan to keep the IVF laboratory suite in specification is a closing item.[10] Chemical filter life can be significantly shorter than the vendor's recommendations. A listing of particulate filter sizes, number, and initial changing schedule should be prepared. A schedule and testing of the IVF laboratory suite before the one year of use is up is wise. This one-year mark is often the end of any component warranty.

References

1. Cohen J, Alikani M, Gilligan A, and Schimmel T. Setting up an ART laboratory. In: Gardner DK, Weissman A, Howles CM, and Shoham Z. (eds.). *Textbook of Assisted Reproductive Techniques*. CRC Press, Boca Raton, FL, 2012, pp. 17–24.
2. Cohen J, Gilligan A, Esposito W, Schimmel T, and Dale B. Ambient air and its potential effects on conception in vitro. *Hum Reprod* 1997; 12: 1742–9.
3. Hall J, Gilligan A, Schimmel T, Cecchi M, and Cohen J. The origin, effects and control of air pollution in laboratories used for human embryo culture. *Hum Reprod* 1998; 13: 146–55.

4. U.S. Department of Health and Human Services, AIA Academy of Architect for Health. *Guidelines for Design and Construction of Hospital and Health Care Facilities*. The American Institute of Architects Press, Washington, DC, 2006, Table 2.1–2, pp. 130–1.
5. Standard Test Methods for Determining Formaldehyde Levels from Pressed Wood Products under Defined Test Conditions using a Large Chamber. Formaldehyde Release from Wood Products: ASTM 1333-90.
6. U.S. Environmental Protection Agency. Analysis Procedure for Chemical Air Contaminants: The TO-14/TO-15/TO-11 procedures is outlined in Compendium of Methods for the Determination of Toxic Organic Compounds in Ambient Air, EPA 600/4-84-041, April 1984/1988.
7. Molhave L. Volatile organic compounds. Indoor air quality and health. *Indoor Air* 1991; 1(4): 357–76.
8. Bearg D. Air contaminant standards. In: Bearg D. *Indoor Air Quality and HVAC Systems*. CRC Press, Boca Raton, FL, 1993, pp. 72–77.
9. Foster RW and Roberson CS. Monitoring indoor air in the laboratory building. *Chem Health Safety* 2001; 8(3): 24–28.
10. Liu RT. Use of activated carbon absorbers in HVAC applications. In: Teichman KY (ed.). *Operating and Maintaining Buildings for Health Comfort and Productivity*. American Society of Heating, Refrigerating and Air Conditioning Engineers Inc. 1994, pp. 209–17.

chapter five

What is HEPA? How to achieve high efficiency particulate air filtration

Raul A. Sadir, Cesar J. Velardez, and Raul I. Sadir

Contents

Abstract

High efficiency particulate air (HEPA) is a type of particulate air filter designed to trap the vast majority of very small particulate contaminants from an air stream. HEPA filtration has many applications, including medical and biomedical facilities, pharmaceutical manufacturing, electronic microcircuits (computer chips), automobiles, and the aerospace industry. HEPA filters are composed of a mat of randomly arranged fibers. The fibers are typically composed of fiberglass and possess diameters between 0.5 and 2.0 μm. Key factors affecting its functions are fiber diameter, filter thickness, and face velocity. HEPA filters are critical in biomedicine applications requiring prevention of the spread of airborne bacterial and viral organisms such as in vitro fertilization.

5.1 Introduction

The Manhattan project, in addition to creating the atomic bomb in the 1940s during World War II, contributed to important technological advancements in the area of air filtration. Due to the high concentration of radioactive particles in the air of their laboratories, the scientists developed a method for removing those harmful particles by filtering the air using HEPA air filtration.

Table 5.1 HEPA filter equivalence according to ASHRAE and Eurovent standards

Particle range size (0.3 to 1 μ)	ASHRAE (types A through D yield efficiencies at 0.3 μ)[a]	EN 1822 (2012)
≥99.95%	MERV 17	H13
≥99.995%	MERV 18	H14

[a] IEST (Institute of Environment Sciences and Technology test methods).

5.2 Definitions

HEPA stands for high efficiency particulate air. A filter has to be able to remove at least 99.95% of particles that are 0.3 μ or larger to be rated HEPA class. A filter's percent efficiency can be calculated using simple equation.

$$E = (1 - \boldsymbol{D/U}) \times 100 \tag{5.1}$$

where:

E = percent efficiency
D = downstream concentration (of contaminants)
U = upstream concentration (of contaminants)

HEPA filters are usually rated according to one of the two most common classification systems, the EN-1822 standard issued by Eurovent,[1] and the minimum efficiency reporting value (MERV) standard issued by the American Society of Heating, Refrigerating and Air-Conditioning Engineers (ASHRAE)[2] (Table 5.1).

In practice, MERV 17 filters can replace H13 filters, the only difference being the type of tests to which they are subjected to ensure efficiency. The ASHRAE classification is widely used in North America while the rest of the world uses the Eurovent classification. Nevertheless, there are other similar standards that follow different test procedures.

HEPA standard usage of 0.3 μm particles to describe efficiency is based on the fact that particles of this size are actually the most difficult to filter.

5.3 Applications

HEPA filters are used in applications requiring very efficient filtering of airborne particulate matter, including pathogens. These filters are also useful in manufacturing environments that require very clean air. The main applications include:

- Airline cabin air purifiers
- Biomedical air filtration
- Electronics manufacturing
- Pharmaceutical manufacturing
- Vacuum cleaner filters
- Heating, ventilation, and air conditioning (HVAC) systems

5.4 Health issues

Some of the most harmful particles to human health measure between 0.3 and 10 μ, which include pathogens like bacteria (Figure 5.1).[3]

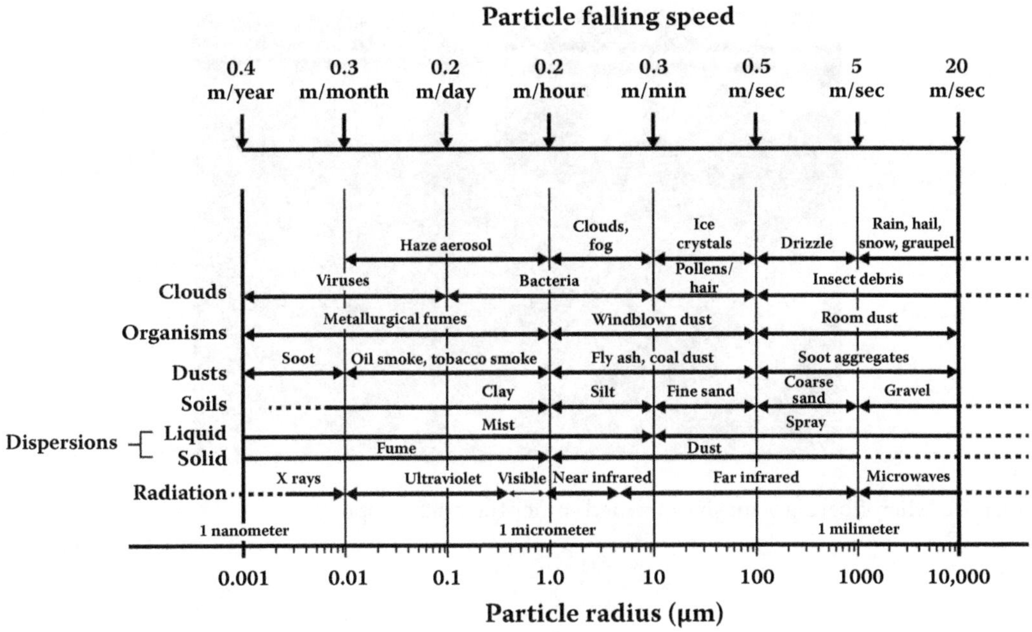

Figure 5.1 Airborne particle distribution in the atmosphere.

A variety of respiratory problems are associated with particles in air suspension ranging between PM2.5 and PM10 (particulate matter measuring between 2.5 and 10 µ in diameter, respectively).[4,5] An excessive exposure to such particles has been associated with the following health issues:

- Breathing problems
- Worsening of asthma symptoms
- Adverse birth outcomes, such as low birth weight
- Decreased lung growth in children
- Lung cancer
- Early deaths

It has been hypothesized that the aforementioned particles would be even more detrimental to critically ill patients as well as other conditions sensitive to contaminations, such as those involving the handling of gametes and embryos.

5.5 *Physics*

Air filters are designed to arrest and retain particles, preventing them from returning to the air stream. HEPA filters do so by means of microfiberglass media intertwined in microscopic meshes (Figure 5.2).

To pass through a HEPA filter, the air requires considerable energy. And due to the limited space for the air to go through the microfiberglass mesh, such filters also require a larger contact area or otherwise particles clog up the filter very quickly.

Diffusion, inertial impaction, interception, and sieving are the four known methods for trapping particles, as shown in Figure 5.3.

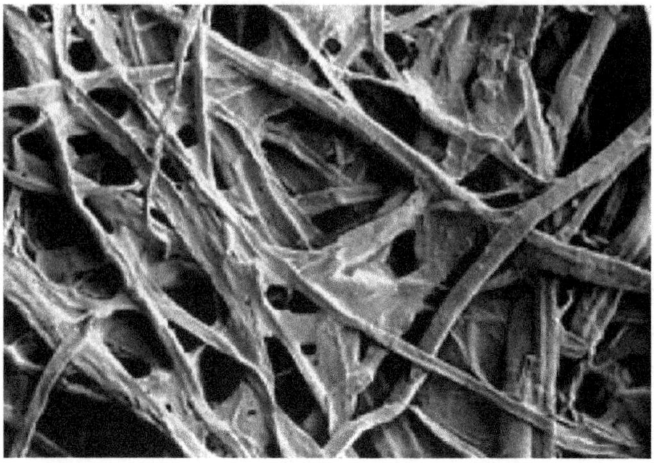

Figure 5.2 Microfiberglass mesh examined under the microscope.

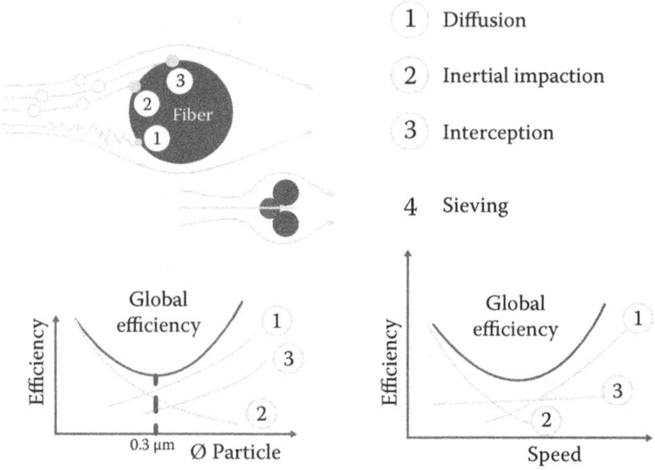

Figure 5.3 Methods for trapping particles.

Diffusion relates to the impact of Brownian motion on air particles. As the air diffuses throughout the filter, small particles (typically 0.1 µm or less) tend to travel on a streamline in an erratic fashion, making random motions as they interact with gas molecules. This erratic motion causes the contaminant particles to become stuck to the filter fibers.

Impaction occurs when a large particle, unable to adjust to the change in air direction near a filter fiber, becomes trapped on the fiber. The particle's inertia ensures that it continues along its original path instead of circumventing the fiber, resulting in its capture.

Interception takes place when a contaminant particle passes within the distance equal to one particle's radius of a filter fiber, resulting in it touching the fiber and being removed from the airflow. Particles passing beyond that of one particle radius from a fiber will not be trapped.

Last, particles captured by sieving are generally larger in size and are removed because they cannot trespass the filter.

The lowest "global efficiency" point in the efficiency versus particle diameter chart in Figure 5.3 represents the hardest point to capture airborne particles. That specific point relates to particles of 0.3 μ, hence another reason for HEPA filters to be tested for this particle size. Particles smaller than 0.1 μm are easily trapped due to diffusion while particles larger than 0.4 μm are trapped by inertial impaction. Particles between 0.1 and 0.4 μm are too large for effective diffusion and too small for inertial impaction and efficient interception, so that the filter's efficiency drops within this range.

Figure 5.3 can also explain why HEPA filters can capture viruses. Despite being smaller than 0.3 μ, viruses can be trapped because both diffusion and interception efficiency increase for low-sized particles.

5.5.1 Construction

The most important characteristics for selecting HEPA filter media are:

- Stiffness, which determines pleatability
- Airflow resistance, which determines how much air can pass per square meter of media
- Dioctyl phthalate (DOP) smoke penetration, which determines media efficiency

Once the proper media is chosen, it can be pleated basically in three different configurations based on the method utilized to separate the pleats and the actual configuration of the filter (Figures 5.4 through 5.6). The functionality of either type is similar but applications vary due to temperature, environment, space constraints, and ultimately cost.

Support frames for HEPA filters include galvanized steel, aluminum, stainless steel, and plastic. Some customers still require wood frames for certain applications. Filter frames can be arranged in plain or "V" shaped configurations, as shown in Figures 5.7 through 5.9.

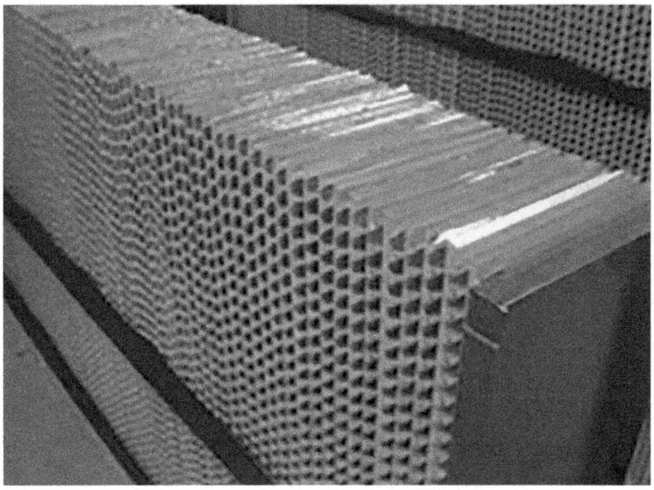

Figure 5.4 Pleated filter media using aluminum separator.

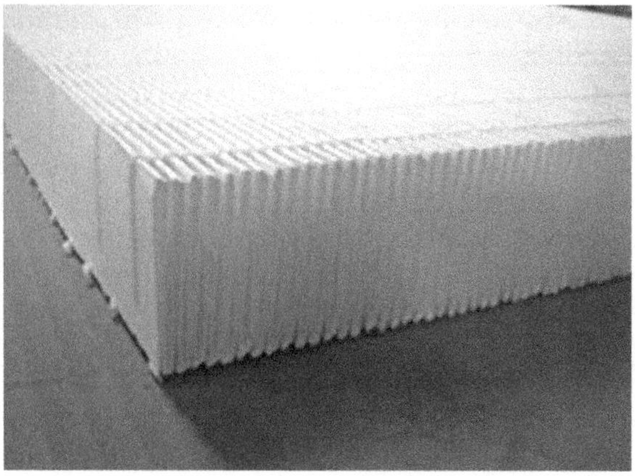

Figure 5.5 Pleated filter media using resin separator.

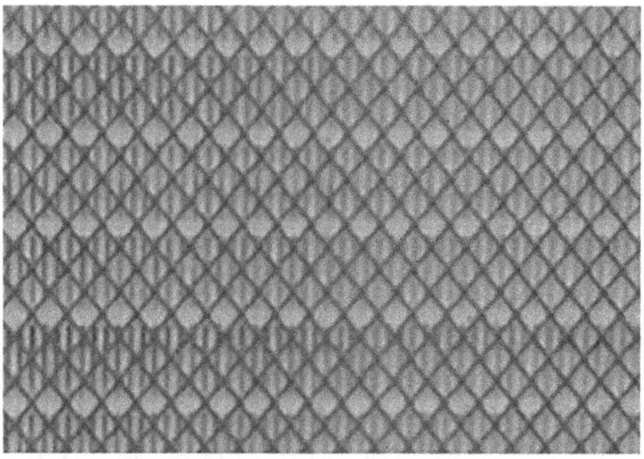

Figure 5.6 Pleated filter media using ribbon separator.

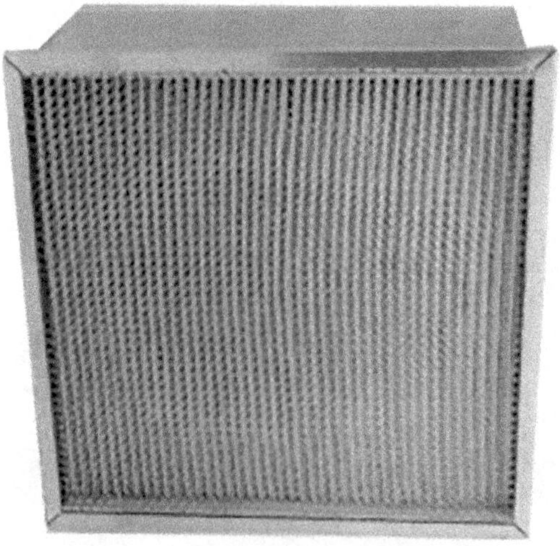

Figure 5.7 Aluminum separator, stainless steel frame, and flat surface.

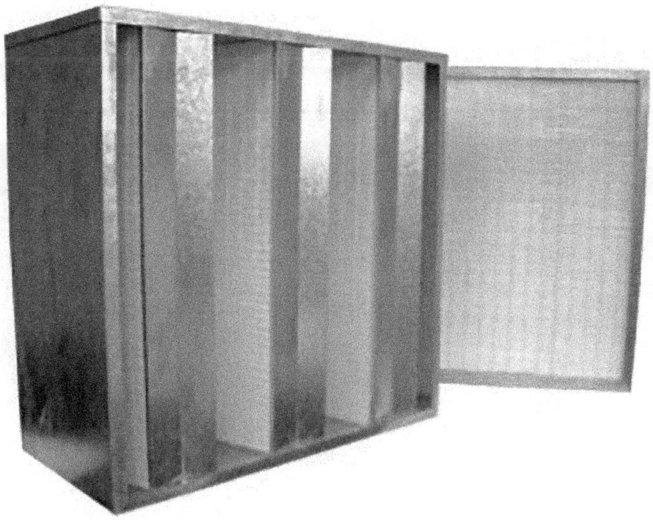

Figure 5.8 Resin separator, galvanized steel frame, and "V" shaped surface.

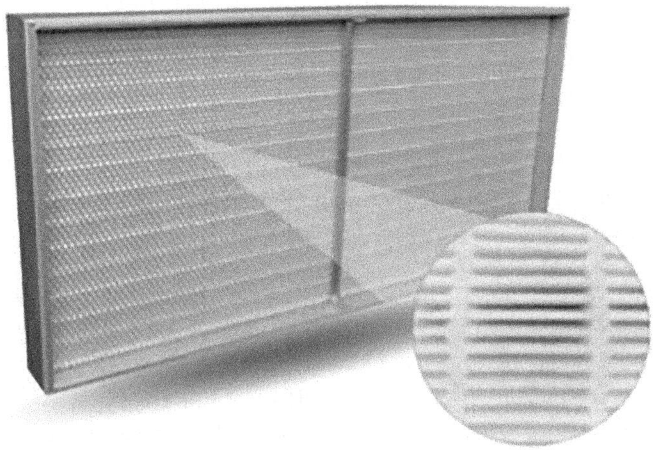

Figure 5.9 Ribbon separator, aluminum frame, and flat surface.

5.6 Installation considerations

When designing or specifying a system or device that incorporates HEPA filters, it is important to take into account that airflow resistance will increase due to the tightness of the microfiberglass media. It is unlikely that existing fans and HVAC systems-not designed to operate with HEPA filters-will have enough capacity to surpass the resistance generated by HEPA filter media.

The specific application for which the filter is utilized can affect its service life and possibly its actual selection for the application. In general, suppliers have the technical skills to design new installations or adjust existing ones to comply with the standards of high efficiency air filtration.

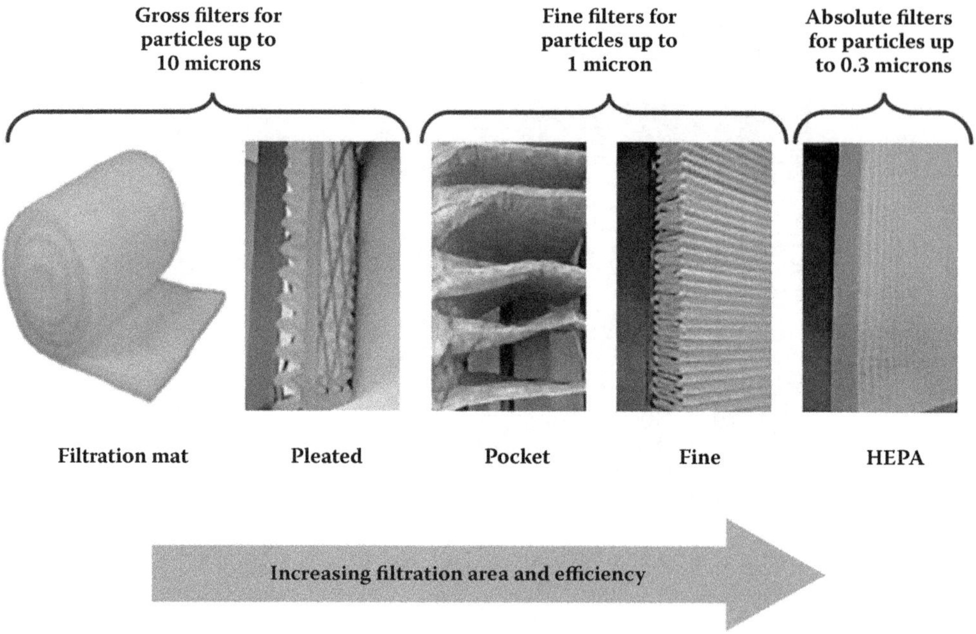

Figure 5.10 **(See color insert.)** Particulate air filtration design for increased efficiency. Pre-filters and fine filters (less expensive) should be placed in series upstream the HEPA filter (more expensive).

5.7 Costs

In order to optimize air filtration and enhance HEPA filter life, and therefore minimizing costs, pre-filters and fine filters should be placed in series upstream from the HEPA filter. This strategy will protect the HEPA filters from saturation. The cost of a filter is inversely proportional to its efficiency, so a high efficiency filter is more expensive than a lower one. Essentially, a cheaper filter is always protecting a more expensive one.

Figure 5.10 shows a good rule of thumb when designing air filtration for better efficiency. Instead of replacing a standalone HEPA filter every two months, it is better to "protect" the HEPA filter with lower class filters. The system will then require more frequent changes of the cheaper filters, but will in turn require that the HEPA filter be changed less often (every six months or even longer intervals). Although the initial investment is higher, the long-term investment will be lower.

5.8 Conclusions

High efficiency air filtration, when properly designed, has proved its long-term benefits. Although it may require a higher initial investment, HEPA air filtration should be an integral element of in vitro fertilization air filtration systems to avoid contamination and ensure safety.

References

1. BS EN 1822-1 2009 Edition. High efficiency air filters (EPA, HEPA and ULPA) Part 1: Classification, performance testing, marking. British Standards Institution, December 31, 2009. https://global.ihs.com/doc_detail.cfm?item_s_key=00304197&rid=GS. Cited September 20, 2015.
2. American Society of Heating, Refrigerating and Air Conditioning Engineers (ASHRAE). Handbook—HVAC Systems and Equipment, Chapter S29, 2012 ASHRAE. http://www.techstreet.com/ashrae/products.
3. Meteorology Course at Penn State University. http://www.ems.psu.edu/~lno/Meteo437/Ptclcat.jpg. Cited September 29, 2014.
4. Stone, SL. How air pollution is affecting our health. http://www.epa.gov/airnow/teachers/ss_airpollhealtheffects.pdf. Cited July 8, 2014.
5. Centers for Disease Control and Prevention (CDC). Air and health. http://ephtracking.cdc.gov/showAirHealth.action#pm. Cited September 28, 2014.

chapter six

Volatile organic compounds

Mechanisms of filtration

John T. Fox

Contents

Abstract

Volatile organic compounds (VOCs) can be removed from the air phase via sorption. Adsorption is a mass transfer process from the gas phase (air) to the solid phase (adsorbent). The process of adsorption is dependent on the properties of both the adsorbate and the adsorbent. The affinity of the adsorbate for the adsorbent is modeled by isotherms that are widely used to predict the removal capacity of organic compounds. The application of adsorption is commonly performed with activated carbon due to both a high surface area and the availability of diverse surface functionality, which enables the sorption of a wide range of organic compounds. When targeting certain adsorbates, activated aluminas, molecular sieves, and impregnated sorption materials can be utilized. Herein, the discussion within this chapter covers fundamentals of adsorption, properties of VOCs relevant to adsorption, adsorption isotherms, adsorbent materials, system design considerations, and competitive adsorption.

6.1 VOC sorption fundamentals

Volatile organic compounds (VOCs) are chemical constituents found in the gas phase—but with a change of pressure or temperature could become a liquid. Therefore, VOC behavior is similar to gases, but most VOCs can be defined as vapors.[1] For example, when a pure organic liquid is in an enclosed system, some liquid will volatilize, exerting a pressure on the system. This volatized liquid is dependent on the vapor pressure. As such, when a compound exerts higher vapor pressure, the pure compound contains a higher affinity for the gas phase than a compound with a lower vapor pressure. As an example of this, medical facilities often use alcohols as sanitizing agents. The alcohol sanitizer is in the liquid form during application; however, the alcohol component will volatilize. Vapors, unlike gases, can often be transferred from the gas phase into the liquid phase or solid phase. The affinity to volatize is attributed to the vapor pressure of the organic compound. Removal of organic vapors can be achieved via sorption, including both absorption and adsorption.

Once VOCs are in the gas phase, interactions with liquids and solids are governed by gas–liquid and gas–solid equilibrium. Gas–liquid equilibrium is defined as absorption, where the vapor enters into the absorbing liquid. The fundamental process of absorption is governed by the two-film theory, where two films of stagnant gas and stagnant liquid exist at the interface of the two phases. During absorption the vapor enters into the stagnant gas film, where the vapor can now undergo a mass transfer process of absorption into the liquid stagnant film. Diffusivities of the organic compound in the gas phase and liquid phase govern the mass transfer rate.[2] The concentration of gas–liquid equilibrium is modeled by Henry's law, which is a linear relationship.

A gas–solid equilibrium is defined as adsorption, where the vapor sorbs onto the surface of the adsorbent media. Vapors with an affinity for the solid adsorbent will be transferred from the gas phase to the solid phase. The amount of vapor adsorbed is dependent on both the properties of the sorbent and the properties of the vapor. Adsorption occurs via physisorption, which is reversible, and chemisorption, which forms a chemical bond to the carbon.[3] The amount of vapor adsorbed is modeled by isotherms, which provide the ultimate loading (mass of vapor per mass of adsorbent) with respect to the partial pressure or concentration of the VOC.

Adsorbent materials are widely utilized for air phase applications such as industrial solvent recovery, pollution abatement, automotive or other transportation cabin air cleaning, indoor ventilation system air cleaning, odor removal, and air purification. The specification and engineering of an adsorbent system are based on the source of VOCs, concentration of vapors, environmental conditions, and treatment requirement. Activated carbon is the most widely utilized air phase adsorbent material, and is also the oldest technology available.[1] Activated carbon possesses incredible surface area, and this large surface area provides sorption sites for vapors to sorb. Specific application of adsorbent materials includes air phase treatment of VOCs laden air streams.

6.2 Properties of VOCs relevant to adsorption

Organic vapors possess chemical and physical properties determined by chemical composition, atomic architecture, and electron sharing between atoms. Herein, specific properties of interest are vapor pressure, melt and boil temperatures, chemical structure, polarity, molecular weight, and K_{ow}. Table 6.1 provides common organic vapors with respect to chemical and physical properties. A few trends are evident based on common properties. In general, as molecular weight increases, the vapor pressure decreases. Therefore,

Table 6.1 Common VOCs, molecular weight, chemical structure, vapor pressure, log K_{ow}, melting point, and boiling point

Compound	MW (g/mole)	Structure	Vp mmHg	Log K_{ow}	Kw solubility mg/L	Tm °C	Tb °C
Acetone	58.1	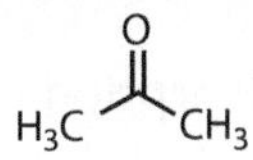	270	–0.24	Total	–94.7	56.1
Benzene	78.1	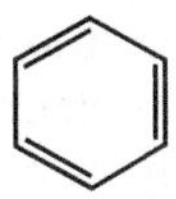	95.2	2.14	1780	5.5	80.1
Ethanol	46.1	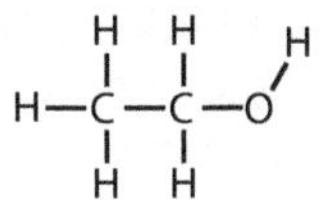	75	–0.32	65,200	–114.1	78.3
Formaldehyde	30.0	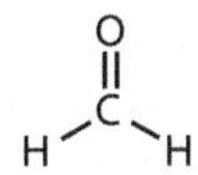	3880	0.35	400,000	–92	–19.1
Isoprene	68.1	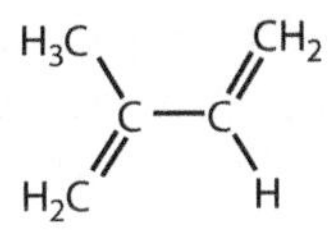	493	2.05	621	–146	34
Methanol	32.1	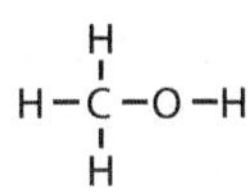	100	–0.77	Total	–97.7	64.6
Toluene	92.2	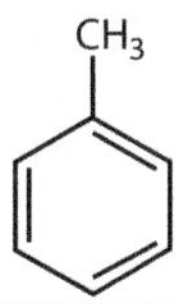	22	2.73	515	–95	110.6

Source: Adapted from Schwarzenbach RP, Gschwend PM, and Imboden DM. *Environmental Organic Chemistry*. 2nd ed. John Wiley & Sons, Hoboken, NJ, 2003.

this vapor pressure is perhaps the most important indicator of VOC adsorption efficiency. Increased vapor pressure contributes to increased affinity for the gas phase; therefore, the energetic favorability of adsorption decreases.[4] Additionally, vapor pressure decreases with increasing polarity, and compounds in the atmosphere will be in the gas phase if their vapor pressure at ambient temperature is $>10^{-5}$ atm.[5]

The melting and boiling points are important parameters to understand whether the compound is a liquid or vapor at the temperature range of interest. Adsorption of compounds at temperatures below the boiling point is more energetically favorable than adsorption above the boiling point. The chemical structure contributes to the chemical properties of organic vapors. As seen in Table 6.1, short chain aliphatic compounds generally possess higher vapor pressures and lower boiling temperatures than longer chain aliphatics or aromatics. In general, short chain aliphatics are difficult to adsorb, whereas aromatic compounds generally adsorb more favorably to carbon adsorbents. The polarity of compounds influences the surface groups that compounds may favorably adsorb, as well as influence the compatibility with water vapor.[4] Water solubility, or K_w, defines the maximum concentration of an organic compound dissolvable into water. Relevant to vapor phase adsorption, when water vapor is present on the surface of adsorbents, compounds with higher water solubility are generally more resilient to increased levels of humidity.[6]

6.3 Adsorption isotherms

VOCs can adsorb to sorption media via physical adsorption or chemisorption. Physical adsorption, or van der Waals adsorption, involves weak bonding due to attraction by charge. The surface charges available for sorption are due to the variations in surface chemistry. The charges can be partial charges due to electron imbalance in surface functional groups. As the forces of this attraction are relatively weak, and the bonds holding these compounds to the media are low energy, physical adsorption can be overcome with heat, reduced pressure, or the application of steam. In fact, heating the media, reducing the pressure on the media, or applying steam to physical sorbed compounds can regenerate adsorption media, whereas chemisorption involves the chemical bonding of gas phase compounds with the adsorption media.[1] As these bonds are chemical, and involve covalent bonds via electron sharing, this type of adsorption bonding is not easily reversed.

The capacity at equilibrium for a specific compound and a specific adsorbent is modeled by an isotherm. The isotherm provides a model to calculate the mass of compound adsorbed per mass of adsorbent, for a given partial pressure of compound and temperature. It should be noted that there are multiple varieties of adsorption isotherm models. Two of the most commonly used isotherm models are the Langmuir isotherm and the Freundlich isotherm. The Langmuir isotherm assumes that adsorption occurs only via a single atomic adsorption layer. Specifically, Langmuir assumes an ideal gas covers the adsorbent in a monolayer of atoms, whereas the Freundlich isotherm model is an empirical model, which thereby accounts compounds sorbing via multiple atomic layers. Both the Fruendlich and Languir isotherms are widely utilized; however, the Fruendlich isotherm often provides more reliable modeling. The Freundlich isotherm used herein is depicted as follows:

Freundlich isotherm

$$q_e = k\bar{P}^n$$

$\bar{P}$ = partial pressure of the adsorbate
q_e = mass of adsorbate adsorbed per unit mass of adsorbent
n = Freundlich exponent
k = Freundlich constants or capacity factor

6.4 Sorbent materials

A wide variety of adsorbent materials are commercially available for organic vapor removal. The specific adsorbent specified for an application should meet the design criteria for removal. Activated carbons, activated alumina, molecular sieves, and other similar materials all provide organic vapor removal capacity. Within each class of sorbent materials, there are products tailored to provide specific properties that optimize removal efficiency for specific organic vapors. The production method within each class of sorbent contributes to the removal efficiency exhibited during application.

6.4.1 Activated carbons

Activated carbons are the most prevalent and oldest adsorbent materials. Activated carbons are widely utilized for both water treatment and air treatment. However, the specific activated carbons utilized in water treatment are different than the activated carbons utilized in air treatment. Therefore, the appropriate carbon must be selected for optimum organic vapor removal efficiency.

Activated carbon production begins with selecting a high carbon content precursor material. Among the most commonly used carbon precursors are lignite coal, bituminous coal, anthracite coal, coconut shells, carbon fibers, walnut shells, wood, coke, agricultural by-products, and bones. The precursor materials are first carbonized at temperatures around 700°C in the absence of air. The carbonization process eliminates low molecular weight compounds, and begins to form the structural matrix for activated carbon. The next step is the activation process. The activation process is performed by introducing a gas, such as steam, at high temperatures (800–1000°C) to the carbonized material. The activation process is a controlled oxidation that fully develops the final pore structure and pore distribution of the activated carbons.[1,3]

Following activation, there are optional post-activation treatment processes for specific functionalities, for example, introduction of silver impregnation for antimicrobial properties, introduction of organic or inorganic functional groups to the surface of the carbon for targeted removal of specific compounds, and treatment to develop catalytic carbon. As evident in the discussion, an array of precursor materials, carbonization and activation processes, and post-activation treatments are available to activated carbon producers. Producers of activated carbon can tailor the final adsorbent properties by selecting precursor materials; varying carbonization temperatures and residence times; changing activation gas, time, and temperature; and selecting post-production chemical tailoring. The characteristics of carbons from various raw materials are cataloged in Table 6.2.

The precursor materials, manufacturing processes, and post-production processes all contribute to the activated carbon material properties. Carbon selection can begin with reviewing carbon properties provided by the carbon manufacturer or supplier. The iodine number, carbon tetrachloride number, and butane pore volume values can all provide insight on selecting the appropriate carbon for organic vapor removal. Also, working closely with carbon suppliers will help product selection as each specific material will have properties desired for specific applications. One aspect of carbon selection is specifying the appropriate activated carbon size distribution. Most carbons available in the United States are sized according to the U.S. mesh sizing. For example, carbons could be supplied as 4 × 6, 12 × 30, or 10 × 30. The sizing indicates U.S. mesh that carbon granules would pass through and be retained. Vapor phase applications generally use

Table 6.2 Characteristics of activated carbons from various raw materials

Raw material	CCl_4 number	Butane pore volume, cc/g	Application
Bituminous coal	60	0.45	Vapor/liquid phase
Coconut	63	0.49	Vapor phase
Subbituminous coal	67	0.48	Vapor phase
Wood	76	0.57	Vapor/liquid phase

Source: Adapted from Cooper DC and Alley FC. *Air Pollution Control: A Design Approach.* 4th ed. Waveland Press, Long Grove, IL, 2011.

sizing to control pressure drop, and therefore specify larger carbons than water treatment applications.[7]

6.4.1.1 Adsorption performance tests

Two conventional tests used to appraise activated carbon for vapor phase applications include the carbon tetrachloride (CTC) number and the butane capacity. The CTC number[8] describes the ultimate loading, or saturation in grams of CCl_4 adsorbed per 100 g of carbon, when the carbon is exposed to a constant stream of CCl_4. The butane capacity measures the ultimate loading of butane for an adsorbent as per ASTM D5228-92.[9] The carbon tetrachloride number may be obtained empirically by multiplying the butane number by 2.25.[1] For each of these appraisal tests, adsorbent materials with higher butane pore volume or higher CTC number generally indicate increased adsorption capacity.

6.4.2 Activated alumina

Activated alumina is produced by thermal dehydration or activation of aluminum trihydrate, $Al(OH)_3$, or gibbsite. The most widely used form is made from Bayer α-trihydrate, which is a by-product of the Bayer process for aqueous caustic extraction of alumina from bauxite. The trihydrate gibbsite is activated in air to ~400°C to form a surface area of ~250 m^2/g, or heated very rapidly at 400–800°C to form an amorphous alumina with a surface area of 300–350 m^2/g.[7] Similar to other sorbents, variations in the heating rate, starting material, gas composition, moisture in the atmosphere, and final temperature are all important components of activated alumina properties. Alumina surface acidity is important for both adsorption and catalysis as Lewis acid sites (i.e., sites that can accept electrons) are abundant on aluminas. These are the Al^{3+} sites on the surfaces.[7]

The most common application for activated alumina is dessication. Total water capacity is greater for activated aluminas than zeolites; however, zeolites are able to remove water vapor at lower concentrations. Desiccation remains a major application for activated alumina.

Tailoring of alumina via variation of the activation process or the use of chemical dopants enables the use for new applications, as well as the conventional applications of removal of acidic gases, sulfur dioxide, and polar organic compounds.[7]

6.4.3 Molecular sieves

Carbon molecular sieves (CMSs) or molecular carbon sieves (MSCs) are less hydrophilic than zeolites and can therefore be used effectively in wet-gas streams.[7] These carbons possess tailored porosity for selective adsorption, and are often used for collecting very small molecular-sized compounds (C2-C5). The effectiveness of CMS depends on the size and shape of the molecule, and the size and shape of the pore entrances in the CMS particle. Most often CMS are prepared from polymers.[10]

6.5 Design considerations

VOC adsorption is widely utilized in applications ranging from treating industrial exhaust gas streams to purifying ambient air for high purity requirements. In general, four key design components govern for both applications: (1) selecting the proper adsorbent material, (2) providing ample contact time for sorption, (3) providing the proper sorption system architecture, and (4) providing adequate mass of sorbent material. There are, however, other factors that influence design, beyond these three factors, such as influent gas concentrations, effluent requirements, environmental factors, pressure drop, etc.

Adsorbent bed breakthrough is an important consideration for adsorption system design. Breakthrough is the function of inlet concentration and effluent concentration. When the effluent concentration exceeds the effluent standard, "breakthrough" has occurred. In the case of VOCs in air, breakthrough occurs because the inlet gas laden with VOCs enters an adsorbent system. As the VOCs sorb to the activated carbon, the first part of the carbon system becomes saturated, and the next part of the carbon bed is the active adsorption zone—where VOCs still sorb to the surface of the activated carbon. The zone following the adsorption zone is clean carbon. When the active adsorption zone exceeds the "clean carbon," breakthrough occurs as VOCs begin to enter the effluent gas. Based on this principle, key design considerations for breakthrough include depth of adsorption zone, influent and effluent concentrations, ultimate capacity of adsorbent, mass of adsorbent, time between adsorbent change out, volumetric flow rate, loss of capacity due to carbon (adsorption zone size, heat wave, moisture in gas, and residual moisture on carbon), and sorption kinetics.

6.6 Adsorption of VOCs at low concentrations

VOC adsorption is widely studied for high concentration scenarios (industrial air treatment, effluent gas treatment, industrial solvent recovery, etc.); however, adsorption of VOCs at lower concentrations is a less studied topic. Low concentrations represent the scenario for the sorption of indoor air pollutants. A few representative studies investigated granular activated carbon and activated carbon fibers for the application of sorbing low concentrations of volatile organics. Work by VanOsdell et al. challenged small scale beds with VOCs ranging from 0.5 to 100 ppm. The conclusion from their work, testing at 25°C, 50% RH, and 0.11 second residence time, was that as the concentration of VOCs decreased the breakthrough time increased. For example, hexane at 107 ppm reached 10% breakthrough in 4.3 hours, as compared to hexane at 0.4 ppm, which reached 10% breakthrough in 376 hours.[11] In general, it is accepted that adsorbent and sorbate performance at high concentrations can be used with caution to predict the performance of adsorbent and sorbate at lower concentrations.

6.7 Competitive adsorption

6.7.1 Competition with organic vapors

Organic vapors compete for loading on activated carbon. Among the complexities of indoor air VOC removal is competitive adsorption between compounds, due to the varying affinity for carbon between compounds. Therefore, VOCs with a high affinity for the adsorbent material will out-compete VOCs with a low affinity for the adsorbent material, resulting in low affinity compounds to not adsorb and potentially desorb from the adsorbent.

6.7.2 Competition with water vapor

The preference of organic vapors over water vapors is a paradigm long plaguing organic vapor adsorbents. Activated carbon's affinity for water vapor is due to oxygen containing functional groups within the carbon's surface. Beyond the specific affinity for water vapor by activated carbon, the adsorption of VOCs in the presence of water vapor has been well

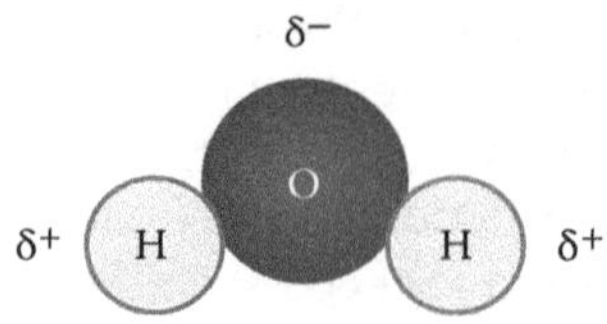

Figure 6.1 Water molecule, depicting polarity.

studied. As a general rule, increased RH decreases VOC adsorption. Researchers investigating the interaction of water soluble compounds found that water miscible compounds (e.g., acetone) exhibits less degradation of capacity when water vapors are present.[6,12] In general, for most organic compounds, researchers decide to account for the effects of RH below 50% as having negligible impact on activated carbon adsorption performance.[13,14]

Certain sorbents including silica gels and activated aluminas can be utilized to selectively remove water vapor from gas streams. Commonly, when adsorbents are used to remove water vapor from gas these adsorbents are called desiccants. However, nearly all gas phase adsorbents demonstrate some degree of affinity for water vapor. Yet, it is important to note that certain adsorbents are more selective in their affinity for water vapors, and can preferentially remove organic vapors (VOCs) from humid gas streams.

The best review of water is to examine the atomic structure of it. Figure 6.1 demonstrates that water is a polar compound. The polarity of water is due to uneven electron sharing. Specifically, the oxygen atom possesses a greater affinity for electrons than hydrogen, which results in partial negativity (due to electron presence) on the oxygen atom. Subsequently, the hydrogen atom develops partial positivity, resulting in a polar water molecule. This polarity contributes to how water interacts with itself as a liquid, but also interactions with dissolved compounds in liquid water, and as pertinent herein, influences the interaction between water and sorbent materials. The partial positive charge of hydrogen produces an affinity for oxygen atoms in surface functional groups (or other partially negative groups) on the surface of adsorbents. Similarly, the partial negative charge of oxygen yields an affinity for partially positive atoms on surfaces of adsorbents.

Each class of adsorbent has a specific affinity for water vapor; within the classification of adsorbents, variations of unique sorbents possess a specific affinity for water vapor. In general, for most adsorbent materials, as the relative humidity increases, the ultimate loading (mass of water/mass of adsorbent) of water also increases. The adsorption of water depends on the polarity of the surface functional groups. As previously mentioned, the surface properties of activated carbon, porosity, and surface chemistry provide activated carbon the mechanisms to be an effective gas treatment technology. Specifically, activated carbon is non-polar or slightly polar due to surface oxide groups and inorganic impurities. This unique property provides activated carbon with the capability to be used in air purification applications without stringent moisture removal, adsorb nonpolar and weakly polar organic molecules better than other sorbents due to internal surface area/large pore volume, and the bond energy of sorbed compounds is relatively low so therefore removal of compounds is easier than other sorbents.[7]

References

1. Cooper DC and Alley FC. *Air Pollution Control: A Design Approach.* 4th ed. Waveland Press, Long Grove, IL, 2011.
2. Logan BE. *Environmental Transport Processes.* John Wiley & Sons, New York, 1999.

3. Heinsohn RJ and Kabel RL. *Sources and Control of Air Pollution.* Prentice-Hall, Upper Saddle River, NJ, 1999.
4. Schwarzenbach RP, Gschwend PM, and Imboden DM. *Environmental Organic Chemistry.* 2nd ed. John Wiley & Sons, Hoboken, NJ, 2003.
5. Goldstein AH and Galbally IE. Known and unexplored organic constituents in the Earth's atmosphere. *Environmental Science & Technology*, March 2007.
6. Cal MP, Rood MJ, and Larson SM. Removal of VOCs from humidified gas streams using activated carbon cloth. *Gas Separation & Purification* 1996; 10.2: 117–21.
7. Yang RT. *Adsorbents: Fundamentals and Applications.* John Wiley & Sons, Hoboken, NJ, 2003.
8. ASTM D3467-99. Standard Test Method for Carbon Tetrachloride Activity of Activated Carbon, ASTM International, West Conshohocken, PA, 2003.
9. ASTM D5228-92. Standard Test Method for Determination of the Butane Working Capacity of Activated Carbon, ASTM International, West Conshohocken, PA, 2000.
10. Verma S. Carbon adsorbents. AnalytiX Volume 9 Article 4. http://www.sigmaaldrich.com/technical-documents/articles/analytix/carbon-adsorbents.html#sthash.goR7AAot.dpuf.
11. VanOsdell DW, Owen MK, Jaffe LB, and Sparks LE. VOC removal at low contaminant concentrations using granular activated carbon. *J Air & Waste Manag Assoc* 1996; 46(9).
12. Rudisill EN, Hacskaylo JJ, and LeVan MD. Coadsorption of hydrocarbons and water on BPL activated carbon. *Indust & Engin Chem Res* 1992; 31(4): 1122–30.
13. Fariborz H, Lee C-S, Pant B, Bolourani G, Lakdawala N, and Bastani A. Evaluation of various activated carbons for air cleaning—Towards design of immune and sustainable buildings. *Atmosph Environ* 2008; 42: 8176–84.
14. Nelson GO, Correia AN, and Harder CA. Respirator cartridge efficiency studies: VII. Effect of relative humidity and temperature. *Am Industrial Hygiene Assoc J* 1976; 37(5): 280–8.

chapter seven

Clean room design principles
Focus on particulates and microbials

Tim Sandle

Contents

Abstract

This chapter describes the design and operation essentials for clean rooms used in IVF centers and the associated operation of clean air devices. The main focus is on the design elements and, as will be stated in the chapter, spending time getting the design essentials right can help to avoid contamination problems and help with cost controls. The key aspect of the chapter are with air. Air is a problem because it carries microbial carrying particles and it can, potentially, direct contamination toward cells. However, good design means that air is also the solution to dealing with contamination, through filtration, dilution, and air movement. Understanding these essentials can help with running an IVF facility that it is at a low risk from microbial contamination.

7.1 Introduction

Clean rooms are highly controlled environments where the air quality is monitored to ensure the required standards of cleanliness are met. This requires high fresh air rates, extensive filtering, temperature, and humidity control. Protection from uncontrolled ingress of external ambient air is achieved by creating a pressure differential between the clean room and its surroundings.

The primary objective of clean rooms is to minimize and control microbial and particulate contamination. There are many sources of contamination. The atmosphere contains dust, microorganisms, condensates, and gases. Contamination control is the primary consideration in clean room design; however, the relationships between contamination control and airflow are not well understood.[1] Contaminants such as particles or microbes are primarily introduced to clean rooms by people, although processes in clean rooms may also introduce contamination.[2]

In vitro fertilization (IVF) centers must make use of clean room technology. This is necessary to protect cells and embryos.[3] It is also required in order to provide the necessary clean air spaces required by European Commission Directive 2006/86/EC.[4] According to the European Union Tissues and Cells Directive (EUTCD), the clean air requirements are for a clean air zone equivalent to EU GMP Grade A (equivalent to ISO 14644 Class 5) within a clean room operating at a minimum of Grade D (there is a proviso for a lower quality clean zone air grade, if such a level of particle cleanliness can be justified through risk assessment. Equally, some centers opt for higher grade clean rooms). This chapter does not make any recommendations as to whether an environment below EU GMP Grade D can be adopted for this is a matter for local managers and their respective regulatory bodies. Aside from European GMP, other regulatory agencies have issued directives stating specific requirements for air quality standards in embryology facilities.[5]

The Grade A air requires the processing of tissues and cells in order to minimize the risk of microbial contamination (either from the air, via operators, or from the cross-contamination between samples), and studies suggest that such an environment leads to lower rates of contamination.[3,5] Grade A quality is defined by the concentration of the permitted maximum number of particles of a given size. For this, EU GMP Annex 1 defines a level of particle cleanliness of not more than 3500 particles of a size ≥0.5 μm and greater and not more than 20 particles of a size ≥5.0 μm and greater.[6] In addition, there are requirements for the number of permissible microorganisms (which must average no more than one colony forming unit). With the surrounding Grade D area, the particle limits are user defined, although EU GMP maximal value recommendations for the viable microorganisms should be applied.

While the technology deployed must produce air quality of the appropriate standard, and ensure that air movement and desired pressure differentials are maintained, the technological requirements for IVF centers need not be to the complexity or cost as used by the electronics sector or those deployed to enable the mass production of sterile pharmaceutical medicinal products. With IVF centers, basic and minimum low cost solutions can be used in order to set up a clean room facility. This chapter describes the clean room technology required to achieve the minimum standards required for IVF centers.

7.2 Clean rooms and clean air devices

Clean rooms and clean air devices are typically classified according to their use (the main activity within each room or zone) and confirmed by the cleanliness of the air though the measurement of particles. Air cleanliness is either based on EU GMP guidance for aseptically filled products, where EU GMP alphabetic notations are adopted, or by using International Standard ISO14644, where numerical classes are adopted. The World Health Organization uses the same cleanliness grades as EU GMP. The cleanliness of the air is controlled by a heating, ventilation, and air conditioning (HVAC) system.

By prescribing a grade or a class to a clean room, the areas are then regarded as controlled environments. A controlled environment means that airborne particulate and microbial levels are controlled to be below specific levels, appropriate to the activities conducted within that environment.[7]

Clean rooms in IVF centers contain clean air devices. The terminology of ISO 14644-7, Clean Rooms and Associate Controlled Environments–Part 7, adopts the term "Separative Devices" to collectively describe clean air hoods, gloveboxes, isolators, and mini-environments. These devices include unidirectional airflow (UDAF) devices, biosafety cabinets (microbiological safety cabinets), and isolators. Such devices normally operate at EU GMP Grade A/ISO Class 5. The term "cabinet" is used more widely within Europe and the term "hood" is used more widely in the United States.

The reader should be aware that UDAF devices were, until the late 1990s, described as laminar airflow devices and this term is still sometimes used. The term should be avoided because "true" laminarity of air movement cannot be easily demonstrated. Unidirectional, instead, refers to a filtered air stream moving within a confined space, along parallel flow lines, with uniform velocity. Both EU GMP and U.S. FDA guidances for aseptic processing require the velocity to fall between 0.36 and 0.54 meters per second. With EU GMP, this air velocity must be verified at the "working height," whereas to meet FDA concerns, the requirement is to take the measurement six inches (around 15 cm) below the filter face.[8]

Whereas most clean rooms operate with a turbulent airflow, clean air devices are designed to minimize turbulence, for turbulence can lead to dust and dirt collecting air pockets. To overcome this, the devices operate with the air blowing in one direction (hence "unidirectional"), where the principle design feature is to move air away from the critical activity to ensure that any contamination is blown away to a less critical area (the surrounding room).

UDAF devices are either constructed with horizontal flow or vertical flow. Specially designed UDAFs are biosafety cabinets. These are "self-contained" enclosures that provide protection by creating an air barrier at the work opening and by filtering the exhaust air. Class I cabinets protect the operation or the product from personnel contamination, whereas Class II cabinets protect personnel, environment, and products.

With some UDAF devices, gloves are fitted in order to restrict the number of personnel interventions. Such devices are described as restrict access barrier systems (RABSs). These stand partway between a conventional UDAF and an isolator. Isolators differ in that they are fully sealed and can be subjected to a decontamination cycle (normally by using a vapor).[9]

7.3 Defining parameters

Before assessing the clean room technological requirements, key parameters such as temperature, humidity, or air quality must be defined.

7.3.1 Clean room design

The performance of a clean room is defined by a set of complex interactions between the airflow, sources of contamination and heat, and the position of vents, exhausts, and any objects occupying the space. Consequently, changes to any of these elements will potentially affect the operation of the clean room and could invalidate aspects of the room design.[10]

The primary objective of clean room design is particle control. Particles are made up of both viable microorganisms and nonviable matter. Particle assessment is important because most microorganisms will be shed by personnel. These will be primarily skin commensurables like *Staphylococcus* and *Micrococcus* species.[11] Moreover, most microorganisms in the air will not be free-floating; instead they are attached to skin, dust, and so on (so-termed microbial carrying particles).

While air is the main vector for contamination in clean rooms, it also stands that with properly designed clean rooms, airflow is also the answer to many contamination problems. There are four principles that apply to the control of airborne microorganisms in clean rooms.[12] These are

- Filtration (through the use of HEPA filters). The air entering a clean room from outside is filtered to exclude dust, and the air inside is constantly recirculated through high efficiency particulate air (HEPA) filters (alternative filters are ultra low penetration air [ULPA] filters). This is controlled through an heating, ventilation, and air conditioning (HVAC) system.
- Dilution (to ensure that particles generated in clean rooms, in addition to those that pass the filters, are carried away by diluting the area with new, "clean" air).
- Directional air flow (to ensure that air blows away from critical zones, as particles and microorganisms cannot "swim upstream" against a directional air flow). This is achieved through pressure differentials.
- Air movement (rapid air movement is important, for as long as particles and microorganisms stay suspended in the air, they are not really a problem; it is only when they settle out that they become an actual cause of contamination).

Thus, the key design consideration for the clean room is the HVAC system. For this, airflow and air changes must be controlled, and the temperature and humidity of the air must be maintained at appropriate levels. In addition, the air must be filtered. The HVAC system operates on the basis of mechanical ventilation.

To design the clean room, the following factors must be accounted for:

- Minimize clean space
- Correct cleanliness level
- Optimize air change rate
- Consider use of mini-environments
- Optimize ceiling coverage
- Consider clean room protocol and cleanliness class
- Minimize pressure drop (air flow resistance)
- Consider location of large air handlers—close to end use
- Provide adequate sizing and minimize length of ductwork
- Provide adequate space for low pressure drop air flow
- Low face velocity

- Use of variable speed fans
- Optimize pressurization
- Consider air flow reduction when unoccupied
- Efficient components
- Fan design
- Motor efficiency
- HEPA filters' differential pressures (ΔP)
- Fan filter efficiency
- Electrical systems that power air systems

The most important aspects of design are discussed next.

7.3.2 Temperature and humidity

A design consideration for air includes temperature and humidity control. High temperatures and humid environments can encourage microbial growth where microorganisms are deposited from the air stream onto surfaces. These parameters are controlled via HVAC systems. HVAC systems normally have two preheat coils. The first coil recovers waste heat from chillers, while the second supplements this as required, followed by a spray humidifier, and finally a chilling battery. The heating and cooling coils are utilized only for temperature control.

7.3.3 Filtration

Filtration removes microorganisms. In clean rooms, this is achieved through HEPA filters. Different classes of HEPA filters are available with different efficiency ratings. The efficiency rating refers to the theoretical level of particle removal. Standard HEPA filters are designed to remove up to 99.97% of particles from air (higher specification filters are available but these should be unnecessary in most situations). What this means is that, in theory, for every 1000 particles of size 0.3 μm that are passed into a filter, no more than three particles will pass through.

HEPA filters are protected from blockage by pre-filters, which remove up to about 90% of particles from the air. Therefore, if air contains about 3×10^8 particles per m^3, and there is one pre-filter and one HEPA filter, the pre-filter removes a sufficient number of particles to leave about 3×10^7 per m^3 as a challenge to the HEPA filter. The terminal HEPA filter will leave about 10^3 per m^3 to enter the clean room. In the EU GMP, this relatively low number is within the limits for Grade A/ISO Class 5 and Grade B/ISO Class 7 "at rest" (Annex 1.4).

In fact, most pharmaceutical air handling systems recirculate up to 80% of the air supplied to clean rooms. Therefore, the initial challenge to HEPA filters is probably only about 10^6 particles per m^3. So, in practice, there are normally no more than 3×10^2 particles per m^3 supplied to pharmaceutical clean rooms. This level is even further within the limits of Grade A/ISO Class 5 and Grade B/ISO Class 7 "at rest" in the EU GMP.

A typical HEPA filter installation is depicted in Figure 7.1.

HEPA filters function through a combination of three important aspects. First, there are one or more outer filters that work like sieves to stop the larger particles of dirt, dust, and hair. Inside those filters, there is a concertina—a mat of very dense fibers—which

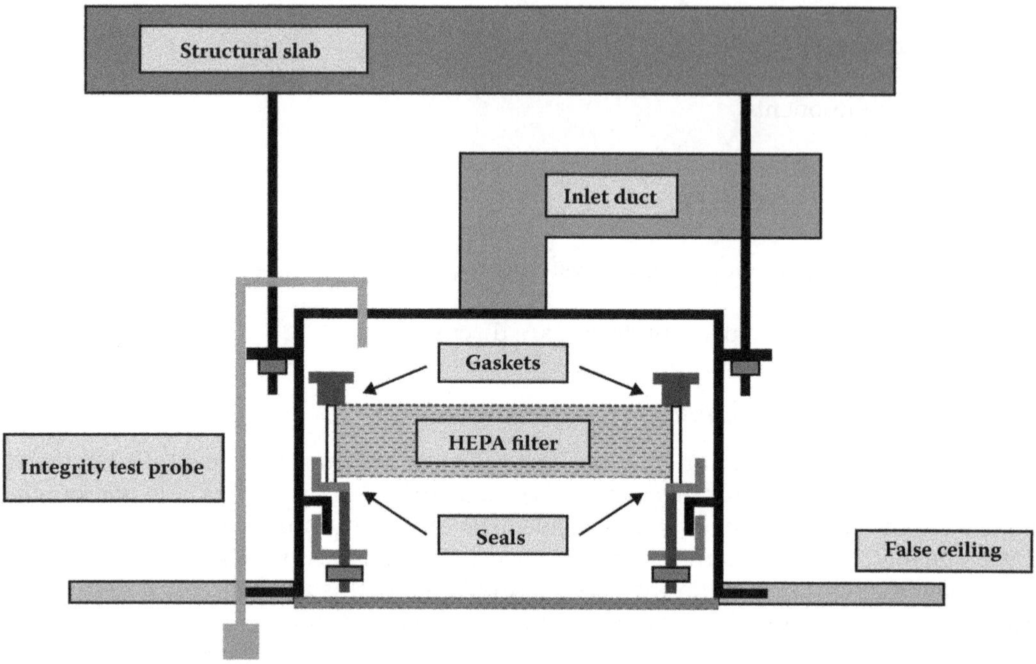

Figure 7.1 **(See color insert.)** Example of HEPA filter installation.

traps smaller particles. The inner part of the HEPA filter uses three different mechanisms to catch particles as they pass through in the moving airstream.

- Impaction, where larger particles are unable to avoid fibers by following the curving contours of the air stream and are forced to embed in one of them directly; this effect increases with diminishing fiber separation and higher air flow velocity. Thus, at high air speeds, some particles are caught and trapped as they smash directly into the fibers.
- Interception, where particles following a line of flow in the air stream come within one radius of a fiber and adhere to it.
- Diffusion, an enhancing mechanism that is the result of a collision with gas molecules by the smallest particles, especially those less than 0.1 µm in diameter, which are thereby impeded and delayed in their path through the filter (via Brownian motion). This occurs at lower air speeds.

Together, these three mechanisms allow HEPA filters to catch particles that are both larger and smaller than a certain target size.

There may be an additional requirement to have filters to remove volatile organic compounds (VOCs), chemical active compounds (CACs), and odors due to risks that such compounds pose to embryos in culture.[5,12,13] With these types of filters, a common adsorbent is activated charcoal, which has a high internal surface area, and the pollutant molecules attach to active sites on these internal surfaces. Such filters can be combined with HEPA filters or act as separate filters.[14]

7.3.4 Dilution

Particles build up in enclosed spaces where there is no ventilation. Therefore, effective clean rooms will have good ventilation. Ventilation is the process by which any particles generated in clean rooms (in addition to those that pass the filters) are carried away, and any particles remaining in the room will be diluted with new "clean" air. The minimum ventilation rate expected in clean rooms is 20 air changes per hour (although it is preferable to design a clean room capable of achieving up to twice as many air changes as this, and an even higher number of air changes per hour is preferable for changing room due to the presence of personnel and changing activities). With 20 air changes per hour, the air in a clean room is replaced at least every three minutes. In comparison, an office with standard air conditioning might have only two to three air changes per hour. Although 20 air changes is the accepted minimum standard, air change rate recommendations were developed decades ago with little scientific research to back them up. For a UDAF device, much higher rates are required to assist with meeting EU GMP Grade A/ISO Class 5 requirements. In terms of air change rates, these are between 250 and 700 air changes per hour.

Recirculation air change rates are an important factor in determining fan and motor sizing for a recirculation air handling system. Air handling sizing and air path design directly impacts the capital costs and configuration of a building. In assessing the requirement of airflow and air supply, airflow modeling is undertaken during the design stage. The key information gathered from such modeling relates to the establishment of appropriate air change rates. Such modeling allows for the performance of the clean room environment to be assessed prior to construction and to thus make changes to the layout of the clean room. The standard modeling approach is computational fluid dynamics (CFD). Spending time on design is one route for achieving optimization and subsequent lower operational costs.

7.3.5 Air movement

In relation to an assessment of air change rates, the clean room requires assessment for airflow. In aseptic processing, it is critical that contamination is avoided. Products or equipment can become contaminated from airborne microorganisms if microorganisms settle out of the air. If particles and microorganisms stay suspended in the air, they are less of a problem; it is only when they settle out that they become an actual cause of contamination. Therefore, controlling air movement is an important control step. Air movement is used in two beneficial ways in clean rooms:

- Turbulent air flow
- Unidirectional air flow (UDAF)

Most clean rooms are of the turbulent air flow type. Here, air is driven in through grills and ducts at ceiling height and removed through low level ducts. While the air is in the room, its initial supply velocity is sufficient to keep it in constant turbulence, which prevents particles and microorganisms from settling out (this is ideal because dead air can occur beneath tables and some large objects). It is important to know where dead areas occur. Where air strikes an object, any contamination in the air can be deposited, or where air becomes trapped, then dead air spots can develop. These air patterns can be shown through airflow visualization studies using smoke; the behavior of the smoke is studied and then captured onto a video camera.[15] If they cannot be avoided, viable environmental monitoring should be targeted at these locations.

An example of airflow visualization is depicted in Figures 7.2 and 7.3.

The idea of unidirectional airflow is that if air is supplied at a very high velocity through specially designed grills, it will flow for quite a distance in straight lines. Unidirectional air flow blows away all the contamination and particles that come into its path. Unidirectional airflow is also capable of sweeping up microorganisms that are sitting on surfaces, thereby cleaning the surfaces up. This can be illustrated as shown in Figures 7.4 and 7.5.

With the clean room, above the UDAF, the air is drawn from the room through high-level returns. The air is then filtered and resupplied to the room through the HEPA filters.

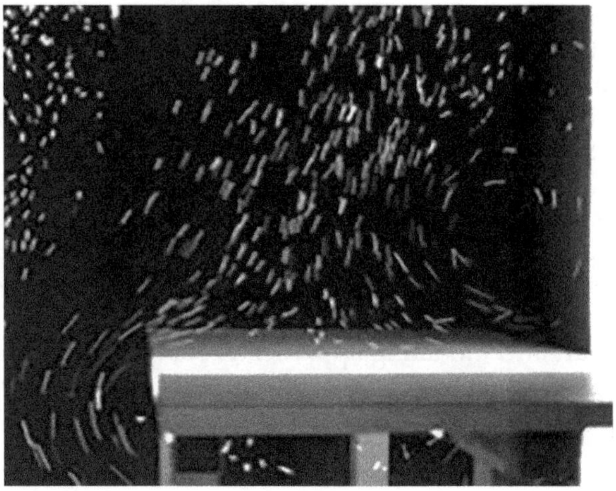

Figure 7.2 An example of turbulent airflow visualization.

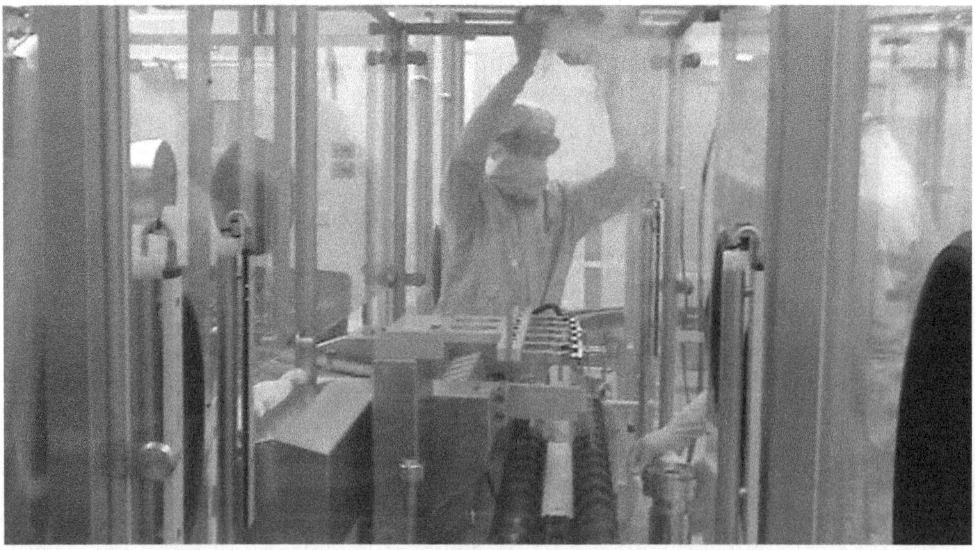

Figure 7.3 **(See color insert.)** An example of turbulent airflow visualization.

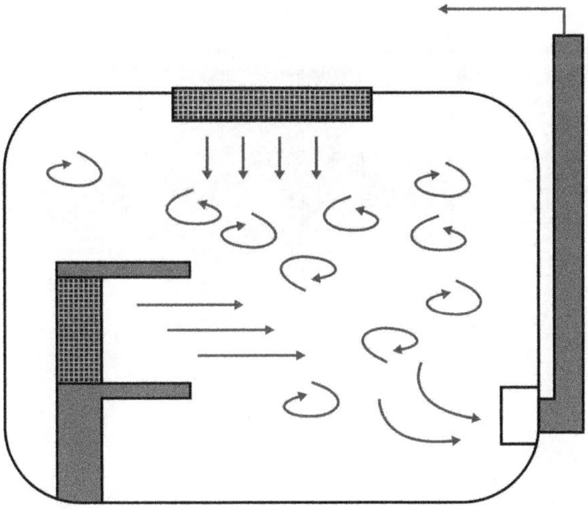

Figure 7.4 Illustration of air movement: UDAF unit (laminar flow) within a turbulent flow clean room.

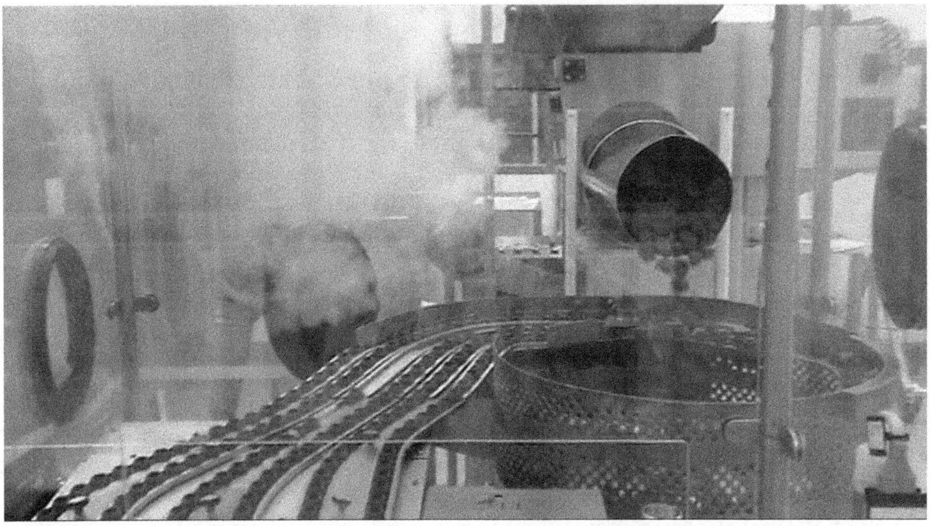

***Figure 7.5* (See color insert.)** Illustration of air movement: UDAF unit (laminar flow) within a turbulent air flow clean room.

7.3.6 Micro-environments or mini-environments

Within the clean room it is common to have a UDAF unit. A UDAF is classified as a mini-environment. This is a localized environment created by an enclosure to isolate a product or process from the surrounding environment. The advantages of using a mini-environment include the following:

- Mini-environments may create better contamination control and process integration.
- Mini-environments may maintain better contamination control by better control of the pressure difference or through the use of unidirectional airflows.
- Mini-environments may potentially reduce energy costs.

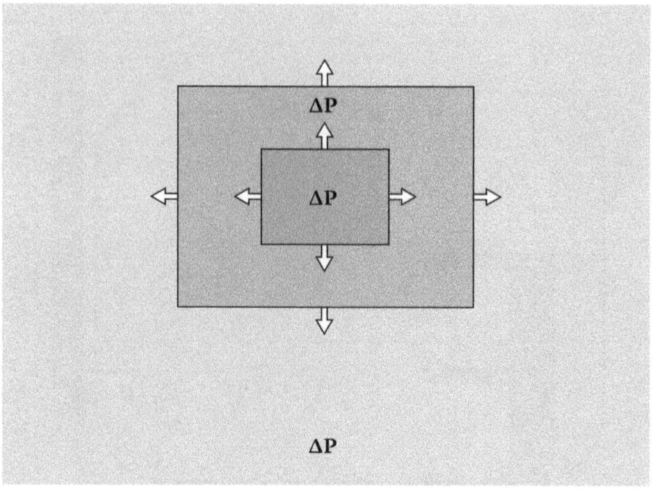

Figure 7.6 Pressure cascade.

7.3.7 Directional airflow

Directional airflow is essential for clean rooms. To illustrate this, imagine there is a room full of "clean" air. Now imagine that personnel have free access to this room from a surrounding area containing normal environmental air. If this were the case, the less-clean air would enter the clean room as personnel accessed it. To avoid this in pharmaceutical manufacturing, systems are designed to prevent "dirty" air from entering the clean room by ensuring that there is always a flow of air in an outward direction.

The way in which the "dirty" air is prevented from entering the clean room is by ensuring a very high rate of air supply to the clean room, thus keeping it at a higher pressure than its surroundings. If there is contact with "outside" air, any mixing of the two types of air takes place outside the clean room because the direction of airflow is from the clean to the dirty area. This directional airflow is measured and monitored through pressure differentials. Thus, air will always move from an area where it is at a high pressure to one where there is a low pressure (this is due to the law of physics). Particles and microorganisms cannot "swim upstream" against a directional air flow.

To protect against pressure being lost too quickly, air locks are placed over the access and exit doors of clean rooms.

An example of a "pressure differential" cascade is depicted in Figure 7.6.

7.4 Cost saving measures

The low cost IVF settings may not have enough resources to install high end AHU units or HVAC systems. Cost-effective design can be achieved through the use of pre-filters, which can remove larger particulates from the air, thereby increasing the life of HEPA and VOC filters. Pre-filters can also be protected when air is recirculated from the room, rather than air being draw from outside since the room air (which has been filtered) will contain less particulates.

Another means of saving costs is with energy savings. Clean room air systems should not be turned off when the room is not being used; however, they can be run at lower settings. The reason that air systems should not be deactivated is because in doing so contaminated air will enter the room. The contamination that can enter the room will settle onto surfaces, and the extent of this is incalculable. To restore a room to clean conditions cannot simply be achieved by restoring clean air supply. Surfaces will need to be cleaned with a detergent and then disinfected. This task is time-consuming and difficult to qualify.[16,17]

As an alternative, running clean rooms at a lower energy level when the rooms are not in use (such as overnight) can be effective. Here a small reduction in the number of air changes per hour can save considerably on energy consumption. The risks are relatively low because the room continues to be supplied with clean air and turbulent airflow is maintained. The primary risk in clean rooms comes from people, as a result of shedding skin detritus. Without people present, the performance requirements of clean rooms can be lowered.

7.5 Validation

The effectiveness of the clean room and its operational technology must be validated. For this the requirements outlined in the ISO 14644 series of clean room standards are normally adopted.

At the end of the design phase, verification should be undertaken by particle counting to assess air cleanliness to ISO 14644 Part 1.[18] At the very end of the qualification process, viable environmental monitoring must be performed. This is to assess how the design measures for clean room control function with operators present within the clean room. Environmental monitoring is typically performed at a high level and then reduced, provided that the data are satisfactory in terms of the avoidance of excursions above action levels. Initially it is commonplace to place an "imaginary" grid over the clean room and to take environmental monitoring samples within each area. Once the initial assessment has been completed, sample locations should be selected by risk assessment.[19]

The types of samples taken are

1. Active air samples: mechanical samplers draw in 1 m^3 of air. Any microorganisms present in the air are deposited onto the surface of an agar plate through direct impaction or by centrifugal force.
2. Settle plates: these are exposed agar plates that when positioned in meaningful locations will capture any microbial carrying particles that gravitate out from the air.
3. Contact plates: these are domed agar plates, containing a disinfectant neutralizer, designed to assess contamination from flat surfaces.
4. Swabs: these are devices that are used to measure contamination from irregular surfaces. They are not as efficient as contact plates due to relative poor recovery from the swab tip to culture medium.

7.6 Ongoing monitoring

The effectiveness of the clean room and its operational technology must be assessed through an ongoing monitoring program. Monitoring should consist of physical measurements, such as pressure differentials between the main preparation area and surroundings areas, and particle counting during processing. As an optional assessment, some facilities also elect to undertake tests to assess the control of VOCs (chemical compounds that evaporate and react with indoor ozone). As well as physical monitoring, viable microbiological environmental monitoring must also be performed.

Ongoing monitoring is not only important for informing about the contamination risk to the cells, it provides useful information for when cost saving measures are implemented and allows a risk-based approach to be adopted.[20] By taking baseline readings before and after the instigation of energy saving, the impact of the reduction in energy, or modification to the air handling system, can be reviewed.

The performance of a clean room is defined by a set of complex interactions between the airflow, sources of contamination and heat, position of vents, exhausts, and any objects occupying the space. Consequently, changes to any of these elements will potentially affect the operation of the clean room and could invalidate aspects of the room design.

7.6.1 Airflows

Airflows are important for two significant aspects of clean room design and operation: the speed (or velocity) of the air and the direction in which the air travels.

With aseptic filling, EU GMP Grade A/ISO 14644 Class 5 zones (unidirectional airflow devices in the EU GMP Grade B/ISO Class 7 rooms, in operation) have a requirement for controlled air velocity and unidirectional air flow (either horizontal or vertical). The specification is 0.45 m/s ± 20%, according to the EU GMP. Airflows are monitored using an anemometer. The air velocity is designed to be sufficient to remove any relatively large particles before they settle onto surfaces. This monitoring should be performed routinely and during requalification exercises.

Within clean rooms the air is normally operating at a turbulent flow (this is where air enters the room with nonuniform velocity). Here, air is driven in through grilles and ducts at ceiling height and removed through low level ducts. While the air is in the room its initial supply velocity is sufficient to keep it in constant turbulence, which prevents particles and microorganisms from settling out (this is an ideal because dead air can occur beneath tables and with other items of equipment). Between clean rooms of different grades or classes, the airflow must be from a higher grade area to a lower grade area.

7.6.2 Air change rates

Each clean room grade should have a set number of required air changes per hour. Air changes are provided in order to dilute any particles present to an acceptable concentration. Any contamination produced in the clean room is theoretically removed within the required time appropriate to the room grade. This is important because particles would otherwise build up in enclosed spaces if there were no ventilation.

Monitoring air changes is necessary because the recirculation of filtered air is important for maintaining control of the clean area. Air change rates stated are the minimum and should be calculated from supply air volume and room volume measurements.

7.6.3 Clean-up times (recovery tests)

Connected to air changes is the time taken for a clean area to return to the static condition, appropriate to its grade, in terms of particulates. Clean-up times are sometimes referred to as "recovery tests." This is assessed by the room being subject to a level of particles above the room class and then measuring, through the use of an optical particle counter, how long the room takes to return to the level of particles required for the room class. The typical target is for a room to "clean up" within 15–20 minutes.

The conducting of clean-up times is an optional test to be considered at the time of room classification, following substantial changes to room design, for newly built clean rooms, or as part of an investigation.

According to the EU GMP Guide these "clean-up" times apply to Grade A and B areas only. They may, however, be used as a guidance for ISO Class 8/EU GMP Grade C and D areas in the course of an investigation. There are no specifications in either the EU GMP or ISO 14644 for the level of particles that is required to be generated above the static limit in order to demonstrate the room clean-up. In the absence of a defined limit, a level of twice the static state limit is recommended. This is considered to be an effective challenge of room clean-up.

Other factors that need to be decided include:

a. The time period at which particles are elevated above the static state.

   In setting a time a balance needs to be struck between raising the level of particles to a sufficiently high level against the risk of damaging the optics of the particle counter and the difficulties in sustaining a high level of particles, especially for Grade C and D areas. It is considered that a minimum of two minutes is a practical time period to set.

b. The number of particle counter locations in the room.

   If a clean room has satisfactorily passed requalification for airborne particles and no location has been shown to be "worst case," then one location at the approximate center of the room is a practical option. Other locations can be added if required.

7.6.4 Pressure differentials

Connected to the measurement of airflow is the maintenance of positive pressure. In order to maintain air quality in a clean room, the pressure of a given room must be greater relative to a room of a lower grade. This is to ensure that air does not pass from "dirtier" adjacent areas into the higher grade clean room. Generally this is set at 15–20 Pascals, although some areas of the same grade will also have differential pressure requirements due to specific activities, such as where dust is generated through the weighting of powders.

Pressure differentials are the relative pressures from a higher grade area into a lower one. Pressurization is defined as a method by which air pressure differences are created mechanically between rooms to introduce intentional air movement paths through room leakage openings. With this, the relative quantities of air are delivered and removed from each space by the ducted air system, air transfer system, and losses. These openings could be either designated, such as doorways, or undesignated, such as air gaps around doorframes or other cracks.

To help achieve the required pressure differential between clean rooms of different grades, airlocks are used. An airlock is an airtight room that adjoins two clean rooms. The airlock acts as a buffer zone between two independent areas of unequal pressure. A pressure differential of ≥15 Pa is typically maintained between the inner room and the airlock and between the airlock and the external.

7.6.5 Sanitization

For some healthcare applications, greater assurance that pathogens have been removed from the air supply is recommended. For this ultraviolet (UV) lighting is incorporated into the HEPA filter design. The total power of the UV lamp is a product to the power of the light source multiplied by the exposure time. A typical specification for a UV light is a 254 nanometer wavelength UV light operating at 6500 mW/cm^2. While the use of UV light is recommended, there are concerns about its effectiveness as a microbiocide.[21]

Another key aspect of sanitization relates to the cleaning and disinfecting of clean rooms. Detergents are used to remove soil (such as grease and protein), and the removal allows disinfectants to be able to reach any microbial cells to inactivate or to kill them. Disinfectant solutions are chemical or physical agents that destroy or remove vegetative forms of harmful microorganisms when applied to a surface. The types of disinfectants selected must be effective for use within clean rooms and must be controlled.

To meet regulatory expectations in the pharmaceutical industry, a cleaning and disinfection program is required. The program should consist of a policy outlining the objectives and the criteria for the selection of materials and cleaning agents; and a procedure, detailing how cleaning is undertaken, along with the techniques and cleaning frequencies. There is an expectation that such programs are regularly reviewed and reflect any changes to clean room design and respond to changes in environmental monitoring data.[22]

7.6.6 Leak testing of HEPA filters

In addition to assessing the efficiency of HEPA filters, they are also subject to leak testing. Because potential leakage is not confined to the filter media, there is a requirement to perform an in situ filter integrity test. This is commonly called the DOP test after di-octyl phthalate, one of the first substances used as an aerosol challenge for this test. Alternative fluids with similar particle-size distributions, such as BP-grade paraffin and poly-alfa-olefins (PAOs), are widely used. The chemical is used in conjunction with an aerosol generator (this is a device used in conjunction with an aerosol photometer, which creates a polydispersed sub-micron aerosol to challenge integrity of HEPA filters and containment of safety cabinets).

The standard is that the tolerable leakage of an aerosol challenge shall be not more than 0.01% (note, this is not the reciprocal of the filter efficiency). This is measured using an aerosol photometer (this is a device that determines particle concentration in air by measuring the mass concentration of scattered light).

7.6.7 Temperature, humidity, lighting, and room design

Certain clean rooms have set requirements for temperature and humidity (such as clean rooms used for aseptic processing). These are monitored for operator comfort and to avoid a high temperature–humidity situation, which may result in the shedding of microorganisms. Within EU GMP, Grade B clean rooms are required to have a temperature of 18 ± 3°C. In ISO 14644 Part 4, the recommended range of humidity is 45 ± 15%. Other clean areas have a temperature appropriate to the process step (such as if the process requires a cold room at 2–8°C).

Lighting should be adequate, uniform, and anti-glare to allow operators to perform process tasks effectively. A range of 400 to 750 lux—units of illuminance and luminous emittance—is recommended (equivalent to typical television studio lighting). In addition, the surfaces of clean rooms should be constructed from materials that do not generate particles and are easy to clean.

7.7 Equipment maintenance

The maintenance, servicing, cleaning, disinfection, and sanitation of all critical equipment must be performed regularly. It is important that these activities are recorded in logbooks, and that any changes, including the replacement of parts, are recorded and justified as necessary.

References

1. Reinmüller B. People as a contamination source—Clothing systems. In: *Dispersion and Risk Assessment of Airborne Contaminants in Pharmaceutical Cleanrooms*. Royal Institute of Technology, Building Services Engineering, Bulletin No. 56, Stockholm 2001, pp. 54–77.
2. Sharp J, Bird A, Brzozowski S, and O'Hagan K. Contamination of cleanrooms by people. *European Journal of Parenteral and Pharmaceutical Sciences* 2010; 15(3): 73–81.
3. Boone WR, Johnson JE, Locke AJ, Crane MM, and Price TM. Control of air quality in an assisted reproductive technology laboratory. *Fertil Steril* 1999; 71(1): 150–4.
4. Commission of the European Parliament, 2004. Directive 2004/23/EC of the European Parliament and of the Council of 31 March 2004 on setting standards of quality and safety for the donation, procurement, testing, processing, preservation, storage and distribution of human tissues and cells. http://eur-lex.europa.eu/LexUriServ/LexUriServ.do?uri=CELEX:32004L0023:EN:NOT/. Accessed January 30, 2014.
5. Esteves SC and Bento FC. Implementation of air quality control in reproductive laboratories in full compliance with the Brazilian Cells and Germinative Tissue Directive. *Reprod Biomed Online* 2013; 26(1): 9–21.
6. Eudralex The Rules Governing Medicinal Products in the European Community (Directive 2003/94/EC), Volume 4, Annex 1, published by the European Commission, Brussels, Belgium, 2014.
7. Sandle T, Saghee MR, and Ramstrop M. Environmental Monitoring and Cleanrooms, IDMA-APA Guideline, Technical Monograph No. 5, Indian Drug Manufacturers Association 2010, Mumbai.
8. Food and Drug Administration. Guidance for Industry: Sterile Drug Products Produced by Aseptic Processing—Current Good Manufacturing Practice. [FDA Website.] September 2004. www.fda.gov/downloads/Drugs/GuidanceComplianceRegulatoryInformation/Guidances/UCM070342.pdf. Accessed January 30, 2014.
9. Midcalf B, Neiger J, and Sandle T. Fundamentals of pharmaceutical isolators. In: Sandle T and Saghee MR (eds.). *Cleanroom Management in Pharmaceuticals and Healthcare*, Euromed Communications, Passfield, UK, 2003, pp. 185–226.
10. Ljungqvist B and Reinmüller B. *Cleanroom Design—Minimizing Contamination Through Proper Design*. Interpharm Press, Buffalo Grove IL, 1997, pp. 1–3.
11. Sandle T. A review of cleanroom microflora: Types, trends, and patterns, *PDA Journal of Pharmaceutical Science and Technology* 2011; 65(4): 392–403.
12. Sandle T. Contamination Control: Cleanrooms and Clean Air Devices. Encyclopedia of Pharmaceutical Science and Technology, 4th ed. Taylor & Francis, London, 2013, pp. 634–43.
13. Worrilow KC, Huynh HT, Gwozdziewicz JB, Schillings WA, and Peters AJ. A retrospective analysis: The examination of a potential relationship between particulate (P) and volatile organic compound (VOC) levels in a class 100 IVF laboratory cleanroom (CR) and specific parameters of embryogenesis and rates of implantation (IR). *Fertil Steril* 2001; 76(1): S15–6.
14. Das D, Gaur V, and Verma N. Removal of volatile organic compound by activated carbon fiber. *Carbon* 2004; 42(14): 2949–62.
15. Sandle T. Airflow visualisation in an aseptic facility. *Cleanroom Technology* 2012; 20(5): 13–17.
16. Halls N. *Microbiological Environmental Monitoring Explained*. Sue Horwood Publishing, Storrington, UK, 2002, p. 11.

17. Sandle T. Application of disinfectants and detergents in the pharmaceutical sector. In Sandle T (Ed.). *The CDC Handbook: A Guide to Cleaning and Disinfecting Cleanrooms*, Grosvenor House Publishing, Surrey, UK, 2012, pp. 168–97.
18. ISO 14644-1. Cleanrooms and associated controlled environments—Part 1: Classification of air cleanliness, ISO, Geneva, Switzerland, 1999.
19. Sandle T. Environmental monitoring: A practical approach. In: Moldenhauer J (ed.). *Environmental Monitoring: A Comprehensive Handbook*, Volume 6, PDA/DHI, River Grove, IL2012, pp. 29–54.
20. Sandle T. Risk management in pharmaceutical microbiology. In: Saghee MR, Sandle T, and Tidswell EC (eds.). *Microbiology and Sterility Assurance in Pharmaceuticals and Medical Devices*, Business Horizons, New Delhi , 2011, pp. 553–88.
21. Pigeot-Remya S, Lazzaronid JC, Simoneta F, Petingab P, Valletc C, Petitb P et al. Survival of bioaerosols in HVAC system photocatalytic filters. *Applied Catalysis B: Environmental* 2014; 144: 654–64.
22. Denny VF and Marsik FJ. Current practices in the use of disinfectants within the pharmaceutical industry. *PDA J Pharm Sci Tech* 1997; 51(6): 227–8.

chapter eight

Modular clean rooms

Patrick J. Traver and George H. Wiker

Contents

Abstract

Modular construction is becoming an important trend in many types of buildings. It has the ability to improve a project from a number of aspects including flexibility, speed of construction, and standardization of materials. These are important advantages in all industries but in particular provide significant benefits when used in clean rooms. Industries that use clean rooms need to follow many regulations and having standardized products provides a substantial head start in meeting these criteria. The modularity also provides owners with the flexibility they need to meet changes in processes and practices. The advantages and details underlying modular clean room construction will be discussed in this chapter.

8.1 Clean rooms—The environment is everything

Maintaining a clean environment is an essential aspect of developing and manufacturing many products as well as ensuring an environment that will not contribute negatively to excellence in processing. This is particularly true for products intended for people, where maintaining tight control of airborne particulates and microbial contamination (bio-burden) is required to a measured degree. The purpose of this chapter is to identify the types of clean room environments available and educate readers to make appropriate decisions in the development and operation of a manufacturing process set in a clean room. The chapter will also go into more detail on new design alternatives used in the industry and discuss trends that help reduce bio-burden concerns, increase customer perception of a facility, and reduce construction timelines.

To safely and consistently process materials, certain process operations must be protected within a clean room environment. A clean room is considered a room, or contained area, in which the environment is controlled to mitigate particulate and bio-burden in the air as well as minimize the potential of accumulation of such contaminants on surfaces. Many steps are taken to ensure that the integrity of the clean room environment remains intact for the protection of any process operation. Any breach in the process or the clean room environment in which it resides offers a major source for potential contamination.

Airborne particulates of concern are invisible to the unassisted human eye. Although the human eye cannot see them, they should not be forgotten. To put things into perspective, a human hair measures 75–100 μ in diameter and a 0.5-μ particulate is approximately 200 times smaller. One such particle can be harmful to a process operation, particularly if it is open to the clean room. Because of this "invisible" particulate characteristic, it is very important to mitigate the possibility of contaminations by taking into consideration certain design elements to ensure that cleanliness is not compromised and that the outcome of the intended process is successful.

In the case of in vitro fertilization (IVF) laboratories, sperm, oocytes, and embryos are exposed directly to the clean room environment, which makes it much more important to protect the process operation, due to their acute sensitivity and intolerance of a suboptimal environment. That is why it is especially important to make sure the IVF clean room environment is free of particulate and submicron airborne contaminants.

The only way to mitigate the risk of contamination in a process operation is to minimize the potential for contamination in the entire environment. That includes taking precautions from the very beginning in the design of a new facility and should occur long before any walls are built. Operational flows, standard operating procedures, cleaning procedures, gowning procedures, air flow, and construction materials are part of the determining factors that contribute to the optimization and success of the environment.

8.2 Clean environment options—Define your process

Developing a clean room environment for a process can be expensive, so it is important to understand which areas actually need to be classified as "clean." Are there multiple functions or one dedicated function? Do people need to be involved or is it something that can be done by machines or robots? The process determines the space needs and the old adage particularly applies here, that *form follows function.*

In process operations where the operator is dealing with the open transfer of product, localized enclosures (or barriers) can be used to separate the open product from the clean room environment to mitigate risk of contamination of the product. Inside the enclosure, filtered air is supplied to the enclosure to provide a clean and protected local environment. This usually works well when the size of the product is minimal.

Another way to deal with a localized clean room environment is to use laminar flow hoods, bio safety cabinets, or fume hoods. Again, it depends on the process and the products that are being developed. For example, when personnel protection is required, fume hoods work best when dealing with chemicals as they remove the fumes and protect the operator. When the product is required to be protected in a local enclosure, laminar airflow units provide an effective ability to wash clean air over the product, which is then transferred into the clean room. Laminar airflow units come in a variety of sizes and configurations, with the ability to have air flow in a laminar pathway either vertically or horizontally. In the case in which both the product and the operator need to be protected, biosafety cabinets are the preferred solution. Several different types of biosafety cabinets are available in the market and are selected based on the degree of cleanliness, protection, and containment that will be required during the process.

Manually operated processes often require larger clean room environments. The clean room needs to be able to provide an adequate area for the required personnel and the equipment that is needed to complete the process. In this type of scenario, the entire room needs to be monitored and controlled as well as the adjacent spaces. These adjacent spaces could be airlocks, labs, anterooms, or any other type of clean room required for gowning or processing. To enter and exit these clean room spaces, a transition strategy must be developed, implemented, and maintained to isolate product-specific process operations as well as maintain the environment of the clean room space. Also required is an air pressurization approach to the clean room design, which helps maintain the integrity of the cleanest rooms and prevents unwanted mixing of air by controlling the direction in which it flows. Airlocks, as an example, provide a separation between two clean rooms. The clean rooms and these airlocks are typically positively pressured compared to the lesser clean room spaces, which prevents dirty air from entering the clean room spaces. These airlocks also act as the transition spaces where gowning is usually added or removed depending on the transition strategy. They also provide the ability to transfer materials from one (often clean room) space to another.

In instances where clean rooms are required, it should be noted that both the product as well as personnel need to be protected from airborne contaminates and hazardous materials. The major feature utilized to achieve such protection is through clean room air changes, and this is measured using air changes per hour, or ACHs. The ACH represents the amount of air added or removed from the clean room space in a given amount of time. It should also be noted that air changes by themselves do not achieve the cleanliness required for the room. The air is filtered as it enters the space typically through high efficiency particulate air (HEPA) or ultra low penetration air (ULPA) filters. The clean room is also closely monitored in terms of airflow, temperature, and humidity.

In order for the airflow to provide a clean environment, the clean rooms need to be designed to be able to manage such conditions. As an example, rooms requiring a higher level of cleanliness will require more air changes. The corresponding amount of air supplied into the room increases the air pressure in the room, thus increasing the possibility of the air trying to escape from the room. This phenomenon can be equated to the principle involved in blowing up a balloon. The more air blown into the balloon, the more air pressure is built up in the balloon. Air will try to escape to equalize the pressure between inside the balloon and outside the balloon. The same applies to a clean room. The air will naturally try to leak out of the room so it is important to take certain design measures to prevent this from happening. Oftentimes a normal tile and grid ceiling will not effectively contain the air within a clean room. Leakage will often occur so it is important to specify in the design a type of ceiling that can maintain the clean room environment. An alternative to this is to use a gasketed ceiling grid with nonperforated vinyl-coated ceiling tiles. This ensures that leakage will not occur and the integrity of the room will be withheld. Completely closed ceilings such as drywall ceilings or modular panel ceilings should be used for cleaner spaces.

Selecting the correct environmental protection system all depends on the process being completed. Whatever the process, large or small, the same considerations need to be taken to ensure that the integrity of the process is not compromised. Overlooking the simplest step could be the difference between having successful outcomes or failures associated with the process.

8.3 Modular clean rooms

Modular construction refers to the use of prefabricated and/or pre-engineered building components that are assembled together, often at the site with other construction components, to create a complete facility. Modular walls, doors, ceilings, and process/utility systems are integrated on site to create an environment like puzzle pieces. These "pieces" are built and manufactured off site and are delivered to the site ready to be installed. There are many advantages to this approach as well as some disadvantages, which will be discussed.

The first advantage of a modular clean room is speed of construction and installation. The traditional method of construction is often referred to as stick-built construction. Stick-built construction is considered to be any construction built on site by putting together pieces to form an object. Unlike stick-built construction, modular components can be manufactured elsewhere while construction progresses on site. As an example, the walls in a stick-built clean room project cannot be installed until other objects are installed and/or constructed. The wall studs are first installed, followed by utilities, and concluding with the wall board. After the wall board is installed, the walls need to be finished with multiple coats of joint compound. Finally, a water-based, low VOC epoxy paint is applied followed by a rubber wall base to finish the installation. Depending on the size of the new clean room, this process could take weeks. With modular construction, the walls are manufactured off site in controlled conditions and delivered to the job site ready to be installed. As a standard, they are engineered to be compliant with all governing agencies to meet clean room requirements. Once they are scheduled to be installed, it takes a matter of days to have them completely installed, with less waste and less mess. Since the construction timeline is shortened, theoretically the facility should be up and running for its intended purpose faster, thus creating revenue earlier.

A second advantage to modular construction is the flexibility and durability of the modular systems. Each system is comprised of puzzle pieces that snap together similar to building blocks. These pieces can, in fact, be removed if needed and relocated or reassembled in another configuration. For example, an original IVF facility design may include only one transfer room. This may have been determined in the initial programming based on location and the potential volume of patients in the area. Based on the success of the space design to meet the needs of the processes and the demand of an increased number of cycles, the facility design may need to be changed or expanded. In this scenario, modular construction systems allow the disassembly and reconfiguration of the walls and ceilings without major disruption to the current process operations. Using modular systems optimizes the flexibility of the IVF program and facility. It is a much easier and less disruptive process over that of demolishing conventional stick-built construction items, and then having to rebuild it. Traditional construction techniques rely on an experienced and qualified workforce to construct and demolish a clean room. This type of process increases operating costs and product contamination risks over time, while modular construction systems leverage a proven and simplified construction technology which mitigates risk to the process operations and gets facilities up and running faster.

Another advantage of modular construction is that the materials selected for each system are designed with clean room process operations in mind. These systems typically utilize materials that mitigate the risk of mold growth or other organisms on surfaces. The connections between the different components are also designed with smooth transitions, which will not accumulate particulate. The smooth surfaces of clean room materials will also not shed particulates over time and in the constant exposure of the environment to the vibrations caused by equipment. Exposed surfaces are designed to withstand the routine use of harsh cleaning chemicals. Over time, traditional construction methods and materials may lose their integrity and ability to provide the resistance and durability needed in a clean room environment. For example, traditional wall board partitions sometimes fail for multiple reasons. The finish material initially used may start to fade or chip due to the use of harsh chemical cleaners or damage from mobile processing equipment. If built traditionally, a water-based, low VOC epoxy paint should be used to give the best possible protection. This method, however, relies on a quality contractor to finish partitions according to the manufacturer's specifications, and to ensure that the environment in which it is installed meets the manufacturer's application recommendations. These site-specific variables many times result in a finished product that will not meet all of the demanding requirements of an operational clean room. If the epoxy paint begins to fail, it has the ability to expose the porous substrate, which is the ideal environment for organisms such as mold to grow. Mold remediation can be costly and could compromise process operations if not captured immediately. Mold resistant nonporous wall board assists in mitigating these facility risks but cannot completely defend against contaminants if the wall finishing system is compromised.

Visual perception and customer awareness are becoming increasingly important as new IVF facilities are being designed and constructed. Owners are educating themselves on current construction trends and are taking note that all facilities are not created equal. With that being said, leveraging modular constructed clean rooms contributes to a perception of a high quality and reliable facility which has been constructed and dedicated solely to the success of a patient's procedure. Compared side by side, the modular clean room looks and feels to be of a higher quality compared to traditional construction techniques. This shows patients that the facility and practice care about their procedure and are trying to provide the best environment possible to promote successful outcomes.

One disadvantage to the modular construction systems is an increased initial capital cost for construction materials. Depending on the facility location, modular construction costs can be 5–10% more expensive for the cost of the material. This must always be considered when planning a facility project and formulating construction estimates. However, it should be noted that this is offset by a faster construction timeline, the ability to initiate IVF cycles sooner, the flexibility of the space to accommodate growth and/or changes in processes, and in the maintenance of the overall clean room system. Over the life of the facility, it is more cost advantageous to use modular construction systems versus conventional construction when taking into account all of the factors included in a facility life cycle analysis.

Once the investment is made on a modular system, the system is owned similar to a piece of furniture or equipment. The system could be disassembled, reconfigured, or relocated to another location if desired. This can become important in scenarios where a facility increases the amount of patient cycles it performs and needs more room for growth. The modular system can be relocated to a new location and new wall panels can simply be purchased and installed to accommodate the new, larger design. There are also some significant financial advantages that are associated with purchasing a modular clean room system. It is essentially a piece of equipment and therefore can be considered capital equipment. A stick-built facility falls under the category of a capital improvement. Since modular construction can be considered capital equipment, it can be depreciated at an accelerated rate which results in an improved financial balance sheet for the owner.

8.4 A new modular design approach

Speed to market is a very important movement. In order to get to market faster, the construction timeline must be shortened and optimized. In order to decrease the construction schedule, the design timeline needs to be improved. One option used to do this is standardized facility designs. There is a design process for every project that is essentially always the same. In pre-design, the facility designer gathers information from the client about what the space needs to be and how it will function. The next phase, schematic design, essentially takes gathered information from the pre-design phase and develops an early concept design. Following this is detail design. During this phase, the design is essentially completed. All aspects needed for the construction of the space are worked through and coordinated such as room dimensions and volumes, construction materials, equipment, and utilities.

What if these design phases could be consolidated? What if designers had a head start? The design timeline could be reduced significantly if the designers have more knowledge and experience with the type of facility that is being designed as well as tools to help develop ideas faster. One major tool would be the utilization of standardized rooms. Most IVF facilities have similar functional requirements in which to perform their process operations. In new facilities, why does the design process need to start at the beginning? Typically, the designer will sit with the owner and figure out what rooms they need in a new or renovated facility. Facility designers typically ask which process operations will be performed in each room followed by equipment requirements, utilities requirements, and furniture preferences if needed. Once the room designs are selected, the designer can then assemble the "blocks" in a manner that fits into the space available. A design process that sometimes takes a significant amount of time can be drastically reduced, saving time and money for both the design team and the client. Most of the time, the client has limited design and construction experience so designing a new facility can become a long and sometimes frustrating process. Using this modular design approach helps them move their ideas to paper with less of their time involved and allows them to spend more time concentrating on their practice and their patients.

8.5 Considerations for IVF facilities

Though there are many considerations when designing a new lab, there should be one primary focus when designing for an IVF facility—providing the optimal environment for the successful growth of a human embryo. There are a number of concepts and ideas that should be included and not overlooked in the design to ensure the most probable outcomes.

Assurance of air quality is paramount in the design of the proper in vitro culture environment. Properly designed HVAC systems and equipment must be used. This is not the area to overlook or reduce quality. Poor air quality can have detrimental effects on IVF pregnancy rates so it is very important to provide an environment that yields the best possible air quality results. Careful considerations need to be taken in order to provide the necessary air change rates, proper air intake points, and air filtration requirements. Making the room positive in pressure to the surrounding rooms is also critical. This assures that contaminants do not enter the space coming from adjacent rooms. Short cuts in any of these areas can significantly reduce pregnancy success rates.

As mentioned previously, construction materials are a significant factor. Using materials with zero VOCs should be a requirement. Materials whose by-products give off harmful gases should be avoided. These types of products include sealants and adhesives which are sometimes overlooked. Simply using alternate materials that are IVF appropriate can allow for less of an "off-gas" period normally required in a project timeline. It also is directly related to overall air quality. Not introducing harmful pollutants into the space is critical to keeping the space free of impurities.

Cleanability is also another major consideration to keep in mind when designing a new IVF facility. Choosing construction materials and methods that are user friendly in terms of cleanability is highly recommended. Reducing the amount of corners and edges helps reduce the amount of surfaces where dirt and pollutants can reside. Using materials that are smooth and nonporous contributes to the overall effectiveness of the facility. Construction techniques such as integral coved floor bases and wall corner coving improve the ability to clean surfaces and reduce the chance of build-up of pollutants. Wall and floor finishes that are resistant to chemicals are also a very important consideration because they need to be cleaned often. Having the ability to withstand regular cleanings is important to the everyday life of the facility and will help contribute to the longevity of the space.

Equipment and furniture need to be carefully introduced into the space. There should be an "off-gas" period planned for these items. New equipment and furniture give off gases that could be potentially harmful to the process if not dealt with properly. The finishes of these items should be "clean room" quality and should not include any wood products. Stainless steel is safe because of its ability to withstand contaminants as well as most chemicals used for cleaning.

The location of the facility could potentially play an important role in how the facility operates. It may not be in the best interest to locate the facility next to operations that could potentially create harmful gases that could leak into the facility. Carefully designed facilities can negate these issues, but strategically locating the facility helps in the overall design. It should also be noted that even locations within the same building could affect the success of the facility. As an example, locating the facility on an upper floor of a building could potentially have an adverse affect on the process because of vibration and swaying of the building. These vibrations could cause problems in the process, and so being on the ground floor is more desirable to reduce the possibility of any vibration-induced perturbations.

The current trend for new facilities (whether it is for IVF, pharmaceutical manufacturing, laboratories, etc.) is speed to market and modularity. Clients want the ability to be flexible and want it yesterday, so the demand for these options is driving the way facilities are designed and constructed. Mechanisms are being developed to meet the demand and they are being implemented into the whole process from start to finish. Using "predesigned" standards as a starting point can really accelerate the design. Recreating the wheel is a thing of the past. Modifying the wheel is a thing of the future. Modular construction is providing the ability to be flexible while adding the value of faster construction. Combining both modularity and standardized design lead to faster, higher quality design which creates a professional and patient-friendly environment for many years to come.

Suggested reading

U.S. Pharmacopeia (USP) General Chapter: Microbiological Evaluation of Cleanrooms and Other Controlled Environments. http://www.pharmacopeia.cn/v29240/usp29nf24s0_c1116.html.

International Organization for Standardization, 1999. ISO 14644-1:2005 on Cleanrooms and Associated Controlled Environments—Part 1: Classification of Air Cleanliness.

International Organization for Standardization, 2001. ISO 14644-4:2004 on Cleanrooms and Associated Controlled Environments—Part 4: Design, Construction and Start-Up.

chapter nine

Gases for embryo culture and volatile organic compounds in incubators

Jayant G. Mehta and Alex C. Varghese

Contents

Abstract

This chapter addresses the importance of medical grade gases and the care needed to handle these gases. Additionally, the importance of the types of cylinders, valves, and regulators required for a safe delivery of the medical gas at the point of use is discussed. Last, the impact of volatile organic compounds (VOCs) in an IVF laboratory and how VOCs originate and enter the IVF laboratory and embryo culture environment are considered.

9.1 Introduction

Over the last decade, in vitro fertilization (IVF) laboratories have witnessed increases in pregnancy and live births rates compared to the early days of IVF. A better understanding of the gamete and embryo physiology has allowed scientists to create an appropriate in vitro culture environment. Two major factors responsible for the improvements in outcomes have been the more physiologically appropriate "culture media" and newer designed top loading "mini culture incubators." With advances in technology, multiple incubator types now exist with varying capabilities and differing methods of regulating their internal environment providing tri-gas combinations, even with the front-loading large incubators.

The detrimental effect of volatile organic compounds (VOCs) within the IVF laboratory has been extensively reviewed.[1–7] In The United Kingdom, the Human Fertilization and Embryology Authority (HFEA)[8] stipulates that the quality of the air within the laboratory should be of "grade C" (see Chapter 18). Centers will be required to have documented procedures for achieving the air quality requirements and monitoring compliance. Equally important is the purity of medical grade gases within the enclosed chambers of an incubator.

This chapter addresses the importance of medical grade gases and the care needed to handle these gases. Additionally, the importance of the types of cylinders, valves, and regulators required for a safe delivery of the medical gas at the point of use is discussed. Last, the impact of VOCs in an IVF laboratory and how VOCs originate and enter the IVF laboratory and embryo culture environment are considered.

9.2 Medical grade gases: An overview

The gases designated for therapeutic or diagnostic purposes must undergo rigorous testing and meet standards before use. The medical gases include gaseous (compressed medical gases: CMG) and liquid (cryogenic) stored in high-pressure cylinders. All the gases used in IVF should be of United States Pharmacopeia (USP) medical grade, but the specifications vary for each of them. Each cylinder is accompanied with a written analysis certificate that states the purity and trace elements contaminations. Incubators ought to be connected to pipelines delivering either carbon dioxide, nitrogen, or a gas mixture containing carbon dioxide, oxygen, and nitrogen (e.g., 6% CO_2, 5% O_2, and 89% nitrogen). Production of medical gases (e.g., processing, filling, trans-filling, mixing, purification, separation, cascading, transfer, packaging, and distribution) follows the current good manufacturing practices (cGMP) set forth in 21 CFR Parts 210 and 211 of the FDA Act.[9–12] Furthermore, all medical gases demonstrate compliance with completion of the finished dosage form and its components, meeting cGMPs to assure drug safety, identity, strength, quality, and purity.

The presence of other chemical substances in any gas or gas mixture determines how pure that gas or gas mixture is. Moreover, purity specification requirements have been categorized in "grades." Chemicals that meet the purity specification requirements of a grade can be labeled with that specific grade. An example of this is the USP grade for medical gases. If the manufacturing methods, facilities, processing, packing, or holding do not conform to cGMP, medical gases are considered adulterated under section 501(a)(2)(B) of the FDA Act (21 U.S.C. 351(a)(2)(B).[9]

In the United Kingdom, all medical gases and some of the associated equipment used are regulated by European Directives and U.K. legislation. As in the United States, the medical gases in Europe are classified as medical products as per the European Pharmacopoeia.[13] The associated equipment is classified as a medical device when used to administer the gas.

The Medicines and Healthcare products Regulatory Agency (MHRA) is aimed at protecting and promoting public health and patient safety. They ensure that drugs, healthcare products, and medical equipment meet appropriate standards of safety, quality, performance, and effectiveness and are used safely. For an in-depth understanding, the reader is referred to the many detailed guidelines and directives published and enforced by MHRA.[14–15] Similar to other medicinal products, medical gases require a marketing authorization (product license) to enable them to be sold. Moreover, the marketing authorization stipulates a safe route of administration must be used when using medical gases. Only medical gases with an appropriate license are to be prescribed for the treatment of patients. As with all medicines, the shelf life of medical gases is mentioned within the relevant marketing authorization. The label on each cylinder will show the expiry date as well as the batch number of the medicinal product (Figure 9.1). It is important that IVF laboratories do not use medical gases once the shelf life has expired. Return the expired cylinders to the vendor, and quarantine them in a separate area while awaiting collection.

The medical gas industry is currently working toward global standardization and meeting the Globally Harmonized System of Classification and Labeling of Chemicals (GHS). To this end, the European authorities along with the FDA have decided to standardize the

Gas	USA	International
Oxygen	Green	White
Carbon dioxide	Gray	Gray
Nitrous oxide	Blue	Blue
Helium	Brown	Brown
Nitrogen	Black	Black
Air	Yellow	White and black

Figure 9.1 **(See color insert.)** Cylinder identification color code chart used for medical gases. In Europe, it is anticipated that the identification color codes will be standardized by 2025. The United States designations are as follows: (i) oxygen USP is a green background with white lettering or white background with green lettering; (ii) carbon dioxide USP is a gray background with black lettering or white lettering; (iii) nitrous oxide USP is a blue background with white lettering; (iv) helium USP is a brown background with white lettering; (v) nitrogen USP is a black background with white lettering; and (vi) air USP is a yellow background with black lettering.

identification colors and color codes on the compressed gas cylinders by 2025. Medical gases should be identified by the label, which is the recommended method for positively identifying the contents of a container.

9.3 Production, filling, certification, and delivery of medical grade gases

Although the manufacturing, filling, and necessary certification of the medical grade gases is the same globally, different regulatory authorities handle overseeing these activities in the various countries. In the United States, the FDA[9] regulates the procedures involved. However, the same procedure in Europe, including the United Kingdom, is regulated under European Directive 2001/82/EC or European Directive 2001/83/EC, including the cGMP requirements on manufacturers.[13–15] These directives are similar but the techniques used for medical gas production vary considerably between various production plants within the same country. The difference is due to the production techniques being updated and newer technology introduced. For example, in 2010, to be consistent, an annex document was added to the above European directives.[16] The FDA has now adapted to these directives.

9.3.1 Production of carbon dioxide

Briefly, carbon dioxide is usually generated as a by-product of the large-scale manufacture of hydrogen or more commonly during the combustion of methane. It can also exist as a liquid under pressure at room temperature and is typically stored and transported in this form in high-pressure cylinders for use by patients or in medical laboratories.[12–13] In most hospital applications, gas from these cylinders is connected to the pipeline distribution system in a manifold arrangement.

9.3.2 Production of nitrogen

In nitrogen production, a three-step adsorptive separation process of air is used, which consists of:

1. Purification: the ambient (inlet) air gets filtered before being compressed by an air compressor and dried by an air drier system.
2. Adsorption: the pre-heated air enters a vessel filled with carbon molecular sieve (CMS). Most of the oxygen gets adsorbed so that nitrogen, with an adjustable purity down to a residual O_2 content of 100 ppm, remains in the gas stream. Before the adsorption capability of the CMS is exhausted, the adsorption process is interrupted.
3. Desorption: the adsorbed gases are released using pressure reduction below that of the adsorption process. As for oxygen, a simple pressure release system is used. The resultant waste stream gets vented into the atmosphere. The regenerated adsorbent will now be used again for generating nitrogen. At equal time intervals, the adsorption and desorption take place alternatively. Constant product flow regarding both purity and quantity is ensured by the connected buffer.

9.3.3 Production of tri-gas (6% CO_2, 5% O_2 balanced by nitrogen)

Tri-gas, as the name suggests, is any combination of CO_2, O_2, and nitrogen. The CO_2 concentration will vary depending on preference, culture media, and atmospheric pressure (altitude). Clinics at higher altitudes require a higher CO_2 concentration to achieve the correct pH for embryo culture. To accommodate the higher percentage of CO_2, the percentage of nitrogen is lowered by the appropriate amount. The mixing takes place at the time of the fill, and the entire cylinder is then certified to contain the prerequisite gas mixture. The tri-gas gets delivered to the end user in a compressed gas mixture form, and the same precautionary steps need to be taken for storage and transportation.

9.3.4 Certification

9.3.4.1 Certification methods

As the end users, it is our responsibility to understand that the information given on the certificate attached to the cylinder is accurate. In the United Kingdom, gas industries use two main ways of assigning a certificate value to a gas/mixture. The first method involves careful measurements of the weight of the gases filled into the cylinder while the second checks the contents of the bottle. The latter is usually done by withdrawing the product from the cylinder for post-fill analysis.

9.3.4.2 Gravimetric certification

A certification by weight, often called gravimetric certification, claims high filling tolerance and high certification accuracy. The "mass comparators" have an accuracy of ±1% and are mentioned on the certificate.

9.3.4.3 Certification by analysis

The process of issuing a certificate of analysis involves analyzing the gas from a cylinder. The analysis results are compared to a known gas standard analyzed on the same instrument. The degree of accuracy of the analysis acknowledges the purity and the grade of the gas in the cylinder tested. As certification of medical gases is critical for the end user, all the manufacturers in the United Kingdom make sure that all the medical gases are certified by both the gravimetric and analysis methods.

9.3.4.4 Certification grades

In the United Kingdom, a label attached to the neck of a cylinder (see Figure 9.2) carries all the necessary information about the gas including the "gravimetric" weight of the cylinder.

9.3.5 Traceability

Traceability is a tool to provide accurate and comparable measurement results at both national and international levels. Furthermore, as per the HFEA Code of Practice,[8] all licensed clinics in the United Kingdom are required to demonstrate an unbroken chain of the origin of all products that are in contact with gametes and embryos. Because the medical gases are certified and are in touch with gametes and embryos, it is necessary to ensure the traceability of the calibrators. Further, it should be established and identified that an unbroken chain of comparison leading to an SI unit of measurement exists. In the case of gases, this will be the kilogram mass.

9.3.5.1 Process of tracing

A traceable gas reference mixture is one whose concentration is known through a chain of direct comparisons to national measurement standards for the particular type of gas

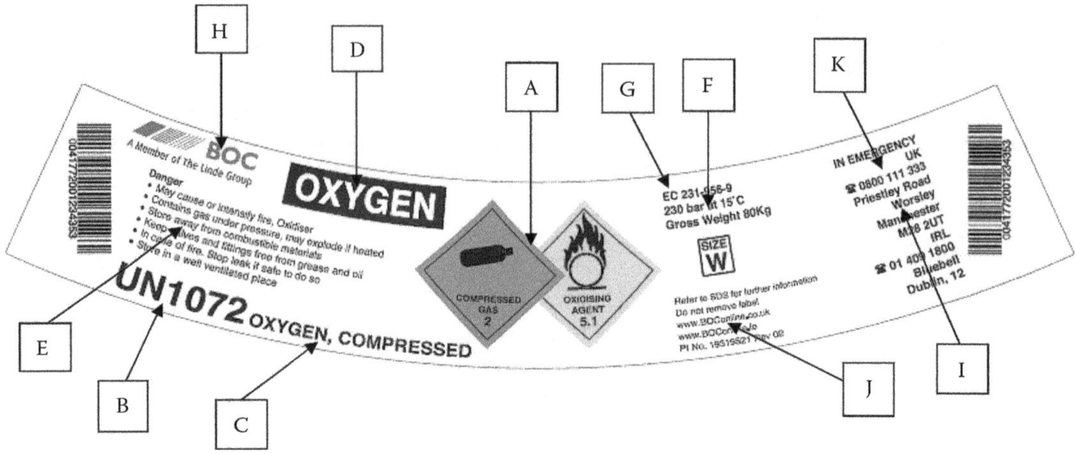

Figure 9.2 **(See color insert.)** A typical label found on the neck of a compressed medical oxygen gas cylinder. The following information is required on a label: (A) a diamond hazard label, displaying the primary hazard with additional hazard labels displaying any subsidiary hazards. These labels will display the dangerous goods classification number. (B) The UN number, preceded by the letters UN. (C) The proper shipping name. (D) Product name (may be omitted if the proper shipping name is identical). (E) Signal word, hazard and precautionary statements. (F) Package size and pressure. (G) EC number, if applicable. (H) Company name. (I) Address of the gas company. (J) Additional company information. (K) A telephone number to call in an emergency. In addition, a bar code on the label identifies the cylinder and is used for inventory purposes and a yellow sticker indicating an oxidizing agent and can be harmful. (Courtesy of British Compressed Gases Association.)

mixture. Because the network of traceable mixtures extends internationally, the national standards, when compared on a regular basis with those of other countries, measurement results are acceptable internationally.

9.3.5.2 Benefits of tracing

Traceable calibrations automatically provide the means to obtain:

1. Consistent data over time with different gas mixtures
2. Comparability of data obtained from similar measurements elsewhere, even internationally
3. A known accuracy in SI units (molar parts per million)

9.4 Things to know about carbon dioxide, nitrogen, and gas mixtures

9.4.1 Carbon dioxide (CO_2)

Carbon dioxide, a colorless and odorless gas, is slightly acidic in taste. Medical grade carbon dioxide is 99.5% v/v (min) pure. Although a waste product of the metabolic process in humans, it is consumed by plants during photosynthesis. Carbon dioxide occurs naturally in the atmosphere at approximately 350 volume per million (vpm). Use of medical grade carbon dioxide is a small fraction of the overall use of the gas throughout the world. Carbon dioxide presents no risk of fire or explosion, as it is not combustible in normal use.

All compressed gases should be stored and transported very carefully. In the gaseous form, carbon dioxide is mildly toxic to humans. Carbon dioxide is known to have negative effects on the human body at concentrations as low as 7%. If accidentally exposed at concentrations approaching 50% for an extended period, it leads to death through asphyxiation in a few minutes.

In IVF laboratories, 100% CO_2 cylinders are connected to IVF front-loading incubators. CO_2 helps maintain the correct pH of the bicarbonate buffered medium and in turn the cellular pH of the gametes and embryos.

9.4.2 Nitrogen

Like carbon dioxide and oxygen, nitrogen is an odorless, colorless gas. Nitrogen has a broad range of uses, ranging from medical research to food packaging. Although highly pure chemicals contain very minute quantities of contaminants, all commercially obtained chemicals are mixtures. Medical nitrogen is a common component in many gas mixtures. It is used as a displacement medium for sterile equipment, a nonoxidizing displacement medium in pharmaceutical vials, and as a propellant in pressurized aerosol dispensers.

9.4.2.1 Nitrogen grade standards

Many industries use nitrogen for different purposes. Despite certain names of grades being very common, the actual grades of nitrogen are not standardized across industries or even within industries. As a result, the manufacturer of the nitrogen chooses the name of the grade to categorize the nitrogen. Consequently, it is likely that different nitrogen products with the same purity specifications may be listed in the same grades with different names. Furthermore, it is also possible for two nitrogen products within the same grade to have different purity specifications. It is, therefore, important to select a nitrogen product based on its purity specifications and not solely on its grade.

9.4.2.1.1 High-purity grades Although "high-purity" grades of nitrogen are composed of greater than 99.998% nitrogen, in the industry the common high-purity grade names include "Research Purity" and "Ultra High Purity." Zero-grade nitrogen is considered as "High Purity" because it meets the specification of having less than 0.5 parts per million of total hydrocarbons. In addition to hydrocarbons, nitrogen contains other impurities like oxygen, carbon dioxide, carbon monoxide, and water. In none of the high-purity grade nitrogen is the concentration of oxygen less than 0.5 parts per million. Carbon dioxide or carbon monoxide is less than 1 part per million and water is less than 3 parts per million.

9.4.2.1.2 Other nitrogen grades On the other hand, "low-purity" grades of nitrogen are composed of up to 90–99.998% nitrogen. The common low-purity grade names in the industry include "High Purity," "Zero," "Pre-Purified," "Oxygen Free," "Extra Dry," and "Industrial." The degree of contaminants in these grades varies widely. Oxygen Free grades contain less than 0.5 parts per million of oxygen. Other grades of nitrogen include high-pressure grades with a purity of 99.998%. It is, therefore, necessary to know the quality of nitrogen required.

9.4.2.1.3 Use of high purity nitrogen High purity grade nitrogen is used by the pharmaceutical industry as a shield gas for some medications. Nitrogen is a nonreactive gas, especially when it contains low levels of impurities. It acts as a protectant for the medicine from contacting and reacting with surrounding oxygen and moisture. Combustion requires oxygen, leading to unsafe fires or explosions in some situations. When there is a danger of combustion "Oxygen Free" nitrogen is used. By coating, it protects the objects and substances. Uses of low-purity nitrogen include tire inflation and industrial uses like heat treatment of furnaces. In IVF laboratories, nitrogen plays a balancing role. When connected to the medical gas pipe sytem (MGPS), nitrogen cylinders along with the carbon dioxide facilitate tri-gas incubators to adjust the inner chamber environment to the desired concentraion of CO_2 and O_2.

9.4.3 Tri-gases

Until recently, the large front-loading incubators used to be set at 5–6% CO_2 or values set as per the pH measurement of the culture media and used atmospheric air containing up to 20% O_2—a nonphysiological concentration.[17–20] Consequently, this meant that the concentration of O_2 within the inner chamber of the incubator was also 20%. Several publications have alluded to the fact that embryo development is better when the culture environment has 5% O_2.

The most common tri-gas cylinders currently employed in IVF laboratories are a combination of 6% CO_2, 5% O_2 and balanced with nitrogen. However, this percentage of combination might vary from lab to lab depending on the culture media pH measurement of each lot of media. This combination may also allow a reduction in the levels of reactive oxygen species (ROS). The gas mixture, transported as compressed gas in cylinders, comes with a certificate of purity and percentage of each gas as discussed earlier.

9.5 Gas regulators, cylinders, and maintenance

9.5.1 Regulators

All compressed gas cylinders come with a gas-specific valve connection, and each gas has a specific regulator type. European medical devices Directive 93/42/EC regulates the use of such regulators and classifies them as "Medical devices." All medical devices carry a CE marking that is the manufacturer's declaration that the equipment complies with the "Essential Requirements" of the relevant medical devices Directive.

There are several types of regulators available on the market. The construction and material used for construction is restricted to their reactivity with any particular gas and the pressure required to operate those cylinders. Figure 9.3 depicts some typical regulators currently used in IVF laboratories. Each regulator connects to a different gas cylinder. The user should confirm the materials used in the construction of the regulators to ensure they are compatible with embryo culture. For example, some regulators contain neoprene diaphragms, which may release VOCs. Stainless steel diaphragms may be better suited to IVF applications.

9.5.2 Construction of carbon dioxide cylinders

The material used for constructing all compressed gas cylinders is the same. They should withstand the pressure under which the cylinder is filled and maintained (Figure 9.4). High tensile steel is used in the construction of many of the larger high pressure CO_2 cylinders. It has a designed working pressure of at least 137 bar (g). There are other materials used in the construction of carbon dioxide cylinders (i.e., aluminum). The color-coding on the

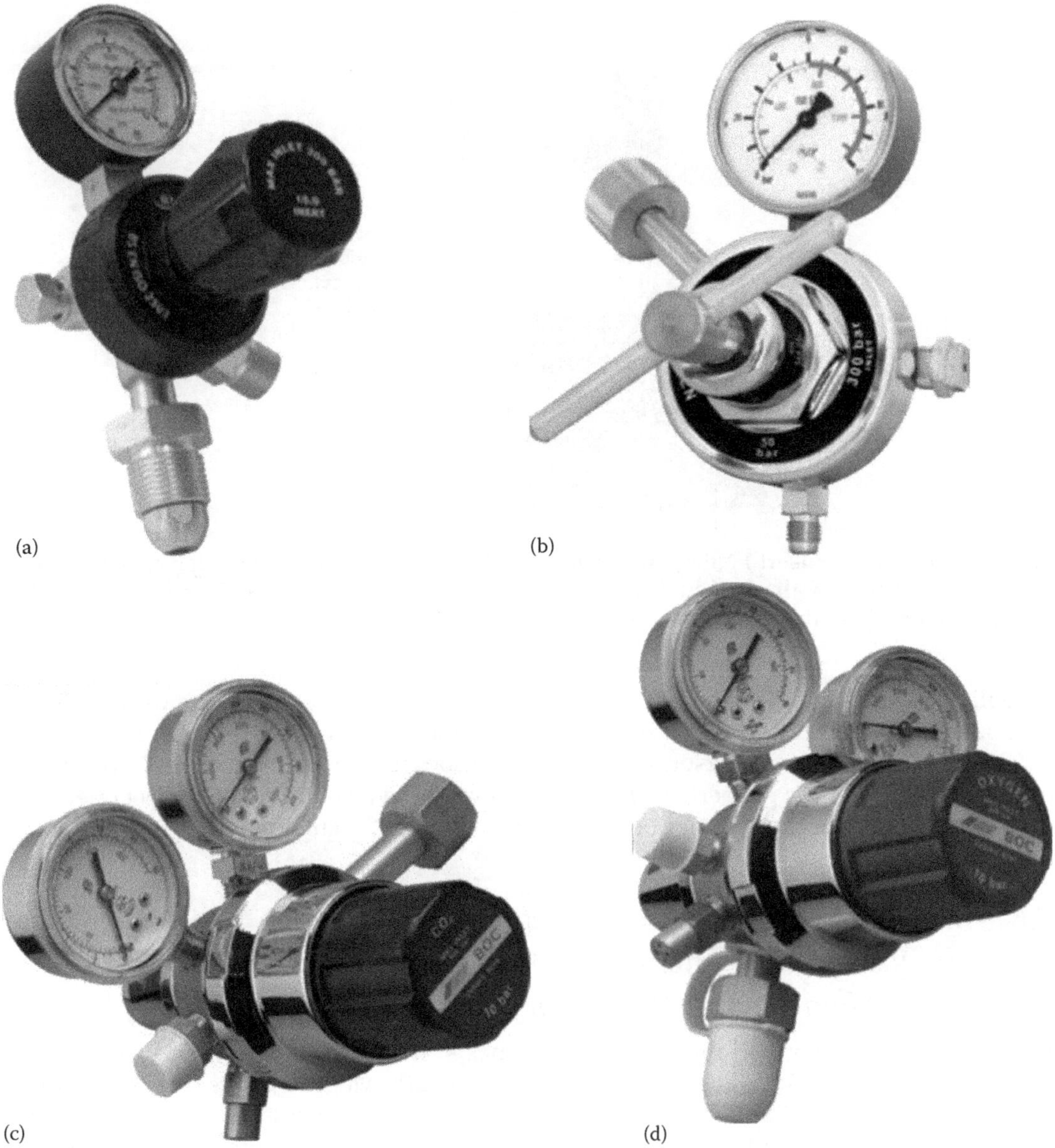

Figure 9.3 Regulators commonly used in IVF laboratories. (a) SSIG INERT 10 bar RYO2010006 regulator; (b) EVOS nitrogen 50 bar flare high-pressure single stage nitrogen regulator; (c) BOC series 8500 carbon dioxide (CO_2) multi-stage regulator. These regulators come in 2-, 4-, and 10-bar pressure. (d) BOC Series 8500 multi-stage regulator used with O_2 and related mixture cylinders. (Courtesy of BOC Health Care, UK.)

shoulders of medical carbon dioxide cylinders is gray (RAL 7037), while the color-coding of the cylinder body should be white (RAL 9010). European union directives require all color coding of all medical gases to be standardized by 2025. It is, therefore, likely that for a limited period, cylinders may have gray bodies. Additionally, cylinders carry the carbon dioxide name printed on the body of the bottle, which may be missing during the

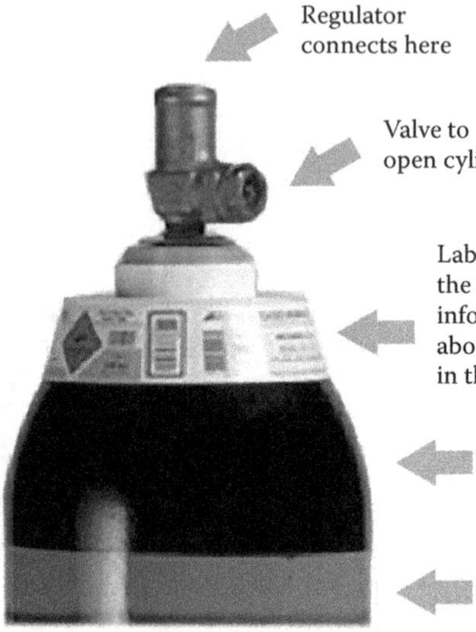

Figure 9.4 **(See color insert.)** Nitrogen (oxygen free) 230 bar cylinder. Note the typical label that is attached to the neck of all certified medical gas cylinders. The cylinder identification color on the neck is different from that on the body. (Courtesy of BOC Health Care, UK.)

transition period. Since it is the primary method for identifying medical gases, cylinders without a label should never be used and immediately returned to the supplier.

It is necessary that all personnel handling carbon dioxide cylinders should have adequate knowledge of the properties of the gas. They should also know the correct operating procedures for the bottle, precautions, and in the event of an emergency.

9.6 Installation and construction of medical gas lines and use of inline filters (HEPA and VOCs) in compliance with clean room facility norms

In the United Kingdom, all medical gas pipelines systems (MGPS) have to be compliant with the standards required by the Department of Health, Medical Gases Health Technical Memorandum 02-01:HTM02.[21] For an IVF laboratory, an MGPS provides a safe, convenient, and cost-effective system for the provision of medical gases to the laboratory at the point-of-use. Additionally, it helps with the safe storage of various compressed gas cylinders away from the laboratory and helps to maintain a clean-air environment needed for the IVF laboratory.

The safety of the patient's gametes and embryos in the laboratory incubators is paramount in the design, installation, commissioning, and operation of MGPS. The fundamental principles of security are achieved by ensuring the quantity of supply of various gases, the identity of supply, continuity of supply, and quality of supply. The design of the pipeline should ensure ease of installation and capacity of the supply to the required flows of the necessary gases, based on the intended number of incubators to be connected within a laboratory at any one time. Moreover, adequacy of supply is established during commissioning of the systems. It is necessary that the identity of supply be achieved by ensuring all points to which the user can connect the incubators (terminal units), and

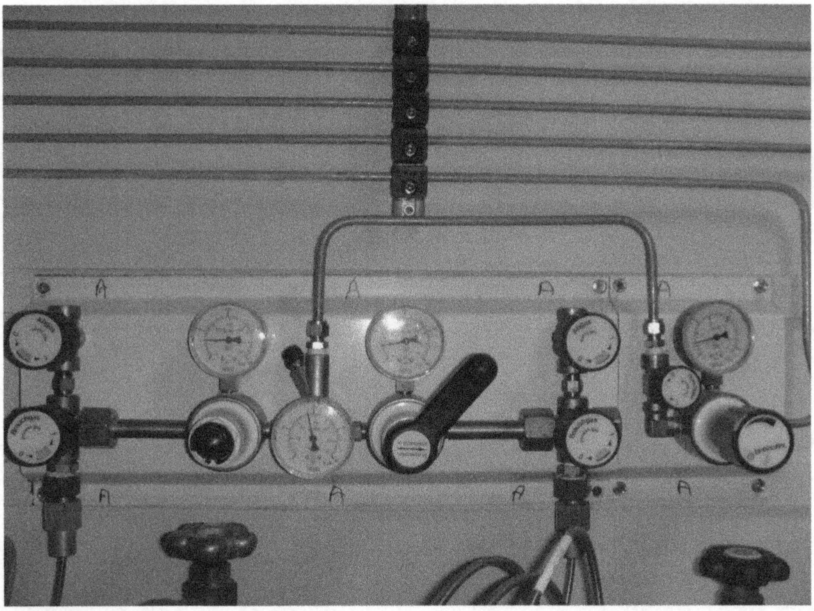

Figure 9.5 Automatic changeover unit connected to a minimum of two cylinders of the same gas. (Courtesy of Giles Palmer, London Womens Clinic, UK.)

user-replaceable components are provided with gas-specific connectors. Usually such connectors are identified by symbol and color.

Comprehensive tests and checks can maintain the gas specificity during installation and commissioning and during any work or maintenance on the systems. To ensure that when one cylinder runs empty the other one takes over, installing an automatic change-over unit connected to a minimum of two cylinders of the same gas will suffice (Figure 9.5). It is necessary that MGPS be connected to the essential electrical supply. Confirmation of the quality of the gases is assured by the certification of an appropriate product specification, usually recognized by a European Pharmacopoeia monogram or a UKAS logo in the United Kingdom. Additionally, the tag on the cylinder should specify the date of filling and an expiry date (see Figure 9.4). To ensure that no gas is adulterated in the MGPS, pipeline installations and components are required to meet specifications.[21]

9.6.1 *Medical gas piping*

In the United Kingdom, the Department of Health guidelines stipulate the use of only seamless types "K" and "L" copper piping for the distribution of medical gas (Figure 9.6).[21] Additionally, copper piping should be manufactured to the ASTM standard B819[22] and only "hard temper copper" size 1/2″ or larger should be used for all installations. Soft copper may be permitted if the pipes are run underground to reduce the total amount of concealed joints.

However, in Scandinavian countries the medical grade for gas lines is mostly of stainless steel put together via argon welding. In Europe, copper gas lines are being faded out for inox seamless pipes (Figure 9.7). Either a blue or a green marking is present on all medical gas copper pipes and tubes. These markings specify that the copper tubing is for medical gas use (i.e., TYPE K MED ASTM B819).[22] A medical gas pipe is shipped and stored with protective plugs or caps placed over the ends and with a nitrogen atmosphere in the

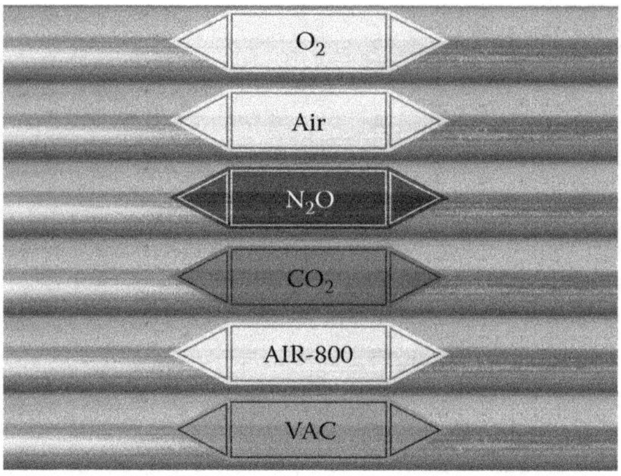

Figure 9.6 **(See color insert.)** Labeling of each pipe of the medical gas pipelines system (MGPS). Although the color-coding may vary, the importance is to note that each pipe has a label.

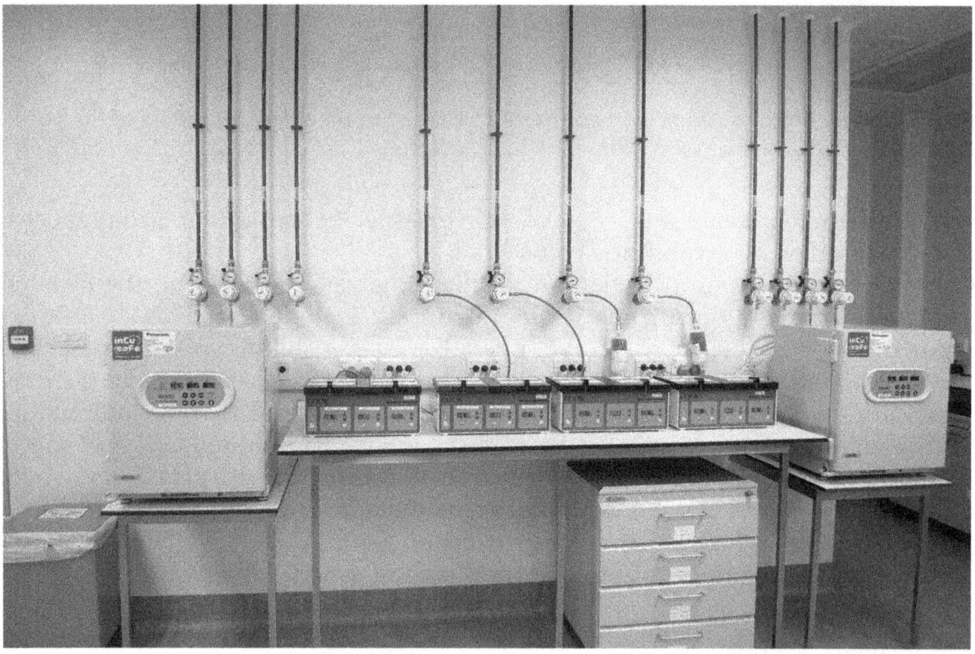

Figure 9.7 **(See color insert.)** Individual gas pipe lines to IVF lab incubators. Each terminal can be connected to an inline filter to remove VOCs from gas bottles. (Courtesy of Magda Carvalho, Cambridge IVF, UK.)

tubing to prevent contamination from entering the tubing. Common contaminants are oils and lubricants used in the manufacturing process, solvents and particulates from the cleaning and abbrading processes, and odors from any one of the primary contaminants. Some of these contaminants, if exposed to pure oxygen, could possibly cause a spontaneous combustion. Oxygen pipelines have to be 1/2 inch inside diameter, and that of other gases can be of 3/8 inch of inside diameter.

Care should be taken to ensure the correct installation of all pipes. It is standard practice that the main line pipe should connect to the source including the riser vertical pipe or branch lines. The riser pipes usually connect with the main line and the branch lines at various levels off the risers. Branch lines, in turn, terminate within the IVF laboratory to be serviced. The terminal units may consist of different connection types depending on the equipment to be used (Figure 9.8). The piped distribution system is connected to a base unit, consisting of primary valves, which automatically shut off and act as self-sealing devices and also are primary check valves. These valves open and permit the gas to flow when the male probe gets inserted and closes automatically when the connection is broken (Figure 9.9). The advantage of quick connectors is that it allows apparatus to be connected or disconnected by a single action. Each quick connector has a pair of gas-specific male and female parts and a releasable spring mechanism that locks the components together.

Another embryo-safe option is to use polytetrafluoroethylene (PTFE) tubing for delivering medical gas. This inert, non-embryo toxic material is ideal for special mix gases as it is not permeable to CO_2. Of the many types of plastic available, even those recommended as food or medical grade, PTFE is the most inert and has less extractable elements such as plasticizers (e.g., phthalate) that can cause embryo toxicity. Silicone is another inert plastic but is permeable to CO_2, and so is not suitable for premixed gases as the CO_2 concentration will drop proportionately with the length of the tubing leading to wrong gas concentrations entering the incubator. PTFE tubing has the added advantage that, being flexible, it can be easily rerouted in the event that the lab requires reconfiguration. It can be purchased as plain tubing or covered in braided stainless steel for protection (e.g., Swagelok®). The addition of Swagelok fittings allow it to be readily attached to regulators, taps, and other gas supply fittings.

Gas line pressure from cylinders to incubators depends on the distance between them and a reliable pressure is needed to be able to supply the incubators. A distance of 10–15 m keeps a pressure of 2 bar. There is always a need for a second regulator close to the incubator (this depends on manufacture's instructions to avoid damage and correct use and

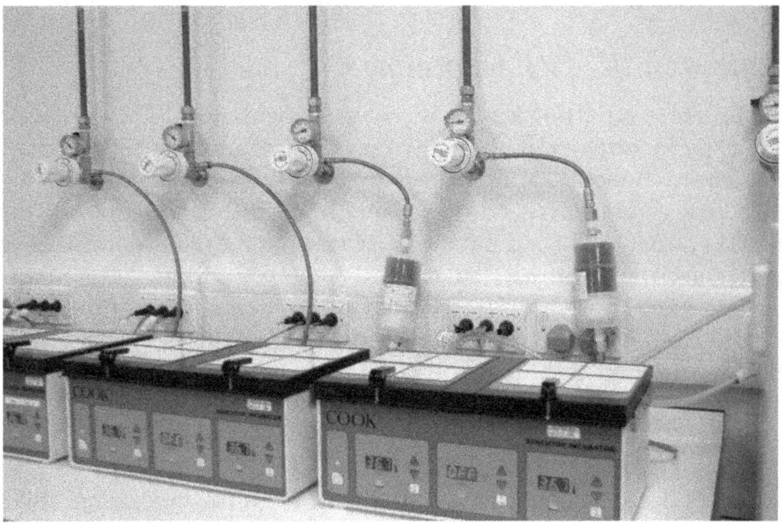

Figure 9.8 **(See color insert.)** Terminal pipeline units may consist of different connection types depending on the equipment to be used. (Courtesy of Magda Carvalho, Cambridge IVF, UK.)

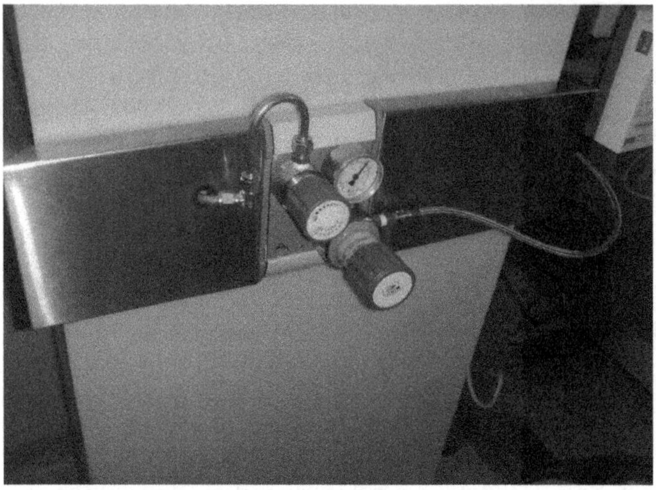

Figure 9.9 Inside the IVF lab: second regulator connecting to the incubator. (Courtesy of Giles Palmer, London Womens Clinic, UK.)

recovery time). For example, Forma Thermo requires 0.8 bar, Galaxy Micro requires 0.4 bar while Planar Bench Top BT37 requires 1.5 bar.

9.6.2 *How to identify medical gas piping*

Medical gas piping must be clearly identified using nonremovable stickers that are color-coded according to the gas. Colors are standardized for a given region. Standardize colors by spacing along the pipe, 6 cm apart. Additionally, they should be visible at every valve, at each access door, and at each service connection.

9.7 *Incubators in the IVF laboratory*

Modern IVF laboratories harbor a wide variety of incubators. These may include large, traditional box type incubators, having a tri-gas environment or CO_2 and air mixture, or bench top incubators. Bench top incubators may be humidified. Additionally, they may run on premixed gas or create their own gas mix by blending CO_2, N_2, and air. Users need to provide mixed gas (CO_2, O_2, and balance nitrogen) or a separate input of CO_2 and N_2 to feed the chamber environment. ART labs are increasingly adopting time-lapse technology for embryo monitoring. These are dry gas, bench top incubators with time-lapse systems. These incubators also have an inbuilt gas mixer to control the gas concentrations. Many of them have inbuilt activated carbon as inline filters for gas purification.

9.7.1 *Culture environment in an incubator*

Box type incubators derive a major chunk of the air from the laboratory and the rest from the CO_2 gas bottles. This may lead to contamination of the culture environment with VOCs present in the room air. Gametes/embryos placed in the culture media are exposed to the gaseous environment of the inner chamber. Hence, any chemically active compounds present in the gaseous inner chamber have the potential to diffuse into the culture media and thereby into the gametes/embryos resulting in perturbation of developmental synchrony at the molecular level.

Sources of VOCs inside an incubator are a wide variety of hydrocarbons and CACs from gas bottles, cleaning agents used inside the lab and oocyte recovery room, lab furnishings, paint, anaesthetic gases, aromatic compounds, refrigerants, consumable packaging, and even sterile Petri dishes used for embryo culture.[2] Cohen and colleagues have shown that routine medical grade (USP Grade) materials can contain low concentrations of VOCs. USP grade carbon dioxide from their IVF unit in Matheson, New Jersey, showed the presence of approximately 18 VOCs amounting to 552 mcg/m^3 including benzene (100 mcg/m^3), Freon (100 mcg/m^3), alcohols, and chlorinated organics. Some of these compounds were found at lower concentrations in incubators and traces could be detected in other areas of the ART laboratory.[23] Many manufacturers of gas inline filters conduct a challenge test using a known cocktail of VOCs or toluene (as representative VOC) to check the efficacy of activated carbon to trap the organic molecules.

Ronny Janssens from the Dutch-speaking Brussels Free University (personal communication) noted that VOCs (measured with an RAE VOC meter, sensitivity 0.1 ppm) were not present in his laboratory incubators (Heracell 240), but added that CODA incubator units and CODA inline filters had been installed and they took extreme care not to use any detergents that had strong smells for cleaning. On a personal note, I was asked to troubleshoot in another lab in Belgium (mid-1990s) and there I found quite high VOC levels originating from the decontaminant they used to clean their incubators. Since 2013, we implemented new clean rooms with VOC filtration in the HVAC (active carbon and chemical oxidation with permanganate) and have continuous VOC measurement in air. VOC measurements results were negative except a short peak while doing deep cleaning of the clean room. Subsequent VOC measurements carried out during validation studies of G185 incubators, embryoscope, G210 and MIRI time-lapse incubators were all negative.

9.7.2 Reduction of VOC in the inner chamber of the incubator

How can we protect the in vitro cultured embryos from the detrimental effects of VOCs? To reduce the concentration of VOCs inside the incubator, strict clean room disciplines along with installation of AHU units must be done. The embryology laboratory should be positively pressured compared to adjacent rooms and with more air exchanges. Additionally, the use of recirculating plus outside air is desirable depending on the outside air quality. Special care should be taken in the cleaning procedures to avoid any alcohols and use embryo-safe disinfectants such as Oosafe/Fertisafe or hydrogen peroxide. Regular cleaning can be performed with deionized water alone. Another option is steam mops, which can efficiently disinfect the floors and walls and as this uses water steam it is not detrimental as other volatile disinfectants. Cohen et al. suggest that a new incubator releases 100 times more VOCs than an old incubator.[24] Hence, care should be taken while introducing new incubators in the embryology laboratories and it seems therefore ideal to culture only a few inseminated oocytes from the cohort in the new incubators until the safety of the system is satisfactorily tested.

Because many of the CAC contaminants are oil solubile, embryologists can prevent VOCs from coming into contact with gametes/embryos to some extent by having an oil overlay culture. In this case, oil acts as a sink for many of these organic chemicals.[25] Anecdotal evidence from batch IVF units in some developing countries exemplifies this fact. In some of these units, visiting embryologists conducting IVF batches instruct the lab to keep the culture media bottle for gasssing overnight as part of media equillibration.

This practice has been shown to have a negative impact on the embryo quality and pregnancy rate. However, the same labs where the embryologist makes the oil overlay dishes the previous day observes a better grade of embryos and pregnancy rate plus less early miscarriages (personal communication).

Placement of an incubator-filter-box (Labotect, Germany or CODA Incubator unit) inside a front-loading incubator may help to filter the VOC inside the incubator atmosphere (see Chapter 23). In one study, Merton and colleagues investigated the effects of an intra-incubator carbon-activated air filtration system during in vitro culture (IVC) on embryonic development and the subsequent pregnancy rate of bovine embryos.[26] Bovine zygotes were placed either in a normal CO_2-O_2-N_2 incubator (control group) or in an identical CO_2-O_2-N_2 incubator with an intra-incubator air purification unit (study group) for IVC. The embryo production rate at culture day 7 was not affected by the availability of an air purification unit (23.4% and 24.7% morula and blastocysts per oocyte for control and study groups, respectively). In addition, there was no effect on embryo stage or quality. However, the pregnancy rate was improved for both fresh (46.3 vs. 41.0%; $p = 0.043$) and frozen/thawed embryos (40.8 vs. 35.6%; $p < 0.05$). These results suggest that atmospheric purification by the activated carbon intra-incubator air purification unit increased pregnancy rate following the transfer of in vitro produced bovine embryos.

In a similar experiment to test the effectiveness of similar incubator air purification units in a tri-gas box incubator, VOCs were measured at defined time intervals after deliberate exposure to isopropanol in the incubator chamber. The author wiped his hands with pure isopropanol and kept them for five seconds in a 150-L 5% O_2, 5% CO_2 incubator, once with and once without the incubator filter. VOCs were reduced to less than 25% after 60 minutes of filtration and to less than 10% of initial value after 165 minutes of filtration in comparison to the tri-gas incubator without a filtration unit, where 30% of the initial value remained even after 180 minutes.[27] Interestingly, such a small pump of the incubator's filter unit needs eight hours to circulate once the entire volume of a 150-L incubator. There are two considerations about this experiment. First, the use of reduced O_2 causes a flow of nitrogen and decreases the percentage of VOCs inside the incubator. Second, oil can be a major source of VOCs. Though the majority of IVF labs use commercially available oil as such for overlay of culture dishes, a precautionary measure may be to wash all the oils before using the culture media once the new lot arrives at the laboratory. This might help to remove any residual toxins.

New generation benchtop incubators provide a constant flow of bottled mixed gas with virtually no exposure to room air. Morbeck and colleagues compared mouse embryo development in different culture media in a traditional CO_2 incubator versus a benchtop incubator.[28] Ten 1-cell mouse embryos from inbred mice were cultured in single step media (SS) or sequential media from three different suppliers (Seq1, Seq2, Seq3). Embryos were cultured in microdrops in a conventional CO_2 incubator (Forma 3130) or a benchtop incubator (Planer BT-37). Eight cell/morula rates (8C) and blastocyst rates (BRs) were calculated at 48 and 96 hours of culture. Although early embryo development rates were similar between the incubators, the BRs were lower for Seq2 and Seq3 compared to SS and Seq1 in the conventional incubator. In contrast, the BR improved for these two media in the benchtop incubator. The BRs in the benchtop incubator were similar across all media. The authors concluded that benchtop incubators provide several advantages over traditional water-jacketed incubators, including provision of a controlled air source distinct from room air that may potentially augment embryo development. Their results show that some sequential culture media may interact adversely with ambient air, likely resulting in increased in vitro stress on developing embryos. By alleviating air quality associated stress, new generation incubators are suggested to improve embryo development.[28,29]

Bench top incubators derive 100% of the gases in the embryo culture chambers from the gas mixtures with negligible contribution of lab air inside the culture chamber. Hence, any organic chemical contaminant present in the gas bottles can negatively affect the embryo development. One report looking at the seasonal variation on implantation rate found that toluene at 2.2–2.7 parts per billion (ppb) in room air affected implantation.[30] When acrolein, a reactive aldehyde that is a common air pollutant, was added to embryo culture media, mouse embryos arrested at the 8-cell stage at 2.1 parts per million (ppm; 0.0375 mM) and the live birth rate was reduced in as little as 0.58 ppm.[2] Karagouga and colleagues used a mouse embryo model to study short-term VOC exposure and found that 0.5 ppm acrolein in air for just 24 h during the zygote stage inhibited mouse embryo development.[31] This effect was dependent on the concentration of albumin present in the culture media. Zygotes degenerated in protein-free medium, developed to the morula stage in medium containing 1 mg/mL albumin, and developed to blastocysts at a high rate in 5 mg/mL albumin. Since laboratory conditions are variable among clinics, a fourth group was included to test if the effects of VOCs are exacerbated by suboptimal conditions. Mouse zygotes were cultured under mineral oil with known sublethal toxicity.[32] Zygotes lysed after reaching the 4-cell stage in medium containing 1 mg/mL albumin but, again, development was protected when 5 mg/mL of albumin was included. Developmental competence was not tested in the study, so it is possible that cell numbers or implantation rates were decreased in the latter group. Protein protects embryos from VOCs in a concentration dependent manner within the range used by clinical IVF labs. Toxicity from oil peroxides and VOCs may be additive, illustrating how air quality may alter lab-to-lab observations when a suboptimal batch of oil or protein is used for clinical IVF. Collectively, the aforementioned results illustrate the multifactorial nature of air quality and its relationship with culture conditions, especially the protein concentration in the media.

Last, a word of caution is needed about inline gas filters that have been used to trap VOCs from gas cylinders or MPGS. Such filters' lifetime is calculated based on the maximum average amount of gas flow passed through. Most inline filters available on the market guarantee to trap the toxic compounds for three months. After three months, trapped toxic compounds may be released to the environment depending on the passed through gas volume. Therefore, keeping inline filters connected to the gas pipe longer than three months is not recommended. In case filters cannot be replaced, it is better to remove and dispose of them.

9.8 Conclusion

The pioneering achievements of Steptoe and Edwards have benefited millions of couples worldwide and advancements in the IVF area in the past decades improved live birth rates from IVF treatments. These improvements are not only due to better understanding of the culture environment but also to better ovarian stimulation protocols. Despite the importance of the correct gaseous environment, only recently has the purity of this environment been properly understood. Regulatory authorities in the United States and Europe have insisted that the manufacturers of various medical gases follow regulatory guidelines. To this end, the regulatory bodies encourage all IVF laboratories worldwide to demand a certified medical gas with a purity of more than 99%. In this chapter, different medical gas production mechanisms were discussed. The importance of gravimetric and sample analysis of the medical gas ensures that the end user subjects the embryos only to correct gas or gas mixtures. The stringent regulatory guidelines for MPGS need to be followed to avoid any deleterious effects on embryos. Advances in engineering technology and the need to better manage patient treatment through providing a more stable and controlled environment for embryo culture has led IVF laboratories to consider investing in newer incubators that better meet the increasing quality standards demanded in the IVF field.

References

1. Cohen J, Gilligan A, Esposito W, Schimmel T, and Dale B. Ambient air and its potential effects on conception in vitro. *Hum Reprod.* 1997; 12: 1742–49.
2. Hall J, Gilligan A, Schimmel T, Cecchi M, and Cohen J. The origin, effects and control of air pollution in laboratories used for human embryo culture. *Hum Reprod.* 1998; 13 (Suppl.4): 146–155.
3. Brown SK. Chamber assessment of formaldehyde and VOC emissions from wood-based panels. *Indoor Air* 1999; 9: 209–15.
4. Chang JC, Fortmann R, and Roache N, Lao HC. Evaluation of low-VOC latex paints. *Indoor Air* 1999; 9: 253–58.
5. De Bortoli M, Kephalopoulos S, Kirchner S, Schauenburg H, and Vissers H. State-of-the-art in the measurement of volatile organic compounds emitted from building products: Results of European inter-laboratory comparison. *Indoor Air* 1999: 9: 103–16.
6. Worrilow KC, Huynh HT, Gwozdziewicz JB, Schillings WA, and Peters AJ. A retrospective analysis: The examination of a potential relationship between particulate and volatile organic compound levels in a class 100 IVF laboratory cleanroom and specific parameters of embryogenesis and rates of implantation. *Fertil Steril.* 2001; 76 (Suppl. 1): S15–16.
7. Esteves SC and Bento FC. Air quality control in the ART laboratory is a major determinant of IVF success. *Asian J Androl.* 2015 Nov 10. doi:10.4103/1008-682X.166433. [Epub ahead of print.]
8. Human Fertilization and Embryology Authority. HFEA code of practice, 8th ed. http://www.hfea.gov.uk/docs/HFEA_Code_of_Practice_8th_Edtion_(Oct_2015).pdf.
9. Food and Drug Administration. FDA guidance for industry. Current good manufacturing practice for medical gases. http://www.fda.gov/OHRMS/DOCKETS/98fr/03d-0165-gdl0001.pdf.
10. Compressed Gas Association. CGA Handbook of Compressed Gas. http://www.cganet.com/.
11. Compressed Gas Association. CGA Pamphlet P-2.6. Transfilling of liquid oxygen used for respiration. http://www.cganet.com/.
12. Compressed Gas Association. CGA Guide P-8.2. Guideline for validation of air separation unit and cargo tank filling for oxygen USP and nitrogen NF. http://www.cganet.com/.
13. European Pharmacopoeia, 8th ed. https://www.edqm.eu/en/european-pharmacopoeia-8th-edition-1563.html.
14. The Human Medicines Regulations 2012 (SI 2012:1916). http://www.legislation.gov.uk/uksi/2012/1916/contents/made.
15. Medicines & Healthcare Products Regulatory Agency (MHRA). https://www.gov.uk/government/organisations/medicines-and-healthcare-products-regulatory-agency.
16. Gouveia BG, Rijo P, Gonçalo TS, and Reis CP. Good manufacturing practices for medicinal products for human use. *J Pharm Bioallied Sci.* 2015; 7: 87–96.
17. Dumoulin JCM, Vanvuchelen RCM, Land JA, Pieters MHEC, Geraedts JPM, and Evers JLH. Effect of oxygen concentration on in vitro fertilization and embryo culture in the human and the mouse. *Fertil Steril.* 1995; 63: 115.
18. Schoolcraft WB, Gardner DK, Lane M, Schlenker T, Hamilton F, and Meldrum DR. Blastocyst culture and transfer: Analysis of results and parameters affecting outcome in two in vitro fertilization programs. *Fertil Steril.* 1999; 72: 604–9.
19. Catt JW and Henman M. Toxic effects of oxygen on human embryo development. *Hum Reprod.* 2000; 15 (Suppl 2): 199–206.
20. Bontekoe S, Mantikou E, van Wely M, Seshadri S, Repping S, and Mastenbroek S. Low oxygen concentrations for embryo culture in assisted reproductive technologies. Cochrane Database Syst Rev. 2012; 7: CD008950.

21. Department of Health, Medical Gases Health Technical Memorandum 02-01: (HTM02). http://www.bcga.co.uk/assets/HTM_02-01_Part_A.pdf.
22. ASTM Standards B819. http://www.astm.org/standards/b819.htm.
23. Cohen J, Gilligan A, Esposito W, Schimmel T, and Dale B. Ambient air and its potential effects on conception in vitro. *Hum Reprod.* 1997; 12: 1742–49.
24. Cohen J, Gilligan A, and Willadsen S. Culture and quality control of embryos. *Hum Reprod.* 1998; 13: 137–44.
25. Balaban B and Urman B. Embryo culture as a diagnostic tool. *Reprod Biomed Online.* 2003; 7: 671–82.
26. Merton JS, Vermeulen ZL, Otter T, Mullaart E, de Ruigh L, and Hasler JF. Carbon-activated gas filtration during in vitro culture increased pregnancy rate following transfer of in vitro-produced bovine embryos. *Theriogenology.* 2007; 67: 1233–8.
27. Elder K, Van den Bergh M, and Woodward B. Gases, air quality and volatile organic carbons (VOCs). In: Elder K, Van den Bergh M, and Woodward B (Eds.). Troubleshooting and Problem-Solving in the IVF Laboratory. Cambridge: Cambridge University Press, pp. 117–37, 2015.
28. Morbeck DE, Fredrickson JR, and Walker DL. Impact of oxygen, air source and incubator design on mouse embryo development. *Fert Steril.* 2013; 100 (Suppl.): S255.
29. Morbeck DE, Fredrickson JR, and Walker DL. Factors that affect mineral oil toxicity: Role of oxygen and protein supplement. *Fertil Steril.* 2012; 98: S29.
30. Worrilow KC, Huynh HT, Bower JB, Schillings W, and Peters AJ. A retrospective analysis: Seasonal decline in implantation rates (IR) and its correlation with increased levels of volatile organic compounds (VOC). *Fertil Steril.* 2002; 78(Suppl. 1): S39.
31. Karagouga G, Fredrickson JR, and Morbeck DE. Interaction of air quality and culture environment: Role of protein concentration and oil quality on effects of volatile organic compounds (VOCs) on embryo development. *Fertil Steril.* 2014; 102: e212.
32. Wolff HS, Fredrickson JR, Walker DL, and Morbeck DE. Advances in quality control: Mouse embryo morphokinetics are sensitive markers of in vitro stress. *Hum Reprod.* 2013; 28: 1776–82.

chapter ten

Air disinfection for ART clinics using ultraviolet germicidal irradiation

Normand Brais

Contents

Abstract

Many mistakenly assume that by following applicable building code guidelines, they are providing sterilized air. And, although the HEPA filter remains the best filter available for ventilation systems, like all filters there exists a determinable inefficiency zone that belies the myth that HEPA is the ultimate answer for air decontamination. In order to complete the air disinfection process initiated by filtration, ultraviolet germicidal irradiation (UVGI) needs to be added. UVGI has a long history of being used for the disinfection of drinking water in all major cities around the world since its first use in Marseille, France, in 1909. For close to two decades, UVGI has been used to disinfect the air streams within ductwork and air conditioning cooling coils. Public health agencies such as the Centers for Disease Control and Prevention (CDC) recommend the use of UVGI as a control technology to interrupt the transmission of pathogens in building ventilation systems and to prevent the formation of biofilms that can severely impair the efficiency of air conditioning cooling coils. This chapter provides an overview of how UV germicidal light sterilizes microorganisms and the dosage that is required in conjunction with the best available filtration practice to obtain an aseptic environment suitable for ART clinics. The chapter concludes with a brief review of common safety precautions as well as ultraviolet system maintenance requirements.

10.1 Introduction

Several guidelines, codes, and standards provide abundant details for designing healthcare facility ventilation systems.[1–4] However, many mistakenly assume that ventilation systems designed and installed according to these codes will supply sterile air. For all practical purposes, sterility is often considered as 6 Log reduction or 99.9999% of a population of microorganisms. In reality, 6 Log reduction means that one in a million will survive whereas absolute sterility implies that there are no surviving microorganisms. As defined, airstream sterility may be quite difficult to achieve and almost impossible to prove in current practice.

Traditional air filtration using high efficiency particulate air (HEPA) filters has been the standard in hospital and clinic ventilation systems to control airborne pathogens for more than 50 years. Multiple studies have demonstrated that despite the presence of HEPA filters, viral and bacterial contamination is still found in ventilation systems.[5–7]

Besides the all too common filter rack bypassing deficiencies, filter puncture leakage, and typical maintenance (or lack thereof) and disposal concerns, the shortcomings of HEPA filtration when it relates to medical applications are essentially caused by the fact that all filters demonstrate a significant drop in their capture efficiency for particulate sizes in a certain range. This is inherent to the fundamental underlying principles of filtration physics.[8] HEPA filters are no different and also display a weakness at a critical particle size between 0.1 and 0.5 μ as shown in Figure 10.1. The HEPA filter efficiency drops to a minimum value at a critical point called MPP (most penetrating particle), which is approximately 0.2 μ. Although the capture rate falls to a still impressive 99.94% to 99.95% at this size range, if a HEPA filter is challenged with a concentration of only 10,000 particles per cubic feet within the size range of 0.1 to 0.5 μ, it means that for a flow of 1000 cubic feet per minute, as many as 5000 particles every minute will pass through the HEPA filter. During the course of a single day, a total of 7.2 million particles will penetrate the filter and contaminate the aseptic zone.

Within the vulnerable size range of 0.1 to 0.5 μ, a variety of undesirable microorganisms may be found in Figure 10.2, starting from the influenza virus up to the legionella bacteria.

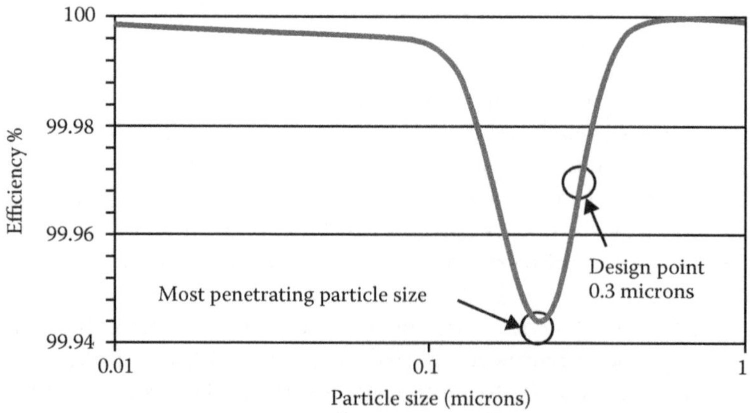

Figure 10.1 Typical performance of a HEPA 99.97% filter.

Microorganism	Type	Size in micron	Note
Influenza A virus	virus	0.098	Causes flu. Can cause epidemia inside buildings.
Vesicular stomatis virus	virus	0.104	Originates from farm animals: causes flue-like illness in infected humans.
Coronavirus	virus	0.113	Common colds and lung infections.
Mycoplasma pneumoniae	bacteria	0.177	Causes pneumonia in 20% of cases.
Neisseria catarrhalis/meningitidis	bacteria	0.177	Second leading cause of meningitidis, also causes pharyngitis.
Francisella tularensis	bacteria	0.200	Tularemia, pneumonia, fever.
Newcastle disease	virus	0.212	Bird origin, can cause mild conjuctivitis and influenza-like symptoms.
Coxiella burnetii	bacteria	0.283	Transmitted from animals to humans. Q fever: causes chills, headache, fatigue.
Haemophilus influenza	bacteria	0.285	Major cause of meningitis. Affects infants, otitis media, sinusitis.
Proteus vulgaris/mirabilis	bacteria	0.291	Pneumonia, opportunistic infections.
Vaccinia virus	virus	0.307	Constituent of the smallpox vaccine. Resistant to interferons.
Measle virus	virus	0.329	Rubeola, affects children, nosocomial. Airbone transmission in school ventilation.
Pseudomonas aeruginosa	bacteria	0.494	Pneumonia, nosocomial, indoor growth in dust, water, humidifiers. Commom HAI.
E. coli	bacteria	0.500	Source: feces. Found in food, meat and water. Causes diarrhea, often deadly.
Legionella pneumophila	bacteria	0.520	Legionnaire's disease. Pontiac fever, pneumonia, deadly in 15% of cases.

Figure 10.2 Viruses and bacteria size falling within the vulnerable size range of HEPA filters (0.1 to 0.5 μ).

Although the HEPA remains the best filter available for ventilation systems, like all filters there exists a determinable inefficiency zone that belies the myth of the HEPA filter as the absolute final answer for air decontamination. In order to complete the air disinfection process initiated by HEPA filtration, ultraviolet germicidal irradiation (UVGI) is introduced. Unlike filtration, UVGI does not capture and retain living microorganisms; it sterilizes them as they pass through the UV irradiated zone. Contrary to a filter that accumulates particulate until the pressure drop increases to a point where it needs to be disposed of and replaced, UVGI systems have a negligible pressure drop and require comparatively very low maintenance. UVGI technology has a long, successful, and documented history of being used for disinfection in ventilation systems and for drinking water in virtually all major cities around the world since its first use in Marseille, France, in 1909.

10.2 *Fundamentals of ultraviolet photochemical disinfection process*

10.2.1 *UV light review*

Much like our familiar "visible light," which extends from 400 nm wavelength called "violet" to the 700 nm that our human eyes perceives as "red," ultraviolet is also an electromagnetic radiation but with a shorter wavelength. The UV light spectrum is not visible to the human eye. The UV spectrum can be conveniently subdivided into four categories:

- UV-A band (400–315 nm)—the most abundant in sunlight reaching the Earth's surface
- UV-B band (315–280 nm)—primarily responsible for skin reddening
- UV-C band (280–200 nm)—the most effective for germicidal effect
- Far or vacuum UV (200–30 nm)—ozone producing and ionizing radiation

As illustrated in Figure 10.3, as the wavelength of light becomes shorter, the amount of energy carried by the light particles called photons increases.

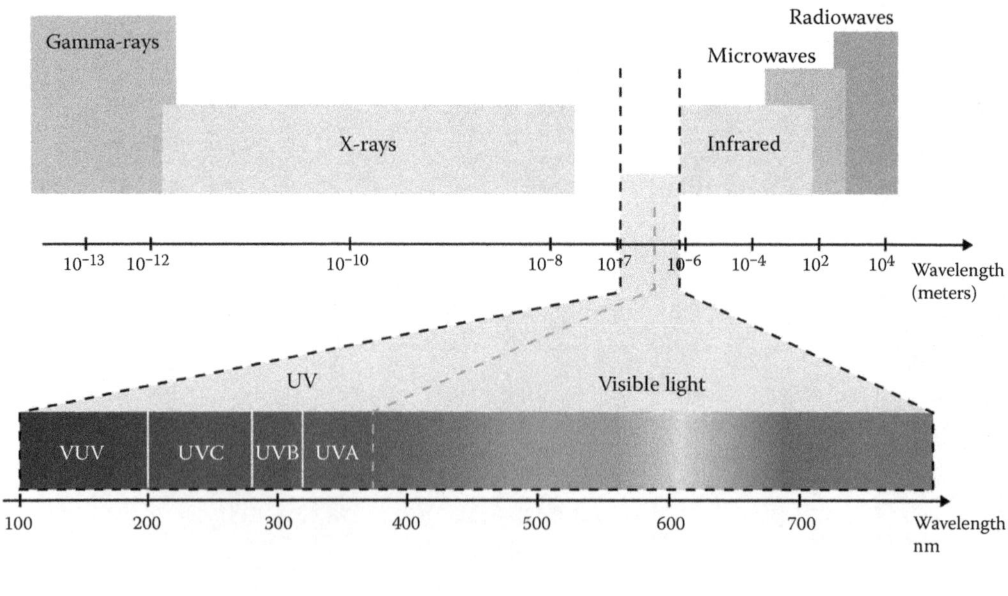

Figure 10.3 **(See color insert.)** Light spectrum.

10.2.2 Photochemistry

Chemical bond dissociation induced by light occurs when a photon's quantum energy is equal to or greater than the energy of the molecular bond. Photochemical damage to a life-sustaining bio-molecular structure can be induced by irradiation with photons having energy levels corresponding to the energy of the chemical bonds. On UV photon absorption, excited states and reactive species are created which interact to form new but non-functional biochemical products.

The history of photochemical microbial inactivation dates back to the discovery in 1877 by Downes and Blunt[9] that UV light can harm microorganisms. Later, in 1928, F.L. Gates[10] made the formal discovery that specific monochromatic wavelengths of UV light are responsible for the observed bactericidal effect. The fundamental physical mechanisms explaining the interaction of specific wavelengths of light with specific molecular bonds were finally revealed by quantum mechanics, developed by Planck, Bose, Einstein, Bohr, de Broglie, Heisenberg, Dirac, Pauli, and others during the first half of the twentieth century.

Then, in the second half of the twentieth century, biochemical research showed that the most effective germicidal wavelengths of 265 nm coincide with the peak absorption spectra of nucleic acids[11] as shown in Figure 10.4. On the basis of this correlation, and the observation that the majority of the damage inflicted to inactivated microbes was found in their genetic material, the primary mechanism in UV-induced microbial inactivation is known today to be molecular damage to DNA and RNA strands. Such disruption of nucleic acids has the ability to affect a wide range of microorganisms, rendering them sterile and consequently unable to infect a host. Within the limits of experimental accuracy, the lethal action of germicidal UV appears to be independent of the nature of the organism and, unlike antibiotics, there has been no signs of adaptive resistance after a century of use for water disinfection.

Most if not all commercially available germicidal light sources are low pressure mercury lamps that emit between 30% and 35% of their input energy at 253.7 nm, a wavelength very close to the peak value as shown in Figure 10.4.

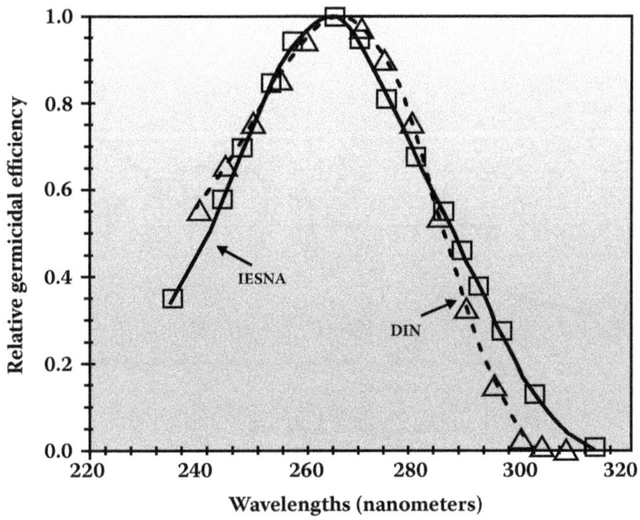

Figure 10.4 Relative germicidal efficiency.

Photochemical sterilization of microorganisms is achieved in practice with the widely available wavelength of 253.7 nm. The quantum energy carried by those UV photons is high enough to dissociate C, H, O, and N single covalent bonds resulting in irreversible molecular damage to nucleic acids leading to a nonviable organism. Among various UV radiation damages to DNA, the formation of cyclobutane pyrimidine dimers (CPDs) and pyrimidine-pyrimidone 6-4 photoproducts (6-4 PPs) are of utmost importance.[12] CPDs are caused by covalent bonding between two adjacent pyrimidines. UV irradiation usually generates thymine dimers in the greatest quantity, cytosine dimers in low quantity, and mixed dimers at an intermediate level.[13] In UV irradiated RNA viruses, the nucleotide uracil forms pyrimidine photoproducts. As shown in Figure 10.5, the movement of DNA/RNA polymerase is stalled when encountering a thymine dimer. At an irradiation dose of magnitude high enough to overwhelm the nucleic acid repair mechanisms, damages result in irreversible alterations, impairment of replication and genetic transcription, and eventual death of the organism.

For a thorough assessment of the photochemistry of UV-induced damages to nucleic acids, and on repair mechanisms, review the in-depth description by Kowalski.[13]

10.2.2.1 UV dose-response mechanism

In order to understand the UV disinfection process, it is helpful to consider UV as the analogue of a bombardment of photon bullets on a microbe. Each photon carries an amount of energy called a quantum $\boldsymbol{E}_\lambda$ of a value connected to the light wavelength according to the Planck-Einstein relation:

$$\boldsymbol{E}_\lambda = \boldsymbol{h}\ \boldsymbol{c}/\lambda \tag{10.1}$$

where

$\boldsymbol{h}$ = Planck's constant, 6.626×10^{-34} Joule.sec
$\boldsymbol{c}$ = speed of light in vacuum, 2.998×10^{8} m/sec
λ = wavelength, m

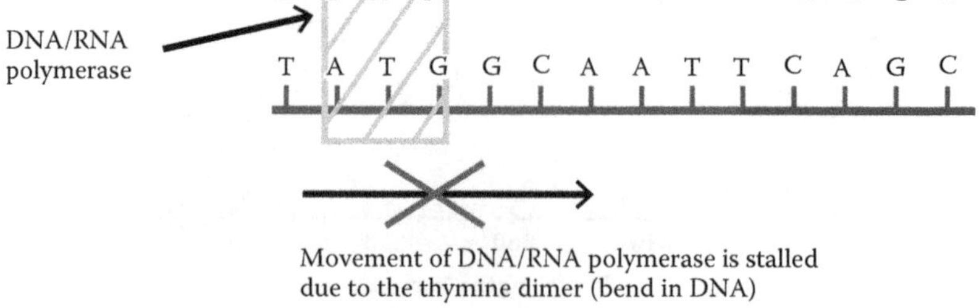

Figure 10.5 UV radiation damages to DNA.

Using the Planck-Einstein relation, the energy conveyed by each UV-C photon at a wavelength of 253.7 nm is equal to 7.83×10^{-19} Joule. Therefore, the number of photons per Joule is the inverse, that is, 1.28×10^{18} photons per Joule. Remember that 1 Watt of power is defined as a rate of 1 Joule of energy per second, and then a UV intensity of 100 Watt/m^2 provides a flow of 1.28×10^{20} photons per second per square meter. Considering that a virus of 0.2-micron diameter has a cross-sectional area of 3.14×10^{-14}m^2, despite its tiny size, this virus will be bombarded by 4 million photons per second. Given a sufficient duration time to this UV photon's assault, photochemical damages will accumulate enough to render the organism biologically dysfunctional. In reality, regardless of the tremendous number of photons shooting at this virus, only a very small number hit their target successfully to initiate the photochemical reactions. The real effective inactivation cross-sectional area of a target microbe is a function of many parameters, among them, the quantum chemical yield, the outside capsid protective layers, and the particular distribution of its DNA sequence. A promising predictive method based on the above-described photon bombardment concept and successful hit probability has been published to predict the UV susceptibility of microorganisms.[14]

Based on the above-described UV bombardment analogy, a mathematical relation can be written to express the UV dose response for a population of bio-organisms. It is reasonable to infer that the rate of decay of a microbial population will vary proportionally to the number of successful hits over a period of time. This rate of successful hits can be described as the product of the UV power per unit area ***I***, the number of bio-organism ***N***, the bio-organism effective UV inactivation cross-section ***k***, also called the bio-organism UV susceptibility constant, and the exposure time ***t*** as follows:

$$\textbf{Hit rate} = \frac{dN}{dt} = k\,N\,I\,t \tag{10.2}$$

Integration of Equation 10.2 yields:

$$N(t) = N_0 e^{-kIt} \tag{10.3}$$

where

N_0 = initial number of microorganisms
$N(t)$ = number of microorganisms surviving after any time t
k = a microorganism-dependent UV susceptibility constant, in m^2/Joule
I = the irradiance UV intensity received by the microorganism, in Watt/m^2
t = exposure time, in seconds

The fraction of the number of microorganisms initially present, which survive at any given time, is called the survival ratio *S* and can be expressed as

$$S = \frac{N_t}{N_0} \tag{10.4}$$

The sterilized fraction, what is called the disinfection rate, is simply 1 minus the survival ratio:

$$\textit{Disinfection} = 1 - S = 1 - e^{-kIt} \tag{10.5}$$

As explained above, we can define the germicidal UV dose by the total number of UV photons emitted per unit area during a time interval, which can be written as

$$\boldsymbol{UVDose} = \boldsymbol{I} \times \boldsymbol{t} \text{ in Joule/m}^2 \tag{10.6}$$

By substituting Equation 10.6 in Equation 10.5, we finally get the well-verified germicidal UV dose-response relation:

$$\boldsymbol{Disinfection} = 1 - e^{-k\,\text{UVDose}} \tag{10.7}$$

Equation 10.7 illustrates that a given dose results in a given disinfection rate, whether the UV dose consists of a low UV intensity for a long exposure time or a high UV intensity for a shorter time. A key difference between surface decontamination and airborne inactivation of organisms is exposure time. The residence time for any in-duct disinfection will be of the order of a few seconds or a fraction of a second depending on airflow velocities. Therefore, the UV intensities for neutralizing an airborne microorganism are required to be orders of magnitude higher than that typically used for stationary surface disinfection such as walls or air-conditioning cooling coils.

Equations 10.3, 10.5, and 10.7 shown in Figure 10.6 describe an exponential decay in time of the number of living organisms as a constant level of UVGI exposure intensity is applied. The very same type of equation is used to describe the effect of chemical disinfectants on a population of microorganisms, with the dose in this example being a chemical concentration multiplied by the contact time.

10.2.2.2 *Susceptibility of microorganisms to UV energy*

Organisms differ in their susceptibility to UV inactivation. A few examples of familiar pathogenic organisms are included in each group for reference. It is important to note that

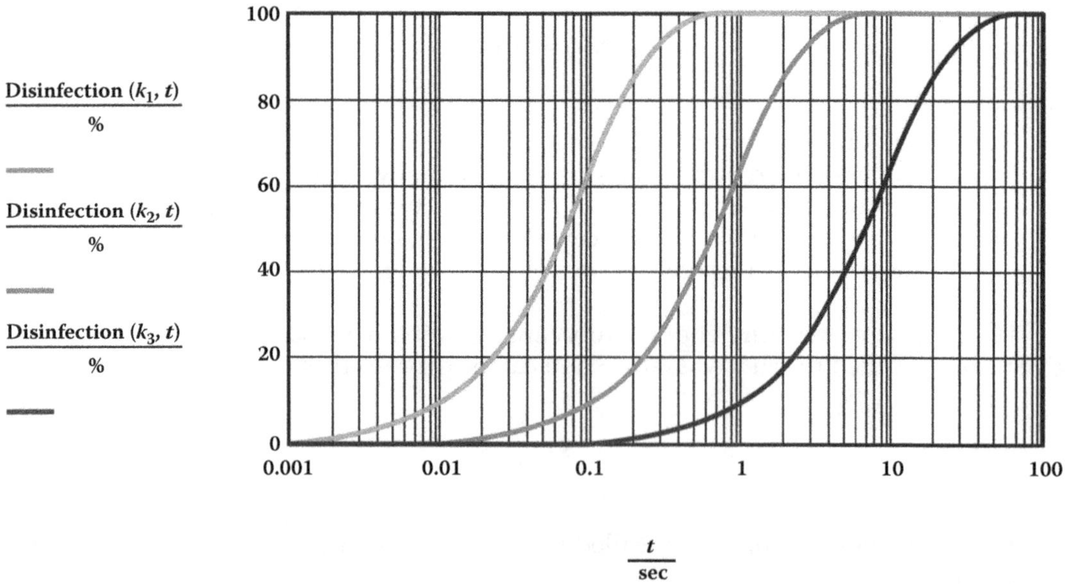

Figure 10.6 Disinfection rate versus UV exposure time for various UV susceptibilities.

it is impossible to list all the organisms of interest in each group. Depending on the application, a public health or medical professional, microbiologist, or other individual with knowledge of the microbial threat or organisms of concern should be consulted.

Within each group of biologicals, an individual species may be significantly more resistant or susceptible, so care should be taken using this ranking only as a guideline. It should be noted that the spore forming bacteria and fungi also have vegetative forms, which are markedly more susceptible to inactivation than the spore forms. Viruses are particularly problematic to categorize, as their susceptibility to inactivation is even broader than that of bacteria or fungi.

Based on Equation 10.5, it is clear that larger values of k represent more susceptible microorganisms and smaller values represent less susceptible ones. Units of k are m^2/Joule, which is the inverse of the units used in UV dose. For example, the value of the UV susceptibility of the Influenza-A virus was measured experimentally by Jensen in 1964 and was found to be 0.0119 m^2/J in air at 68% relative humidity. Based on this value, one can determine the required UV dose to be applied to reach 90% disinfection of a population of Influenza-A virus using the following formula:

$$\boldsymbol{D90} = \frac{\boldsymbol{ln}(10)}{k} = \frac{2.30}{k} \text{ in J/m}^2 \tag{10.8}$$

The **D90** value for Influenza-A virus is therefore equal to 19.3 J/m^2. The **D90** value has a high practical interest as it allows the designer to quickly evaluate the required UV dosage to reach a desired disinfection level. For example, providing a UV dose of twice the **D90** will result in a disinfection level of 99%. Delivering three times the **D90** dose will result in 99.9% disinfection rate, and so on. It can be easily demonstrated mathematically that the number of 9s, also called the disinfection LOG value, is simply equal to the delivered UV dose divided by the **D90** value. To reach sterility, a condition that we have previously defined as a disinfection level of 6 LOG or 99.9999%, at least 6 times the **D90** value of the most resistant microorganism must be delivered. Extensive compilations of published k values can be found in several places in the literature, for example Kowalski.[13]

10.3 UVGI dosage required for ART clinics air disinfection

10.3.1 UVGI system design guidelines

Before examining the various design requirements for a UV system to achieve a homogeneous irradiation level, it is important to note that Equation 10.7 is of no use in determining the actual delivered UV dosage by a given set of UV lamps positioned inside an air duct. In any air duct, the physics is complicated by the movement of the target microorganisms in the turbulent air stream and the fact that the UVGI irradiance is far from being constant within the duct as it varies significantly with the distance from the UV lamps. In addition, the physical geometry of the duct, duct airflow velocity distribution, number of lamps, and UV lamp positions in the duct all have the potential to affect the overall delivered UV dose. Only a computerized program using an integration method and summation of the contribution of all the UV lamps allows the precise calculation of the UV irradiation field inside a duct. Such a calculation also incorporates the important contribution of the UV reflective properties of the duct wall surfaces on the performance enhancement of UV disinfection.

The first design guidelines for UVGI airstream disinfection systems were developed in the 1940s.[15] Systems appeared in commercial catalogs that continue to be reproduced and even used today by some manufacturers such as Philips.[16] These guidelines propose charts and tables to size lamps and reflective surfaces so as to obtain a desired disinfection rate. These sizing methods, though admirably detailed for that time, suffer from several fundamental deficiencies, the most important being:

- The real three-dimensional intensity field is not defined, it is instead simply evaluated based on the lamp power rating or else relying on basic photometric data taken at lamp midpoints.
- Lamps are specified without regard to lamp positioning.
- The correction factors for reflectivity ignore duct dimensions and lengths.

Many manufacturers size systems by rules of thumb, such as filling the available cross-section of ductwork with an array of lamps, or base their designs on limited proprietary testing.

The available computational power of modern-day computers allows for adequate custom sizing of any in-duct UV disinfection system. Proper calculation for predicting the applied UV dose must take into account the relevant input parameters describing a rectangular UVGI system in terms of its geometry, lamp characteristics, lamp placement, lamp orientation, and surface reflectivity.

Kowalski,[17] using computer modeling and taking all these variables into account, has proposed a dimensional analysis to assess the sensitivity of all of the above design parameters on the disinfection performance against the airstream within the duct. An interesting and very useful outcome of Kowalski's work is an elegant, simplified formula correlating the relation of the delivered UV dose as a function of air flow, UV output power, and duct length. The formula is as follows:

$$\boldsymbol{UV\ dose} \sim \frac{\boldsymbol{P}}{\boldsymbol{Q}}\boldsymbol{L} \tag{10.9}$$

where

$\boldsymbol{P}$ = UV output in Watt
$\boldsymbol{Q}$ = Air flow in m^3/sec
$\boldsymbol{L}$ = UV exposure length

For scaling purposes, Equation 10.9 tells us that if the flow rate is doubled in a given duct size, then the UV power or number of lamps must be doubled as well to maintain the same disinfection performances. The same can be said about the duct UV exposure length L, if it is reduced by half to make the system more compact, then the UV output power will have to be doubled to compensate.

By observing in Equation 10.11 that the air flow $\boldsymbol{Q}$ is the product of the duct cross-section $\boldsymbol{A}$ in m^2 by the air velocity $\boldsymbol{V}$ in m/sec and that the UV exposure time $\boldsymbol{t}$ is simply the ratio of the duct length $\boldsymbol{L}$ to the air velocity $\boldsymbol{V}$, we can rewrite Equation 10.9 as follows:

$$\boldsymbol{UV\ dose} = \boldsymbol{P} \times \boldsymbol{t}/\boldsymbol{A} \tag{10.10}$$

This scaling relation concisely expresses the fact that the delivered UV dose in J/m^2 is the product of UV lamps output power in Watts with the exposure time in seconds divided by the duct cross-section area.

10.3.2 *Effect of air velocity, temperature, and lamp aging on UV system output*

Air temperature and velocity may vary over a wide range within a ventilation system, causing tremendous variations in UV lamp output, and must be adequately accounted for in system design and analysis.

UV lamps are designed in such a way that, depending on the lamp type, the cold spot lamp surface temperature must be between 38°C and 50°C to reach the maximum UV output (Figure 10.7). In moving air, the temperature of the UV lamps' cold spot could become too low and the UV output will fall as seen in Figures 10.8 and 10.9. To minimize the chilling effect and allow higher operating efficiency under cold air flow conditions, it is preferable to install the lamps parallel to the flow instead of perpendicular to the flow.

UV lamp output decreases over time. UV lamps are rated in effective hours of UV emission and not in end of electrical life hours. Most UV lamps emit intensity levels at the end of their useful life, that is, 20,000 hours that are 80% or more than those measured at 100 hours of operation. UVGI systems should be designed for UV output at the end of effective life. Modern-day UV lamps will continue to emit blue light long after they have passed their useful germicidal lifespan.

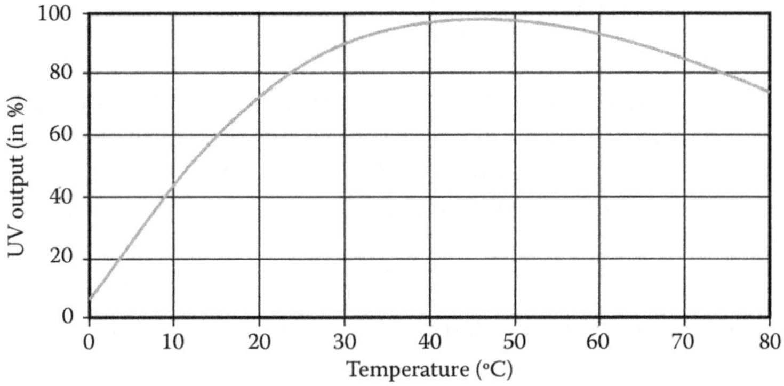

Figure 10.7 Example of lamp efficiency (in %) as a function of cold spot temperature.

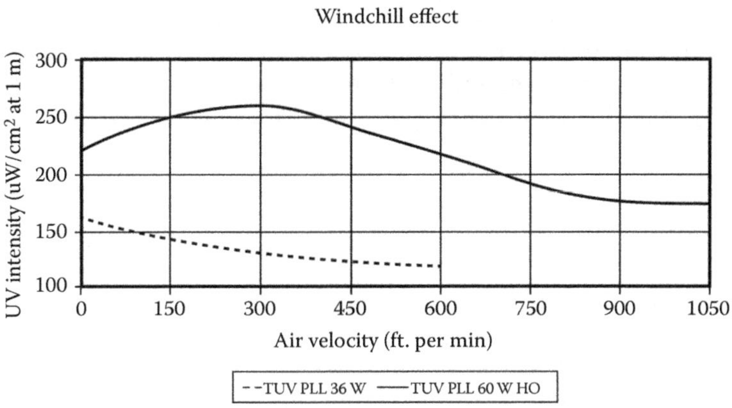

Figure 10.8 Influence of moving air cooling effect on UV lamp efficiency for two types of lamps.

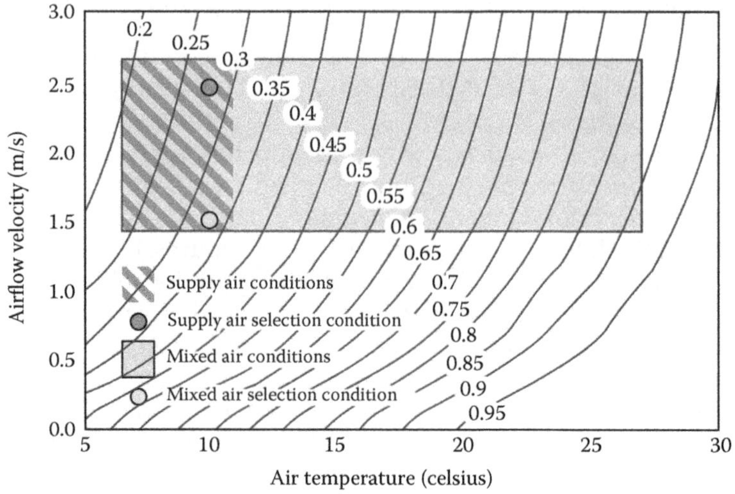

Figure 10.9 Combined effect of air temperature and velocity on UV lamp output. (Adapted from Lee, B. et al., Life cycle cost simulation of in-duct ultraviolet germicidal irradiation system. *Building Simulation*. Glasgow, Scotland, 2009.)

Variations in UV lamp output due to lamp type and ambient conditions can be of equal or greater magnitude than depreciation due to aging. These changes are cumulative and can reduce lamp output by as much as 50% over a range of typical conditions found in ventilation systems.[18] Consequently, design procedures should take these sources of output variation into consideration.

10.4 UVGI system maintenance guidelines

10.4.1 Lamp replacement

UV lamps should be replaced at the end of their useful life based on the recommendation of the equipment manufacturer. Although lamps can operate for as much as two consecutive years, it is prudent to change lamps annually (8760 hours under continuous use) and therefore ensure that adequate UV dosage is always supplied. Lamps can operate long after their useful life but will have greatly reduced output. Switching lamps on and off too often may lead to premature lamp failure. Consult the manufacturer for any specific information regarding expected lamp life in hours and the impact of switching on the lamp life.

10.4.2 Lamp disposal

UV lamps should be disposed in the same way as other mercury-containing devices such as conventional commercial fluorescent bulbs. Most lamps must be treated as hazardous waste and cannot be discarded with regular waste. Low mercury bulbs generally can be discarded as regular waste; however, some state and local jurisdictions classify these lamps as hazardous waste. The U.S. EPA has promulgated "universal waste" regulations for several types of hazardous waste including mercury bulbs. These regulations allow users to treat mercury lamps as regular waste for the purpose of transporting to a recycling facility. This simplified process was developed to promote recycling.

10.4.3 Inspection

UVGI systems must include a feedback component to alert maintenance personnel of UV-C lamp failure. Any failed lamp should be replaced immediately. In the event the lamp becomes dirty or soiled due to inadequate pre-filtration or airborne bio-aerosols, it should be cleaned. A UV lamp may be cleaned with a lint free cloth and commercial glass cleaner or alcohol.

10.4.4 Safety design guidance

In-duct UV systems shall be fully enclosed to prevent leakage of UV light to unprotected persons or materials outside of the HVAC equipment. All access panels or doors with access to the lamp chamber where UV may penetrate either directly or through reflectance shall be affixed with warning labels in appropriate languages. The labels shall be affixed to the exterior of each panel or door in a prominent location visible to persons accessing the system.[19] Lamp chambers shall be equipped with an electrical disconnect device. Positive disconnection devices are preferred over switches. Disconnection devices shall be capable of being locked or tagged out. Disconnection devices shall be located outside of the lamp chamber and adjacent to the primary access panel or door to the lamp chamber. Switches shall be wired in series such that the opening of any access will shut down the UV system. On/off switches for UV lamps must not be located in the same location as general room lighting. Switches must be positioned in such a location that only authorized persons have access to them and should be locked to ensure that they are not accidentally turned on or off.

References

1. American Institute of Architects. Guidelines for Designing and Construction of Hospital and Healthcare Facilities. Washington, DC: AIA, 2001.
2. American Society of Heating, Refrigerating, and Air-Conditioning Engineers. *HVAC Design Manual for Hospital and Clinics*. Atlanta, GA: ASHRAE, 2003.
3. American Society of Heating, Refrigerating, and Air-Conditioning Engineers. *Handbook—HVAC Applications*. Atlanta, GA: ASHRAE, 2003.
4. CDC. *Guidelines for Environmental Infection Control in Health-Care Facilities*. Atlanta, GA: U.S. Department of Health and Human Services Centers for Disease Control and Prevention, 2003.
5. Menzies, D., Popa, J., Hanley, J.A., Rand, T., and Milton, D.K. Effect of ultraviolet germicidal ligths installed in office ventilation systems on workers' health and well being: Double-blind multiple cross-over trial. *The Lancet Medical Journal*, 2003, 362: 1785–91.
6. Gates, F.L. On nuclear derivatives and the lethal action of UV light. *Science*, 1928, 68(1768): 479–480. doi: 10.1126/science.68.1768.479-a.
7. Davidson, J.N. *The Biochemistry of Nucleic Acids*. 5th ed. London: Metheun, 1965.
8. Kowalski, W. *Ultraviolet Germicidal Irradiation Handbook*. Berlin: Springer-Verlag, 2009.
9. Setlow, R.B. Cyclobutane-type pyrimidine dimmers in polynucleotudes. *Science*, 1966, 153: 379–386.
10. Luckiesh, M. and Holladay, L.L. Designing installations of germicidal lamps for occupied rooms. *General Electric Review*, 1942, 45(6): 343–349.
11. Philips. UVGI Catalog and Design Guide. Catalog No. U.D.C. 628.9, Netherlands, 1985.
12. Kowalski, W.J. Design and optimization of UVGI air disinfection systems. A thesis in Architechtural Engineering. Penn State University, Department of Architectural Engineering, University Park, Pennsylvania, 2001.
13. Kowalski, W.J., Bahnfleth, W.P., and Hernandez, M.T. A genomic model for the prediction of ultraviolet inactivation rate constants for RNA and DNA viruses. *IUVA Air Treatment Conference*, Cambridge, MA, May 5. http://www.aerobiologicalengineering.com/Genomic.pdf.

14. Kato, S. and Sung, M. Using UVGI to counter contaminant dispersion. *IFHE Digest*. 2011.
15. Downes, A. and Blunt, T. Research on the Effect of Light Upon Bacteria and Other Organisms. *Proceedings of the Royal Society*, 1877, 26: 488.
16. Lee, B., Bahnfleth, W., and Auer, K. Life cycle cost simulation of in-duct ultraviolet germicidal irradiation system. *Building Simulation*. Glasgow, Scotland, 2009.
17. Kowalski, W.J. and Bahnfleth, W. MERV filter models for aerobiological applications. *Air Media*. 2002, Summer 13–17.
18. Engineers, American Society of Heating Refrigerating and Air Conditioning. *ASHRAE Handbook*, Chapter 16, 2008.
19. Menzies, D., Adhikari, N., Arietta, M., and Loo, V. Efficacy of environmental measures in reducing potentially infectious bioaerosols during sputum induction. *Infection Control and Hospital Epidemiology*, 2003, 24.

chapter eleven

Photocatalytic degradation of volatile organic compounds

Hsin Chu, Yi Hsing Lin, and Ting Ke Tseng

Contents

Abstract

Volatile organic compounds (VOCs) are major sources of indoor air pollution that significantly affect human health and the indoor environment quality. Photocatalytic oxidation is regarded as a promising method to destruct VOCs indoors due to its fast oxidation rate, high decomposition rate, relatively convenient operation at room temperature, good stability, and nontoxicity. In this chapter, we discuss the preparation and doping methods of various photocatalytic catalysts, as well as their operating parameters and kinetic models.

11.1 Introduction

Photocatalytic oxidation of aqueous and gaseous contaminants has been extensively studied in the processes of inorganic and organic pollutants.[1] The technology has drawn considerable interest due to its fast oxidation rate, high decomposition rate, relatively convenient operation at room temperature, stability, and nontoxicity. Semiconductors can provide light-induced charges for redox processes primarily due to their electronic configuration.[2] A photocatalytic reaction is initiated when the illumination of a semiconductor generates photoexcited electrons and positively charged holes that react with adsorbed contaminants on the photocatalyst surface.[3] Among the known semiconductors (TiO_2, ZnO, CdS, Fe_2O_3, WO_3, and $SrTiO_3$), TiO_2 is the most widely used photocatalyst due to its good physical and chemical stability, lower cost, nontoxicity, and high resistance to corrosion.[3] The enormous challenge of novel photocatalysts has been to satisfy growing demands in environmental pollution purification and energy conversion.[4] A number of studies have recently been attempted to overcome these problems, focusing on the surface-modified TiO_2 and change in the operating environment. The advantages of surface modification are (1) nonmetal or transition metal doping into TiO_2 narrows the band gap energy, which enhances the wavelength response range to visible light absorption; (2) efficient separation of photoexcited electrons and holes, thus inhibiting the recombination rate of h^+/e^- pairs during the photodegradation process; (3) increasing the adsorption of surface hydroxyls, which can induce the generation of hydroxyl free radicals; (4) the large specific surface areas can provide more activity sites, in favor of the photocatalytic activity; and (5) changing the selectivity or yield of a particular product.

11.2 Preparation of photocatalyst

11.2.1 Photocatalysis

A semiconductor is a material that has electrical conductivity to a degree between that of a metal (such as copper) and an insulator (such as glass). Semiconductors can be divided into two major types: intrinsic and extrinsic semiconductors. The former is diamond cubic and the latter is zinc blend. The electric conductivity of intrinsic semiconductors can be enhanced by doping metallic oxides, transition metal oxides, or nonmetallic oxides. These methods result in the formation of extra electrons or holes, which can be assigned as N-type or P-type semiconductors.[5]

11.2.1.1 N-type semiconductor

N-type semiconductors have negatively charged electrons, as shown in Figure 11.1, which can be formed by doping a core semiconductor with a group V element such as phosphorus, antimony, or arsenic. These materials have atoms with five valence electrons (pentavalent atoms). These electrons will form covalent bonds with neighboring atoms. There are only four covalent bonds binding with the four neighboring atoms, and the free fifth electron is not part of a covalent bond. ZnO, Fe_2O_3, TiO_2, V_2O_5, CrO_3, and CuO are typically used for N-type semiconductors.

11.2.1.2 P-type semiconductor

The formation of P-type semiconductors is just the opposite of N-type semiconductors. P-type semiconductors have positively charged holes, as shown in Figure 11.2, which are doped with a group III element to produce a hole for each atom. The majority carrier of P-type semiconductors is holes and adsorption of O_2 and the semiconductor increases the

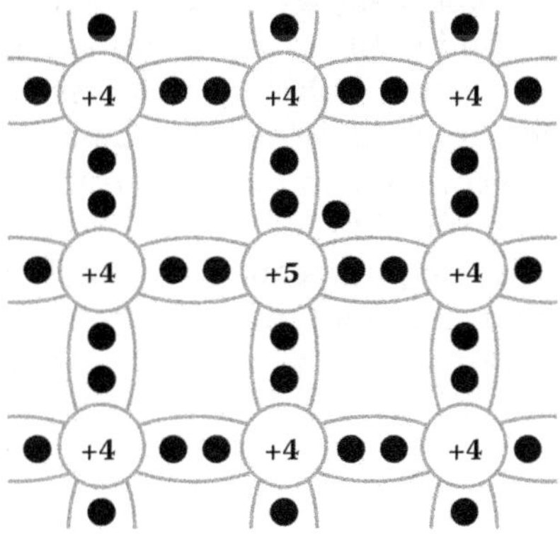

Figure 11.1 N-type semiconductor.

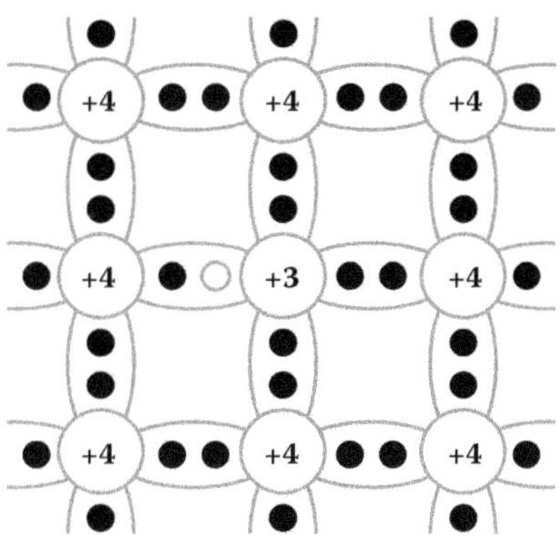

Figure 11.2 P-type semiconductor.

hole conductivity.[6] P-type semiconductors typically include NiO, CoO, Cu_2O, SnO, PbO, and Cr_2O_3.

11.2.1.3 Photocatalyst

When the semiconductor is excited by photons whose energy ($h\upsilon$) is equal or greater than its band gap energy (Eg), it will participate and enhance the chemical reaction, but does not change itself. The material generated from the action of the semiconductor is called photocatalyst. O_2 and H_2O will be converted to highly active free radicals to oxidize organic compounds during the photocatalytic process.[5]

11.2.1.4 Photocatalysis principle

The photocatalytic oxidation process can be divided into five elemental mass transfer processes occurring in series, as shown in Figure 11.3. At the beginning, VOCs and precursor species are carried by airflows (step 1, advection). Then, the reaction species pass through the boundary layer to the photocatalyst surface by external diffusion (step 2). Next (step 3), the species adsorb onto the photocatalyst surface and chemical reactions happen at the surface. Finally, reaction products desorb from the catalyst surface (step 4) and boundary layer to the main flow (step 5).[7]

Figure 11.3 also illustrates the chemical reaction mechanism at the catalyst surface.[7] For photocatalytic oxidation, an important step of photoreaction is the formation of electron–hole pairs. When a photon's energy overcomes the band gap energy ($h\upsilon \geqq Eg$), which is between the valence band (VB) and the conduction band (CB), pairs of electron holes are created in the semiconductor. Within this process, negative charged electrons are displaced to the CB, and positive charged holes are created in the VB. These highly reactive electron/hole pairs can either recombine to produce heat or be used to reduce or oxidize reactants at the semiconductor surface.[8,9]

The elementary mechanisms of photocatalytic transformation include a number of steps.[10,11] The reaction steps for a TiO_2 photocatalyst are listed in the following reactions. In Reactions 11.1 through 11.3, h^+ and e^- are powerful oxidizing and reducing agents, respectively.

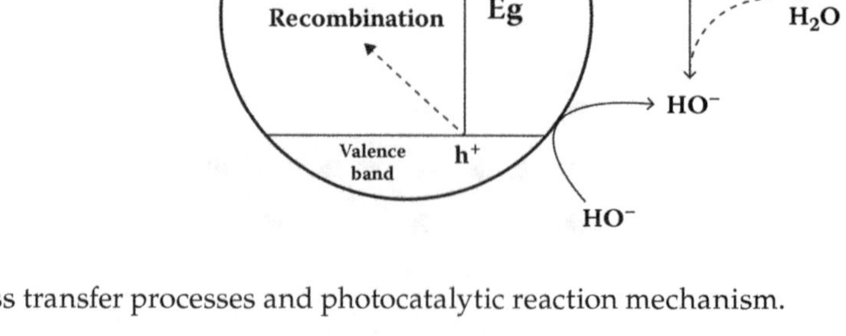

Figure 11.3 Mass transfer processes and photocatalytic reaction mechanism.

$$TiO_2 + h\upsilon \rightarrow h^+_{vb} + e^- \tag{11.1}$$

$$H_2O \rightarrow H^+ + OH^- \tag{11.2}$$

$$h^+_{vb} + e^- \rightarrow \textit{thermal heat or luminescence} \tag{11.3}$$

The oxidation and reduction can be expressed as Reactions 11.4 and 11.5, respectively. The positive charged holes react with adsorbed water to form hydroxyl radicals (•OH), which can initiate the oxidation of the adsorbed organic compounds. In the reduction reaction, the negative charged electrons react with adsorbed oxygen to form super-oxide ions $\left(\bullet O^-_{2ads}\right)$.

$$h^+_{vb} + OH^- \rightarrow \bullet OH \tag{11.4}$$

$$O_{2(ads)} + e^- \rightarrow \bullet O^-_{2\,ads} \tag{11.5}$$

From Reactions 11.1 through 11.5, a series of reactions creates hydroxyl radicals (•OH) and super-oxide ions $\left(\bullet O^-_{2abs}\right)$. Those are highly reactive species that will oxidize VOCs adsorbed on the catalyst surface. A chain of reactions is displayed in the following reactions:

$$\bullet O^-_{2\,ads} + H_2O \rightarrow \bullet OOH + OH^- \tag{11.6}$$

$$2\bullet OOH \rightarrow O_2 + H_2O_2 \tag{11.7}$$

$$\bullet OOH + H_2O + e^- \rightarrow H_2O_2 + OH^- \tag{11.8}$$

$$H_2O_2 + e^- \rightarrow \bullet OH + OH^- \tag{11.9}$$

$$Ti^{4+} + e^- \rightarrow Ti^{3+} \tag{11.10}$$

$$Ti^{3+} + O_{2(ads)} \rightarrow Ti^{4+} + \bullet O^-_{2\,ads} \tag{11.11}$$

Organic pollutants can be completely oxidized to carbon dioxide and water under optimal reaction conditions. Different intermediates will be produced depending on the VOCs, as shown in

$$\bullet OH + VOCs + O_2 \rightarrow \text{Products } (H_2O, CO_2, \text{etc.}) \tag{11.12}$$

11.2.1.5 Band gap

Generally, photocatalysts are nonconductors. When photocatalysts are irradiated by light with high enough energy, they could become conductors. The range of energies between the valence band and conduction band is called band gap. Various semiconductors have different band gaps. Electrons are steadily concentrating in the valence band and vibrating at the same place. When electrons obtain enough energy, they will move to the conduction band and form holes in the valence band. Thus, semiconductors can sometimes be conductors.

TiO_2 is the most important and widely used photocatalyst in recently years. TiO_2 is a well-known photocatalyst for its excellent activity for wastewater treatment and purification of air and other favorable properties including low cost, good stability, and non-toxicity. Other semiconductors such as ZnO, ZnS, CdS, Fe_2O_3, and SnO_2 are also commonly used. Based on the value of the band gap of 3.2 eV, the required wavelength of light excitation for TiO_2 is 385 nm, which is within the UV range.

11.2.2 Photocatalyst preparation

11.2.2.1 Impregnation method

A main method of photocatalyst preparation is impregnation. The active precursor with thermally unstable anions is used in the impregnation process. The support (activated carbon, zeolite, or graphene) is immersed in a solution of the active components under precisely defined conditions. After impregnation, the photocatalyst particles go through drying, calcination, and activation.[12,13] In a previous study, a series of metal-doped (Zn^{2+}, Fe^{3+}, Cr^{3+}, MO^{6+}, or Mn^{2+}) TiO_2 were prepared by a wet impregnation method and examined with respect to the activity for photocatalytic oxidation of nitric oxide.[2]

11.2.2.2 Sol-gel method

The sol-gel process has been used to produce a type of solid materials synthesis procedure, performed in a liquid and at low temperature (typically $T < 100°C$). The process involves the formation of "sols" in a liquid followed by that of a gel. A sol is a stable colloidal dispersion of small particles in the size range from 1 nm to 1 mm, suspended in a liquid. The precursor in a sol-gel preparation can be a metal salt/alkoxide dissolved in a solvent. Metal alkoxides have been used widely due to their high purity and solution chemistry. The preparation steps from taking a precursor to the finished catalyst by the sol-gel method include formation of a gel, aging of the gel, removal of solvent, and heat treatment.[14]

In general, the sol-gel chemistry with metal alkoxides can be described by Reactions 11.13 through 11.15.[13,15]

1. Hydrolysis: metal alkoxides react with H_2O, then –OH substitute –OR to form metal alkoxides that contain –OH and view $M(OH)_x(OR)_n$ as alcohol. For Reaction 11.13, M is metal, R is alkyl group, and n means metal charge value.

$$M(OR)_n + xH_2O \rightarrow M(OH)_x(OR)_{n-x} + xROH \tag{11.13}$$

2. Condensation reaction: dehydration and dealcoholization take place at the same time within a condensation reaction to form bridging oxygen and release H_2O or alcohol.

$$M - OH + RO - M \rightarrow M - O - M + ROH \tag{11.14}$$

$$M - OH + HO - M \rightarrow M - O - M + H_2O \tag{11.15}$$

In previous studies, thin films of TiO_2, Fe-TiO_2, and V-TiO_2 were obtained by a sol-gel method.[2,16] The advantages of the sol-gel method are

1. It is easy and inexpensive.
2. The films are readily anchored on the substrate.

3. It can be used for the deposition of substrates that have complex surfaces or large surface areas.
4. It can be used for preparing several components in a single step at low temperature.

11.2.2.3 Precipitation

The preparation of supported catalysts by precipitation or coprecipitation is commonly used in catalyst manufacture.[14] In the production of precipitated catalysts, the first step is to prepare mixing solutions of materials. Soon afterward, the catalyst particles are converted to the finished catalyst by filtration, washing, drying, forming, calcination, and activation.[6,13] The advantages of precipitation are

1. It generally provides a more uniform mixing on a molecular scale of various catalyst components.
2. The distribution of the active species on the final catalysts is uniform.
3. It is possible to control the pore size and pore size distribution of the final catalysts.

11.2.3 Photocatalyst modification techniques

Titanium dioxide is an N-type extrinsic semiconductor. There are three kinds of crystalline phases in titanium oxide TiO_2, including anatase, rutile, and brookite. Among these, rutile and anatase are generally used in photocatalysis.[9] The properties of rutile and anatase are summarized in Table 11.1.[8,10]

Titanium dioxide photocatalysts can be excited by ultraviolet irradiation, but the large band gap (3.2 eV) of TiO_2 limits its utilization potential and photo-response to visible light.[17] Only 4% of the solar radiation reaching the Earth's surface can be used.[18] Many previous studies have been done to increase the photo-degradation activity by doping metals, non-metal elements, and sensitization to TiO_2. Recent research indicates that sulfur doping into TiO_2 provides defect states in the band gap of TiO_2, causing red shift, promoting photodegradation of VOCs under visible-light, separating electron-hole pairs and inhibiting electron-hole recombination, and decreasing byproducts.[19,20]

11.2.3.1 Doped TiO_2 with metal atoms

A number of research studies indicate that Ag doped into TiO_2 increases the degradation efficiency.[21,22] The phenomena is ascribed to an important change in crystalline structure and surface area. Metal-atom-doped TiO_2 changes the band gap of TiO_2 to promote efficient charge transfer. In addition, the holes react with water molecules to cause the generation of hydroxyl radicals, which increases the degradation of organic compounds and decreases the recombination of electron–hole pairs. The production of $\bullet O^-_{2\,abs}$ and Ti^{3+} was promoted

Table 11.1 The contrast between anatase and rutile

Item	Anatase	Rutile
Density (g/cm^3)	3.78	4.23
Band gap (eV)	3.2	3.0
Index of refraction	2.488	2.903
Hardness (Mohs)	5.0–6.0	6.0–6.5
Melting point (°C)	1560	1640
Photoactivity	High	Low

as shown in Reactions 11.16 through 11.18. If too much dopant is present, Reaction 11.19 takes place and causes recombination of electron–hole pairs.

$$Ag_n + e^- \rightarrow Ag_n^- \quad (11.16)$$

$$Ag_n^- + O_2 \rightarrow Ag_n + \bullet O_{2\,ads}^- \quad (11.17)$$

$$Ag_n^- + Ti^{4+} \rightarrow Ag_n + Ti^{3+} \quad (11.18)$$

$$Ag_n^- + h^+ \rightarrow Ag_n \quad (11.19)$$

11.2.3.2 *Doped TiO_2 with metal ions*

Many studies have described that metal-ion-doped TiO_2 can improve the photocatalytic activity of TiO_2.[23,24] Umebayashi et al. doped 3D transition metal into the lattice of TiO_2, such as V, Cr, Mn, Fe, Co, and Ni, which caused a red shift.[23] Metal ions create defect-induced energy states in the band gap of TiO_2, which reduce the recombination rate of the electron–hole. This is due to metal-ion-doped TiO_2 that causes band gap transition, thus forming a narrow gap between the valence band and the conduction band. Besides, the role of metal-ion dopants (M^{n+}) as h^+/e^- traps promotes photocatalytic activity and alters the recombination of electron–hole pairs. Reactions 11.20 through 11.28 illustrate the reaction steps[11]:

$$TiO_2 + h\upsilon \rightarrow h_{vb}^+ + e^- \quad (11.20)$$

$$Ti^{4+} + e^- \rightarrow Ti^{3+} \quad (11.21)$$

$$M^{n+} + e^- \rightarrow M^{(n-1)+} \quad (11.22)$$

$$M^{(n-1)+} + O_{2(ads)} \rightarrow M^{n+} + \bullet O_{2\,ads}^- \quad (11.23)$$

$$M^{n+} + Ti^{3+} \rightarrow M^{(n-1)+} + Ti^{4+} \quad (11.24)$$

$$M^{(n-1)+} + Ti^{4+} \rightarrow M^{n+} + Ti^{3+} \quad (11.25)$$

$$Ti^{3+} + O_{2(ads)} \rightarrow Ti^{4+} + \bullet O_{2\,ads}^- \quad (11.26)$$

$$M^{n+} + h_{vb}^+ \rightarrow M^{(n+1)+} \quad (11.27)$$

$$M^{(n+1)+} + H_2O_{(ads)} \rightarrow M^{n+} + \bullet OH + H^+ \quad (11.28)$$

M^{n+} in the TiO_2 lattice can also act as recombination sites for holes and electrons, according to

$$h_{vb}^{+} + e^{-} \rightarrow TiO_2 \tag{11.29}$$

$$M^{n+} + e^{-} \rightarrow M^{(n-1)+} \tag{11.30}$$

$$M^{(n-1)+} + h_{vb}^{+} \rightarrow M^{n+} \tag{11.31}$$

$$M^{n+} + h_{vb}^{+} \rightarrow M^{(n+1)+} \tag{11.32}$$

$$M^{(n+1)+} + e^{-} \rightarrow M^{n+} \tag{11.33}$$

$$M^{(n+1)+} + Ti^{3+} \rightarrow M^{n+} + Ti^{4+} \tag{11.34}$$

$$M^{(n-1)+} + M^{(n+1)+} \rightarrow 2M^{n+} \tag{11.35}$$

11.2.3.3 Doped TiO_2 with non-metal elements

Many studies have investigated increasing the photodegradation activity of semiconductors by doping non-metal elements.[25,26] C, N, and S are the most frequently used non-metal elements. Zhou and Yu used UV-visible absorption spectra to observe the performance of the C, N, S-tridoped TiO_2 powders.[13] The results indicated that C, N, S-tridoped TiO_2 exhibited higher photocatalytic activity, which can be attributed to the strong absorption capability in the near-UV and visible-light regions.[13] The absorption shift to the visible-light region could be related to the newly formed orbit O 2p with C 2p, N 2p, and S 3p orbits, respectively. In addition, a high concentration of hydroxyl radicals generated on the non-metal element doped TiO_2 surface could increase the photocatalytic activity dramatically.

11.2.3.4 Co-doped TiO_2

A study has investigated the effect of increasing the photodegradation activity by doping transition metal or nonmetal species to support charge carriers separation.[26] However, metal-ion-doped TiO_2 may increase charge recombination and thermal phase instability.[27] Besides, nonmetal-element-doped TiO_2 would lose ingredients during the annealing process, resulting in its low photocatalytic activity under visible light.[28] A new approach has been developed to improve the photocatalytic activity with a novel multicomponent photocatalyst system.[29] Many previous studies have found that co-doping with nonmetals and transition metals is a highly promising method for second-generation photocatalysts.[11,18,30] The results are attributed to the synergistic effects of dopants to pure TiO_2. Nonmetal species is considered an efficient way to enhance the photocatalytic efficiency under visible light irradiation by forming a defect state in the band gap of titania.[31] Metal ion doping could accelerate the separation of photo-generated electron-hole pairs.[29,30]

11.2.3.5 Coupled semiconductors

A study combined various semiconductors such as CdS, ZnO, and Fe_2O_3 with TiO_2 and performed photodegradation under a variety of conditions of pH and irradiation wavelength. The results show that coupled semiconductors are simultaneously illuminated and their valence and conduction bands are suitably disposed, and both electron and hole transfers occur (as in the ZnO/TiO_2, CdS/TiO_2, TiO_2/Fe_2O_3, ZnO/Fe_2O_3), which would impact the performance efficiency of photo-oxidation.[12]

11.2.3.6 Sensitizations

Recently, considerable attention has been drawn to dye-sensitized photocatalysts. Dye molecules (thionine, eosin Y, rhodamine B, methylene blue, nile blue A, and safranine O) are an effective approach to enhance the photocatalytic activity for the development of visible-light photocatalysts. The light absorption range can be extended by photosensitization by injecting electrons from the lowest unoccupied molecular orbital of excited dye into the CB of the photocatalyst.[8,32] Chatterjee et al. used oxidation and reduction light sensitive agents on the surface of dye-modified TiO_2 semiconductor to degrade various halocarbons and other pollutants under visible light. The conversion of degradation of pollutants could reach 55–72%, and these reaction mechanisms are expounded in the following reactions.[33]

The photochemical reductions of the photosensitizer are shown as Reactions 11.36 through 11.41.

$$TiO_2 - (D^1)_s \xrightarrow{hv} TiO_2 - (D^{1*})_s \tag{11.36}$$

$$TiO_2 - (D^{1*})_s + P \rightarrow TiO_2 - (D^{1-})_s + \bullet P^+ \tag{11.37}$$

$$TiO_2 - (D^{1-})_s \rightarrow TiO_2 - \left(D^1 + e^-_{cb}\right)_s \tag{11.38}$$

$$TiO_2 - \left(D^1 + e^-_{cb}\right)_s + O_{2\,abs} \rightarrow TiO_2 - (D^1)_s + \bullet O^-_{2\,ads} \tag{11.39}$$

$$\bullet O^-_{2\,ads} + H^+ \rightarrow \bullet O_2H \tag{11.40}$$

$$O_2/HO_2 + P/P^+ \rightarrow \bullet OH + VOCs + O_2 \rightarrow \text{Products } (H_2O, CO_2, \text{etc.}) \tag{11.41}$$

where D_1 is thionine, nile blue A, or methylene blue; P is halocarbons; TiO_2-$(D)_s$ is a species of the photocatalysts containing dyes; and TiO_2-$(D^*)_s$ is an excited state after irradiation.

The photochemical oxidations of the photosensitizer are shown as Reactions 11.42 through 11.47.

$$TiO_2 - (D^2)_s \longrightarrow TiO_2 - (D^{2*})_s \tag{11.42}$$

$$TiO_2 - (D^{2*})_s \rightarrow TiO_2 - \left(D^{2+} + e^-_{cb}\right)_s \tag{11.43}$$

$$\mathrm{TiO_2} - \left(\mathrm{D^2} + \mathrm{e_{cb}^-}\right)_s + \mathrm{P} \rightarrow \mathrm{TiO_2} - \left(\mathrm{D^2} + \mathrm{e_{cb}^-}\right)_s + \bullet\mathrm{P^+} \quad (11.44)$$

$$\mathrm{TiO_2} - \left(\mathrm{D^2} + \mathrm{e_{cb}^-}\right)_s + \mathrm{O_{2\,ads}} \rightarrow \mathrm{TiO_2} - (\mathrm{D^2})_s + \bullet\mathrm{O_{2\,ads}^-} \quad (11.45)$$

$$\bullet\mathrm{O_{2\,ads}^-} + \mathrm{H^+} \rightarrow \bullet\mathrm{O_2H} \quad (11.46)$$

$$\mathrm{O_2/HO_2} + \mathrm{P/P^+} \rightarrow \bullet\mathrm{OH} + \mathrm{VOCs} + \mathrm{O_2} \rightarrow \text{Products } (\mathrm{H_2O}, \mathrm{CO_2}, \text{etc.}) \quad (11.47)$$

where D_2 is eosin Y, rhodamine B, or safranine O.

11.3 Characteristics of photocatalysts

The conjunction of characterization and photocatalysis activity is a complex and intimate relationship. The characterization of photocatalysts is generally analyzed by thermogravimetric/differential-thermal analysis (TG/DTA), X-ray diffraction (XRD), UV-Vis spectroscopy, BET surface analysis, Fourier transform infrared spectroscopy (FTIR), and X-ray photoelectron spectroscopy (XPS).

11.3.1 Thermogravimetric/differential thermal analysis (TG/DTA)

In order to estimate optimum calcinations temperatures of photocatalysts, the crystalline behavior can be analyzed by TG/DTA to determine the phase transformation in the temperature range from room temperature to 850°C with a heating rate of 10°C min^{-1}.

11.3.2 X-ray powder diffraction spectroscopy (XRD)

The crystal phase composition and the crystallite size of the TiO_2 nanoparticles can be carried out by a Rigaku X-ray diffraction using CuKα (λ = 1.54056 Å) radiation in the range of 10–80° (2θ) with a scan rate of 1° min^{-1}. The crystallite size is determined by Scherrer's formula, according to[34]

$$D_{\text{Scherrer}} = \frac{k\lambda}{\beta\cos\theta} \quad (11.48)$$

where λ is the X-ray wavelength (nm), k is a shape factor for spherical particles (0.9), θ is the Bragg angle, and β is the full width at half maximum (FWHM). The content of the crystal phase is determined from XRD peak intensities by the Spurr and Myers method, shown as[35]

$$W_R = \frac{1}{[1 + 0.8(I_R/I_A)]} \quad (11.49)$$

$$W_A = 1 - W_R \quad (11.50)$$

where W_A and W_R are the mole fractions of anatase and rutile, respectively. I_A and I_R are assigned to the integrated intensity of anatase (1 0 1) and rutile (1 1 0), respectively, obtained from XRD patterns. Based on Bragg's law (2dsinθ = λ) and a formula for a tetragonal system, the lattice parameters are calculated using

$$\frac{1}{d^2} = \frac{(h^2 + k^2)}{a^2} + \frac{l^2}{c^2} \tag{11.51}$$

where h, k, and l are the Miller indices of a crystal plane (hkl), respectively.

11.3.3 *BET surface analysis*

The specific surface area and pore size distribution of the photocatalysts can be determined on the basis of BET Equation 11.52 through nitrogen adsorption at 77K, and samples dried in an oven at 100°C for 10 h to eliminate moisture on the surface.

$$\frac{P}{V(P_0 - P)} = \frac{1}{CV_m} + \frac{C-1}{CV_m} \times \left(\frac{P}{P_0}\right) \tag{11.52}$$

where P is the equilibrium of adsorbates at the temperature of adsorption, P_0 is the saturation pressure of adsorbates at the temperature of adsorption, V is the adsorbed gas quantity (e.g., in volume units), V_m is the monolayer adsorbed gas quantity, and C is the BET constant.

11.3.4 *Scanning electron microscopy (SEM)*

The surface morphology and surface distribution of elements of synthesized photocatalysts can be observed by the SEM technique. In order to avoid the charge buildup during SEM observations, the samples should be mounted on the copper holder and stubs using double-sided conductive tapes.[36]

11.3.5 *Fourier transform infrared spectroscopy (FTIR)*

Fourier transform infrared spectroscopy is commonly used to identify the gas phase composition in the photo-oxidation process and the major bond formation in the photocatalyst. A blank experiment needs to be performed first with a thin disk of pure potassium bromide (KBr) for the solid-state analysis. The sample powder, ground with KBr (1:100 by weight ratio) and followed by pelletization, is pressed formed in a steel die. The sample is placed on an aluminum-made holder to be measured by the transmission and reflectance spectra. The spectrum is commonly set from a range of 400 to 4000 cm^{-1} with fully computerized data storage and data handing capability. The instrument resolution is usually 4 cm^{-1} and 100 scans are accumulated for each sample. For the gas phase analysis, the measurements are performed at path length gas cells. Prior to analysis, pure dry nitrogen gas is passed through the gas storage chamber to achieve a minimum level of collimation of the beams. The target gas is introduced into the gas cell and the IR absorption spectrum is used to configure a system for the continuous monitoring of fluctuations in gas qualification and quantitation during reactions.

11.3.6 UV-visible spectrometry

The optical absorptions of photocatalysts can be obtained by a UV-Vis spectrophotometer equipped with an integrating sphere. The $BaSO_4$ disc is used as a reference. The spectra are commonly collected at room temperature and standard atmospheric air pressure within wavelengths of 250–800 nm. The band gap of various photocatalysts is determined by[37]

$$E_g = \frac{hc}{\lambda} \tag{11.53}$$

where E_g is the band gap energy (eV), h is Plank's constant, c is the speed of light (m/s), and λ is the wavelength of absorption edges.

11.3.7 X-ray photoelectron spectroscopy (XPS)

X-ray photoelectron spectroscopy can be used for analyzing the binding energy of the samples. The experimental sample is tapped on a sample supporting plate. X-ray photoelectron spectroscopy is commonly measured using Al Kα X-rays with energy of 1486 eV. The binding energies are calibrated with reference to C 1s at 285 eV.

11.4 Effect of operating parameters

The experimental parameters of the main influence factors in photocatalytic activity of VOC conversion include relative humidity, doping type, doping ratio, VOC concentration, residence time, O_2 concentration, and light source. The influences of operating parameters are described as follows.

11.4.1 Relative humidity

Water molecules play a critical role in photocatalytic degradation of gaseous organic compounds. Water vapor is the primary source of hydroxyl radicals, which is the main oxidant in the photocatalysis system.[25] The conversion of VOCs decreases gradually with an increase of humidity content during the photodegradation process. The phenomenon is attributed to the competitive adsorption between water vapor and VOCs on the active sites of the photocatalysts, which would decrease the reaction rates.[18] As a result, water molecules do not dissociate or dissociate to hydroxyl radicals in the reaction. Excessive moisture would block the active sites of the photocatalyst surface and destroy the equilibrium of water vapor between consumption and adsorption. Korologos et al. studied typical indoor air pollution (benzene, toluene, ethylbenzene, and m-xylene) under various concentrations of water vapor. The results indicate the degradation efficiency hinges on the characteristics and structures of the compounds.[19]

The photodegradation of 1,2-dichloroethane (1,2-DCE) with various relative humidity levels is shown in Figure 11.4. Except for the case of 10% RH, the decomposition of 1,2-DCE decreases with increasing relative humidity. This is due to the competitive adsorption between water molecules and 1,2-DCE on the photocatalyst surface. Excessive moisture would occupy the active sites on the surface of photcatalysts, which impedes the degradation of pollutants.

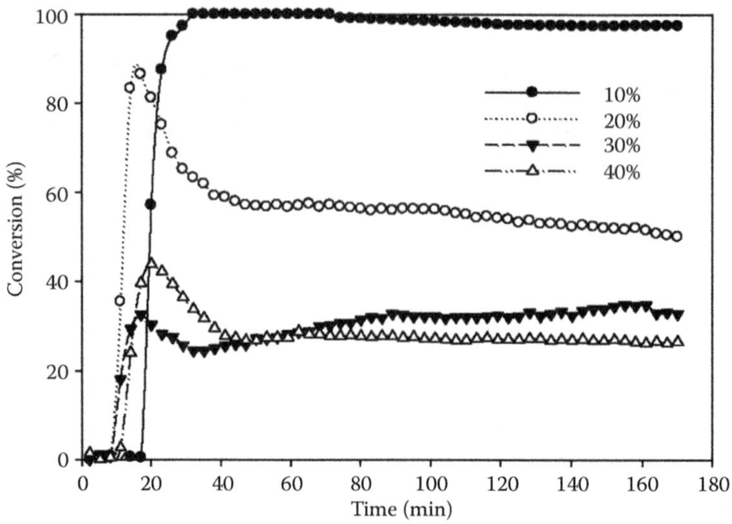

Figure 11.4 Effect of relative humidity on the removal efficiency of 1,2-dichloroethane for TiO_2 (operating conditions: O_2 = 20.8%, 1,2-DCE = 55–60 ppm, residence time = 5 min, UV light source).

11.4.2 Doping type

Previous research indicated that the photo-catalytic activity is limited by the fast charge-carrier recombination lifetime and low interfacial charge-transfer rates of photogenerated electron–hole pairs.[37,38] Recently, studies exhibited that metal-doped TiO_2 is beneficial to reduce the recombination of photogenerated electron–hole pairs and enhance the transfer and transport of charge carriers.[16] The noble metals such as Pt, Au, Pd, and Ru deposited or doped on TiO_2 have been demonstrated to be beneficial for photocatalytic reactions.[11,30] Some investigators have reported that doping with metal ions such as Fe^{3+}, Zn^{2+}, V^{4+}, and Co^{3+} promotes the photocatalytic activity.

Figure 11.5 shows the performance of various photocatalysts on degradation of 1,2-DCE. The degradation results illustrate that the initial efficiencies of all photocatalysts are similar except for TiO_2. After irradiating with UV light for 40 minutes, the degradation efficiencies of all photocatalysts tend to stabilize. However, the photocatalytic activity of $Sr_{0.001}/TiO_2$ is the highest (η = 86%), followed by $V_{0.001}/TiO_2$ (η = 73%) > $Cr_{0.001}/TiO_2$ (η = 62%) > TiO_2 (η = 40%) > $Pd_{0.001}/TiO_2$ (η = 20%) at the end of the experiments. The photocatalytic activity of transition metal is better than those of TiO_2. The photoactivities of various photocatalysts are correlated with factors including crystallite size, lattice parameter, physical characteristics, and chemical structure.[11]

11.4.3 Doping ratio

The activity of a photocatalyst relies on doping species and the amount of doping. Figure 11.6 shows the performance of various doping ratios on degradation of 1,2-DCE. The enhancement of the 1,2-DCE decomposition rate is attributed to Sr atoms doping into the lattice of TiO_2. Among all the photocatalysts, $Sr_{0.0001}/TiO_2$ exhibits the best photocatalytic activity. A lower or highter Sr^{3+} doping ratio reduces the decomposition rate of 1,2-DCE. The lower photocatalytic activities of photocatalysts with high strontium content can be

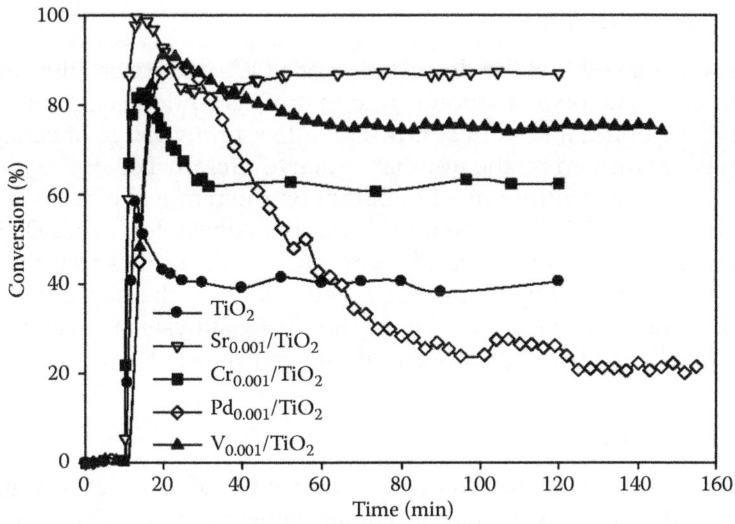

Figure 11.5 The performance of various doped photocatalysts on the removal efficiency of 1,2-dichloroethane (operating conditions: $[O_2]$ = 20.8%, 1,2-DCE = 53–55 ppm, [RH] = 0%, residence time = 1 min, UV light source).

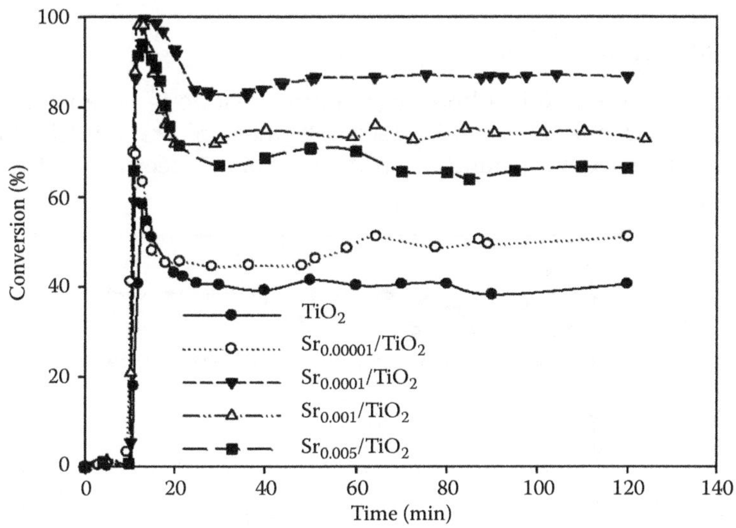

Figure 11.6 Effect of doping ratio on the removal efficiency of 1,2-dichloroethane by Sr/TiO_2 (operating conditions: O_2 = 20.8%, 1,2-DCE = 53–55 ppm, [RH] = 0%, residence time = 1 min, UV light source).

explained by the occupation of the surface active sites by excess strontium. Sr doped into the TiO_2 lattice contributes to the formation of a band gap. The impurity state may increase degradation rate because the impurity states are closer to the valence band. On the other side, the impurity states can also act as recombination centers of photogenerated charge carriers, and thus decrease the photocatalytic oxidation rate.[39]

11.4.4 VOC concentration

Previous studies displayed that the degradation of VOCs decreases with the inlet concentration increasing.[40,41] The phenomenon is due to the adsorption competition between the by-products and the pollutant.[40,42] In contrast, at a low ppmv range of concentrations, the photooxidation is not limited by the number of active sites on TiO_2.[42]

The effect of inlet concentrations of pollutant on the removal efficiency by the $Sr_{0.0001}/TiO_2$ is shown in Figure 11.7. It can be found that the conversion of 1,2-DCE decreases as its concentration increases from 54 to 95 ppm. The result implies that the active sites of the photocatalyst are covered by by-products, especially for the high concentration cases. Other studies also indicate that active sites of the photocatalysts are occupied by pollutant compounds especially for the high concentration conditions.[41,42]

11.4.5 Residence time

Previous studies have shown that the photo-induced oxidation rates of gaseous pollutants are determined by the adsorption step in low concentrations. The decomposition efficiency of pollutant increases with the increasing residence time. Figure 11.8 shows the removal efficiency of 1,2-DCE at various residence times. The photocatalytic activity of $Sr_{0.0001}/TiO_2$ tested at RT = 60 s is the highest (conversion, η = 86%), followed by that tested at 30 s (η = 65%) > $Sr_{0.1}/TiO_2$ at 15 s (η = 35%) at the end of the experiments. The results show that the adsorption capacity is crucial at the short residence time.

11.4.6 O_2 concentration

Oxygen is typically available in photodegradation reactions because it is an effective conduction-band electron acceptor.[43] Oxygen molecules are first adsorbed on the surface of the photocatalyst, and then instantly trap the interfacial electrons of the photocatalyst.

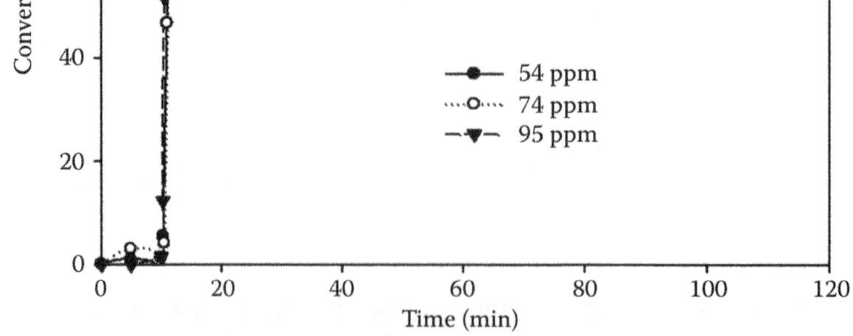

Figure 11.7 Effect of pollutant concentration on the removal efficiency of 1,2-dichloroethane by $Sr_{0.0001}/TiO_2$ (operating conditions: O_2 = 20.8%, [RH] = 0%, 1,2-DCE = 53–55 ppm, residence time = 1 min, UV light source).

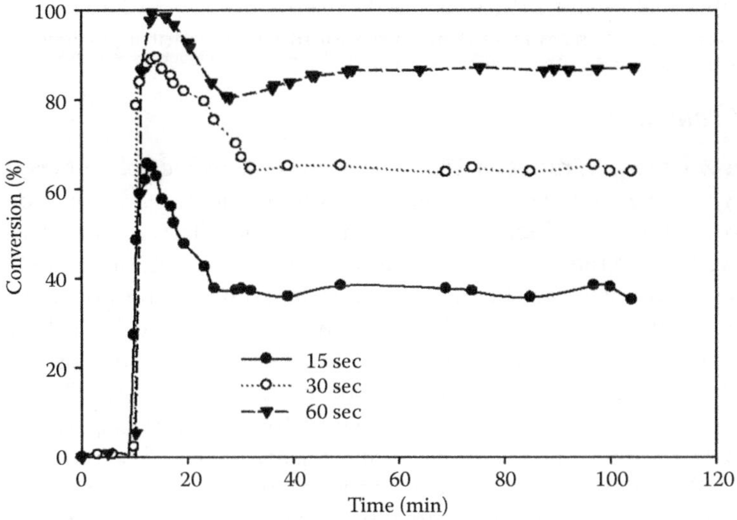

Figure 11.8 Effect of various residence time on the removal efficiency of 1,2-dichloroethane by $Sr_{0.0001}/TiO_2$ (operating conditions: O_2 = 20.8%, [RH] = 0%, 1,2-DCE = 53–55 ppm, residence time = 15–60 s, UV light source).

The presence of residual oxygen can suppress the hole–electron recombination.[44] Figure 11.9 shows the decomposition conversion of 1,2-DCE by $Sr_{0.0001}/TiO_2$ under various oxygen concentrations. The photocatalyst has almost no photocatalytic activity for the decomposition of the organic matter in the absence of oxygen. The photodegradation rate increases with increasing oxygen concentration. The conversions of 1,2-DCE show no significant differences between 1% and 20.8% O_2. These may be due to the saturation of oxygen on the

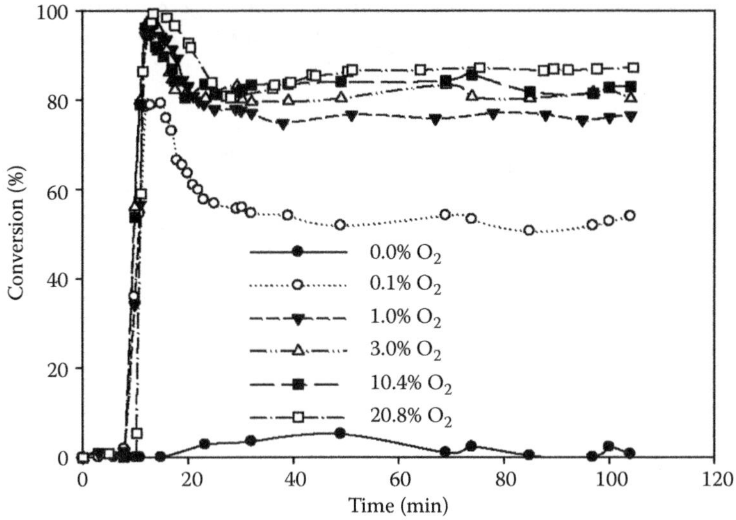

Figure 11.9 Effect of oxygen concentration on the removal efficiency of 1,2-dichloroethane by $Sr_{0.0001}/TiO_2$ (operating conditions: [RH] = 0%, 1,2-DCE = 53–55 ppm, residence time = 1 min, UV light source).

surface of the photocatalyst for the cases with more than 1% O_2. The photodecomposition results imply that oxygen is an essential component in the photocatalytic reaction.

11.4.7 *Light source*

The absorption wavelength range of TiO_2 is less than 5% in the solar energy region, which limits its energy utilization potential and photoreaction rate. Metal/nonmetal species doped TiO_2 is considered an efficient way to improve photoactivity under visible light. The phenomena have been explained by the excitation of electrons of doped metals/nonmetals to the conduction band of TiO_2. The fluorescent lamp is the main light source in buildings; therefore, a fluorescent lamp (370 to 630 nm wavelength ranges) can be a good photon source. The photocatalytic activity of two photocatalysts using various light sources was evaluated by the degradation of 1,2-DCE, as shown in Figure 11.10. The results show the photocatalytic activity of TiO_2 is lower compared to that of $Sr_{0.0001}/TiO_2$. Sr-doped TiO_2 can enhance degradation of 1,2-DCE due to its impurity state. The narrowed band gap is formed between the valence band and conduction band. The role of Sr^{3+} as h^+/e^- traps promotes photocatalytic activity and alleviates the recombination of electron–hole pairs. Both photocatalysts have similar activity under blue light and fluorescent light. The spectra of two different lamps are shown in Figure 11.11.

11.5 *Chemical reaction kinetics*

The photocatalytic oxidation is a series of surface reaction processes. First, VOCs are transferred to the surface by diffusion, and then chemical reactions occur on the photocatalyst surface. Therefore, the mass transfer rate, the kinetic reaction rate, and the photocatalyst properties are the most pertinent performance factors for a photo-oxidation continuous flow reactor.

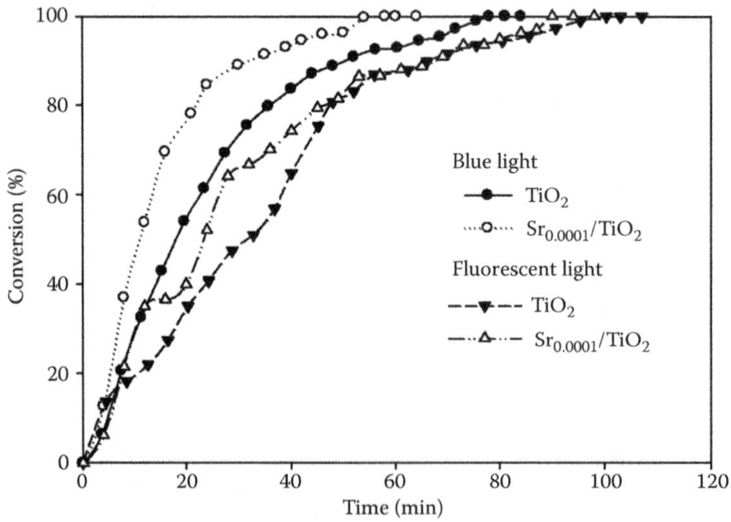

Figure 11.10 Effect of light source on the removal efficiency of 1,2-dichloroethane by various photocatalysts (operating conditions: O_2 = 20.8%, [RH] = 0%, 1,2-DCE = 55–60 ppm, batch reactor).

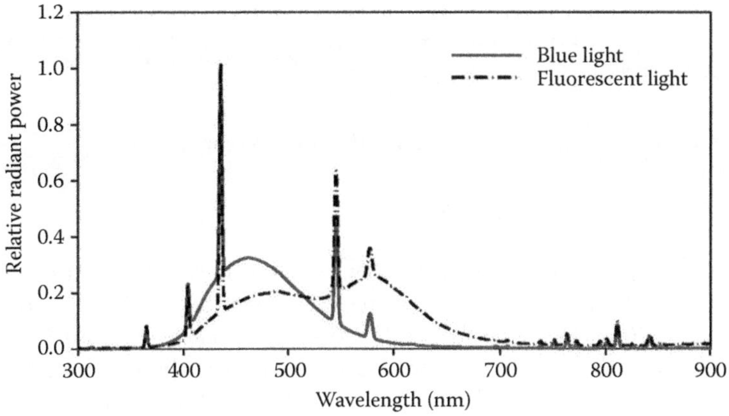

Figure 11.11 Spectra of blue and fluorescent light.

11.5.1 Reactor

Many photooxidation reactors have been reported in the literature, including annular,[3,45] plate,[46,47] pilot unit,[47] packed-bed,[48] fluidized-bed,[49,50] honeycomb,[51,52] and optical fiber.[53] These reactors were assigned according to the configuration of the lamps with respect to the reaction area.[10] The different configurations cause different properties of the reaction surface area, mass transfer rate, quantity of absorbed photons, and photocatalytic degradation rate.[54]

The reactor apparatus typically includes the reaction structure and the light source. The reaction structure supports not only the photocatalyst but also the airflow channels.[10] Packed-bed reactors are normally used to photocatalyze oxidation reactions, but the photodegradation is restricted by the ability of light to penetrate opaque. Besides, a high pressure drop will result in poor system performance.[19] When installing a honeycomb support in a photocatalytic reactor, it is not easy to direct the light to irradiate the surface of the photocatalyst.[19] However, the plate, honeycomb, and annular reactors are three representative types among these reactors.

11.5.2 Photocatalytic oxidation

The conversion χ (%) of VOCs is calculated as

$$\chi = \frac{(C_{in} - C_{out})}{C_{in}} \times 100\% \tag{11.54}$$

where C_{in} is the inlet concentration and C_{out} is the outlet concentration at steady state.[21] The assumptions of an ideal plug flow reactor (PFR) normally satisfy the following properties[32,55]:

1. Mass transfer can be neglected by diffusion or mixing.
2. There are no inter-substrate interactions.

Figure 11.12 shows a plug flow reactor. In the PFR, the composition of fluid varies with reactor location. A differential volume dV can be used to develop a mass balance equation. For reactant A, mass balance can be developed as

$$in - out = accumulation + removal \tag{11.55}$$

$$\mathrm{A_{in}} = \mathrm{A_{out}} + \mathrm{A_{removed}} + \mathrm{A_{acc}}, \tag{11.56}$$

where A_{in} is the amount of A input to the system, A_{out} is the amount of A outflow from the system, $A_{removed}$ is the amount of A removed by reaction, and A_{acc} is the amount of A accumulated in the system. We assume the reaction is in steady state with no accumulation in the reactor. The oxidation rate for a continuous reactor is the product of the conversion observed with the molecular feed in the inlet of the reactor, as shown in the following equations:

$$F_A = (F_A + dF_A) + (-r_A) \times dV \tag{11.57}$$

$$dF_A = r_A \times dV \tag{11.58}$$

$$dF_A = d[F_{A0}(1 - X_A)] = -F_{A0} \times dX_A = r_A \times dV \tag{11.59}$$

$$\frac{dV}{F_{A0}} = \frac{dX_A}{-r_A} \tag{11.60}$$

Equation 11.60 is the reaction rate formula of reactant A in dV. In order to obtain the equation of a full reactor, we have to integrate Equation 11.60 into Equation 11.61. Equation 11.61 is suited for isothermal state.

$$\frac{V}{F_{A0}} = \int_{X_{A_{in}}}^{X_{A_{out}}} \frac{dX_A}{-r_A} \tag{11.61}$$

where F_A is molar flow rate of A (mol s^{-1}), $-r_A$ is reaction rate of A in reactor (mol s^{-1} cm^{-3}), V is reactor volume (cm^3), F_{A0} is molar flow rate of A in reactor inlet (mol s^{-1}), and X_A is conversion (%).

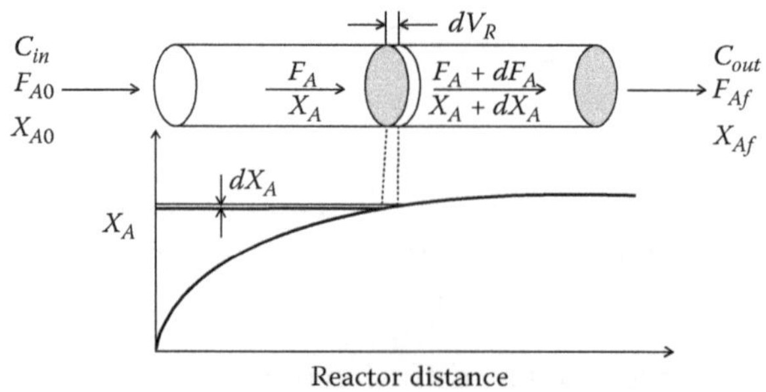

Figure 11.12 Plug flow reactor.

The differential reactor assumes that the concentration change is small enough so that the plug flow equation can be approximated. A large flow rate corresponding to a short residence time reduces the conversion rate in the plug flow reactor. Reactors operated in this circumstance are named differential reactors. Differential flow reactors are typically applied to determine the kinetics of catalytic reactions. In the differential reactor, the reactor inlet concentration is almost equal to the outlet concentration, $C_i \fallingdotseq C_f$, and we may use 0.5 $(C_i + C_f)$ to represent the concentration of the reactor. Thus, the reaction rate equation can be presented by

$$\frac{V}{F_{A0}} = \int_0^{X_A} \frac{dX_A}{-r_A} = \frac{1}{-r_A}\int_0^{X_A} dX_A = \frac{X_A}{-r_A} \tag{11.62}$$

$$-r_A = \frac{F_{A0}}{V} X_A = \frac{F_{A0}}{V}\left(\frac{C_{in} - C_{out}}{C_{in}}\right) \tag{11.63}$$

When $X_A < 25\%$, the conversion is measured for nearly the same test conditions, and it performs with an experimental error less than 5% by Equation 11.63. The flow rates and concentrations at the inlet and outlet pipes of the reactor can be measured and easily calculated. The rate is assumed to correspond to the average of the inlet and outlet concentrations.[56] The main advantage of this differential method of operation is the ease of extracting reaction rate data.[57] Another advantage is that a relatively small quantity of heat is released due to the low conversion. Thus, this method is conducive to maintain isothermal operation. Two drawbacks to the method are[56]

1. The accuracy and precision of parameter measurement is necessary to keep the measurement errors within acceptable limits.
2. It requires a large number of parameters to obtain sufficient data to illustrate the effect of the reaction.

When the conversion is higher, reaction rate is not a constant anymore. In this situation, conversions continue to occur at different positions along the reactor, and the reaction rate is calculated by an integration equation (11.61). We also can use the reaction time to calculate the reaction rate, as shown in the following equations.

$$\tau = \frac{V}{v_0} \tag{11.64}$$

$$\frac{V}{F_{A0}} = \int_0^{X_{Af}} \frac{dX_A}{-r_A} = \frac{\tau}{C_{in}} \tag{11.65}$$

$$\tau = C_{in}\int_0^{X_{Af}} \frac{dX_A}{-r_A} \tag{11.66}$$

$$X_A = 1 - \frac{C_A}{C_{in}} \tag{11.67}$$

$$dX_A = -\frac{dC_A}{C_{in}} \tag{11.68}$$

$$\tau = C_{in} \int_0^{X_{Af}} \frac{dX_A}{-r_A} = -\int_{C_{in}}^{C_{out}} \frac{dC_A}{-r_A} \tag{11.69}$$

where τ is the reaction time (s) and ν_0 is the gas flow rate ($cm^3\ s^{-1}$).

11.5.3 Kinetic model

The Langmuir–Hinshelwood (L–H) rate expression has been widely used to describe the gas-phase and liquid-phase photocatalytic reactions.[4,18,33,58] Some assumptions are suggested as follows:

1. The number of surface adsorption active sites is a constant.
2. An adsorption site combines with a substrate only.
3. This model predicts a nearly constant heat of adsorption and does not seem to be influenced by surface coverage.
4. There is no interaction between each adsorbed substrate.
5. The rate-limiting step is the surface adsorption.
6. The adsorption of reactant and product on active sites is a reversible reaction.

According to the adsorption and reaction behaviors, reactants and water are competitively adsorbed on the same adsorption sites, or adsorbed on different types of surface sites with or without competitiveness. There are seven forms of L–H bimolecular models, as shown in Table 11.2.[10,21,59–61]

11.5.4 Arrhenius equation

Temperature generally influences the rate of a chemical reaction. The reaction temperature affects not only the rate constant of decomposition, but also the adsorption of contaminants. The temperature dependence of the rate constant can be calculated by the Arrhenius equation, which can be expressed as the following equation:

$$k = A\exp\left(-\frac{Ea}{RT}\right) \tag{11.70}$$

where A is the frequency factor (s^{-1}), Ea is the activation energy ($kJ\ mol^{-1}$), T is the temperature (in Kelvin), and R is the gas constant ($8.31 \times 10^{-3}\ kcal\ mol^{-1}\ K^{-1}$).

Table 11.2 The rate expressions of Langmuir–Hinshelwood model applied for the experiments with water present

Model	Kinetics rate expression	Assumption
1	$-r = k \times \frac{K_A C_A}{1 + K_A C_A}$	Reaction of VOCs adsorbed on catalyst surface but water does not take part in the reaction
2	$-r = k \times \frac{K_A C_A K_W C_W}{1 + K_A C_A}$	Reaction of VOCs adsorbed on catalyst surface and react with water
3	$-r = k \times \frac{K_A C_A}{1 + K_A C_A + K_W C_W}$	VOCs and water adsorbed on catalyst surface but water does not take part in the reaction
4	$-r = k \times \frac{K_A C_A K_W C_W}{(1 + K_A C_A + K_W C_W)^2}$	Reaction of VOCs and water adsorbed on catalyst surface
5	$-r = k \times \frac{K_A C_A}{1 + K_A C_A} \times \frac{K_W C_W}{1 + K_W C_W}$	Reaction of VOCs and water adsorbed on different active sites
6	$-r = k \times \frac{K_W C_W K_A C_A}{1 + K_W C_W}$	Reaction of water adsorbed on catalyst surface and gas-phase VOCs
7	$-r = k \times \frac{(K_A C_A K_W C_W)^{1/2}}{[1 + (K_A C_A)^{1/2} + (K_W C_W)^{1/2}]^2}$	Reaction of VOCs and water dissociatively adsorbed on catalyst surface

Note: r is the reaction rate (mol cm^{-3} s^{-1}), C_A is the pollution concentration (mol cm^{-3}), C_w is the water concentration (mol cm^{-3}), k is the reaction rate constant (mol cm^{-3} s^{-1}), K_A is the adsorption equilibrium constant of pollutant (cm3 mol–1), and, K_W is the adsorption equilibrium constant of water vapor (cm^3 mol^{-1}).

11.6 Summary

Indoor air pollution has received increasing attention in recent years since people spend almost 80% of their time indoors. VOCs, which are usually emitted from construction materials, household products, and office furnishings, are the main indoor air pollutants. Photocatalytic oxidation (PCO) is regarded as a promising method for air purification due to its fast oxidation rate, high decomposition rate, relatively convenient operation at room temperature, good stability, and nontoxicity. TiO_2 requires high-energy irradiation at wavelengths shorter than 385 nm for photocatalytic reaction via the absorbance of photons. However, the traditional photocatalysts may have limitations on the exclusive use of UV light sources, and the intermediates which are produced from photocatalytic reactions are more poisonous and carcinogenic.

Recent studies have reported that progress has been made in developing visible-light-activated photocatalysts toward practical applications. However, doping TiO_2 may increase the visible light response of the photocatalyst. The intermediate compounds are vital due to the fact that some of the intermediates can be more toxic than the original compound. Besides, the intermediates, which have potential threats of leakage, can trigger deactivation of the photocatalysts by occupying the active sites on the photocatalysts' surface. The phenomenon is attributed to the instability of these photocatalysts and the operating environment. Previous studies indicate operational parameters affect the conversion and degradation pathway. The operational parameters include light intensity, nature of photocatalyst, humidity, pollutant concentration, temperature, and oxygen concentration. Therefore, the products and byproducts were adopted for further analysis to optimize the operational parameters. Final products and by–products must comply with environmental laws and regulations, for protecting the public health and decreasing risk.

References

1. Pelaez M, Nolan NT, Pillai SC et al. A review on the visible light active titanium dioxide photocatalysts for environmental applications. *Appl Catal B Environ* 2012; 125: 331–49.
2. Liu Y, Wang HQ, and Wu ZB. Characterization of metal doped-titanium dioxide and behaviors on photocatalytic oxidation of nitrogen oxides. *J Environ Sci* 2007; 19: 1505–9.
3. Hagen J. *Industrial Catalysis: A Practical Approach.* 2nd ed. Weinheim: Wiley-VCH, 2006.
4. Wang L, Shang J, Hao W et al. A dye-sensitized visible light photocatalyst-$Bi_{24}O_{31}Cl_{10}$. *Sci Rep 4* 2014; 7384: 1–8.
5. Kisch H. *Semiconductor Photocatalysis: Principles and Applications.* New York: John Wiley & Sons, 2014.
6. Yurish S. *Modern Sensors, Transducers and Sensor Networks.* Intel. Frequency Sensor Association (IFSA) Publishing, Barcelona, Spain, 2012.
7. Zhong L, Haghighat F, Blondeau P, and Kozinski J. Modeling and physical interpretation of photocatalytic oxidation efficiency in indoor air applications. *Build Environ* 2010; 45: 689–97.
8. Wang S, Ang HM, and Tade MO. Volatile organic compounds in indoor environment and photocatalytic oxidation: State of the art. *Environ Int* 2007; 33: 694–705.
9. Klauson D, Portjanskaya E, Budarnaja O, Krichevskaya M, and Preis S. The synthesis of sulphur and boron-containing titania photocatalysts and the evaluation of their photocatalytic activity. *Catal Commun* 2010; 11: 715–20.
10. Mo J, Zhang Y, Xu Q, Lamson JJ, and Zhao R. Photocatalytic purification of volatile organic compounds in indoor air: A literature review. *Atmos Environ* 2009; 43: 2229–46.
11. Lin YH, Tseng TK, and Chu H. Photo-catalytic degradation of dimethyl disulfide on S and metal-ions co-doped TiO_2 under visible-light irradiation. *Applied Catalysis A: General* 2014; 469: 221–8.
12. Twigg MV and Twigg M. *Catalyst Handbook.* 2nd ed. London: Wolfe Publishing, 1989.
13. Zhong M and Yu J. Preparation and enhanced daylight-induced photocatalytic activity of C,N,S-tridoped titanium dioxide powders. *J Hazar Mater* 2008; 152: 1229–36.
14. Goyer N and Lavoie J. Emissions of chemical compounds and bioaerosols during the secondary treatment of paper mill effluents. *Am Ind Hygi Assoc* 2001; 62: 330–41.
15. Brinker CJ and Scherer GW. *Sol-Gel Science: The Physics and Chemistry of Sol-Gel Processing.* San Diego, CA: Academic Press, 2013.
16. Hung WC, Fu SH, Tseng JJ, Chu H, and Ko TH. Study on photocatalytic degradation of gaseous dichloromethane using pure and iron ion-doped TiO_2 prepared by the sol–gel method. *Chemosphere* 2007; 66: 2142–51.
17. Niu Y, Xing M, Zhang J, and Tian B. Visible light activated sulfur and iron co-doped TiO_2 photocatalyst for the photocatalytic degradation of phenol. *Catal Today* 2013; 201: 159–66.
18. Lin YH, Chou SH, and Chu H. A kinetic study for the degradation of 1,2-dichloroethane by S-doped TiO_2 under visible light. *J Nanopart Res* 2014; 16: 1–12.
19. Korologos CA, Nikolaki MD, Zerva CN, Philippopoulos CJ, and Poulopoulos SG. Photocatalytic oxidation of benzene, toluene, ethylbenzene and m-xylene in the gas-phase over TiO_2-based catalysts. *J Photochem Photobiol A: Chem* 2012; 244: 24–31.
20. Nasir M, Xi Z, Xing M et al. 2013. Study of synergistic effect of Ce- and S-codoping on the enhancement of visible-light photocatalytic activity of TiO_2. *J Phys Chem C* 2013; 117: 9520–8.
21. He C, Yu Y, Zhou C-H, and Hu X-F. Structure and photocatalytic activities of Ag/TiO_2 thin films. *J Inorg Mater* 2002; 5: 019.
22. Liu SX, Qu ZP, Han XW, and Sun CL. A mechanism for enhanced photocatalytic activity of silver-loaded titanium dioxide. *Catal Today* 2004; 93–5: 877–84.

23. Umebayashi T, Yamaki T, Itoh H, and Asai K. Analysis of electronic structures of 3d transition metal-doped TiO_2 based on band calculations. *J Phys Chem Solids* 2002; 63: 1909–20.
24. Zhang Y, Shen Y, Gu F, Wu M, Xie Y, and Zhang J. Influence of Fe ions in characteristics and optical properties of mesoporous titanium oxide thin films. *Appl Surf Sci* 2009; 256: 5–89.
25. Lin YH, Chiu TC, Hsueh HT, and Chu H. N-doped TiO_2 photo-catalyst for the degradation of 1,2-dichloroethane under fluorescent light. *Appl Surf Sci* 2011; 258: 1581–6.
26. Zhang G, Zhang YC, Nadagouda M et al. Visible light-sensitized S, N and C co-doped polymorphic TiO_2 for photocatalytic destruction of microcystin-LR. *Appl Catal B: Environ* 2014; 144: 14–621.
27. Gu DE, Yang BC, and Hu YD. V and N co-doped nanocrystal anatase TiO_2 photocatalysts with enhanced photocatalytic activity under visible light irradiation. *Catal Commun* 2008; 9: 1472–6.
28. Chen Q, Jiang D, Shi W, Wu D, and Xu Y. Visible-light-activated Ce–Si co-doped TiO_2 photocatalyst. *Appl Surf Sci* 2009; 255: 7918–24.
29. Sasikala R, Shirole AR, Sudarsan V et al. Enhanced photocatalytic activity of indium and nitrogen co-doped TiO_2–Pd nanocomposites for hydrogen generation. *Appl Catal A: Gen* 2010; 377: 47–54.
30. Song H, Zhou G, Wang C, Jiang X, Wu C, and Li T. Synthesis and photocatalytic activity of nanocrystalline TiO_2 co-doped with nitrogen and cobalt (II). *Res Chem Intermed* 2013; 39: 747–58.
31. Liu SY, Tang QL, and Feng QG. Synthesis of S/Cr doped mesoporous TiO_2 with high-active visible light degradation property via solid state reaction route. *Appl Surf Sci* 2011; 257: 5544–51.
32. Pankaj C, Hassan G, and Ajay KR. Dye-sensitized photocatalyst: A breakthrough in green energy and environmental detoxification. Sustainable nanotechnology and the environment: Advances and achievements. Symposium Series, Washington, DC. American Chemical Society 2013; 1124: 231–66.
33. Chatterjee D, Dasgupta S, and Rao N. Visible light assisted photodegradation of halocarbons on the dye modified TiO_2 surface using visible light. *Sol Energy Mater Sol Cells* 2006; 90: 1013–20.
34. Ogawa H, Abe A, Nishikawa M, and Hayakawa, S. Preparation of tin oxide films from ultrafine particle. *J Electrochem Soc* 1981; 128: 685–9.
35. Bangkedphol S, Keenan HE, Davidson CM, Sakultantimetha A, Sirisaksoontorn W, and Songsasen A. Enhancement of tributyltin degradation under natural light by N-doped TiO_2 photocatalyst. *J Hazard Mater* 2010; 184: 533–7.
36. Hemmati Borji S, Nasseri S, Mahvi AH, Nabizadeh R, and Javadi AH. Investigation of photocatalytic degradation of phenol by Fe(III)-doped TiO_2 and TiO_2 nanoparticles. *Iran J Environ Health Sci Eng* 2014; 12: 101.
37. Yoneyama H, Haga S, and Yamanaka S. Photocatalytic activities of microcrystalline titania incorporated in sheet silicates of clay. *J Phys Chem* 1989; 93: 833–7.
38. Jacoby WA, Blake DM, Penned JA et al. Heterogeneous photocatalysis for control of volatile organic compounds in indoor air. *J Air Waste Manage Assoc* 1996; 46: 891–8.
39. Li D, Ohashi N, Hishita S, Kolodiazhnyi T, and Haneda H. Origin of visible-light-driven photocatalysis: A comparative study on N/F-doped and N-F-codoped TiO_2 powders by means of experimental characterizations and theoretical calculations. *J Solid State Chem* 2005; 178: 3293–302.
40. Ertl G, Knözinger H, and Weitkamp J. *Preparation of Solid Catalysts*. New York: Wiley-VCH, 2008.
41. Katz HS and Mileski J. *Handbook of Fillers for Plastics*. 1st ed. New York: Van Nostrand Reinhold, 1987.
42. Sleiman M, Conchon P, Ferronato C, and Chovelon JM. Photocatalytic oxidation of toluene at indoor air levels (ppbv): Towards a better assessment of conversion, reaction intermediates and mineralization. *Appl Catal B: Environ* 2009; 86: 159–65.
43. Zhang M, An T, Fu J et al. Photocatalytic degradation of mixed gaseous carbonyl compounds at low level on adsorptive TiO_2/SiO_2 photocatalyst using a fluidized bed reactor. *Chemosphere* 2006; 64: 23–31.
44. Hussein FH, Obies MH, and Drea A. Photocatalytic decolorization of bismarck brown R by suspension of titanium dioxide. *Int J Chem Sci* 2010; 8: 2736–46.

45. Wijngaarden RI, Westerterp KR, Kronberg A, and Bos A. Industrial Catalysis: Optimizing Catalysts and Processes. Weinheim: Wiley 2008.
46. Zhang Y, Yang R, and Zhao R. A model for analyzing the performance of photocatalytic air cleaner in removing volatile organic compounds. *Atmos Environ* 2003; 37: 395–9.
47. Assadi AA, Bouzaza A, Wolbert D, and Petit P. Isovaleraldehyde elimination by UV/TiO_2 photocatalysis: Comparative study of the process at different reactors configurations and scales. *Environ Sci Pollut Res* 2014; 21: 11178–88.
48. Pestana CJ, Robertson PKJ, Edwards C, Wilhelm W, McKenzie C, and Lawton LA. A continuous flow packed bed photocatalytic reactor for the destruction of 2-methylisoborneol and geosmin utilising pelletised TiO_2. *Chem Eng J* 2014; 235: 293–8.
49. Nam W, Kim J, and Han G. Photocatalytic oxidation of methyl orange in a three-phase fluidized bed reactor. *Chemosphere* 2002; 47: 1019–24.
50. Hajaghazadeh M, Vaiano V, Sannino D, Kakooei H, Sotudeh-Gharebagh R, and Ciambelli P. Heterogeneous photocatalytic oxidation of methyl ethyl ketone under UV-A light in an LED-fluidized bed reactor. *Catal Today* 2014; 230: 79–84.
51. Wu YT, Yu YH, Nguyen VH et al. Enhanced xylene removal by photocatalytic oxidation using fiber-illuminated honeycomb reactor at ppb level. *J Hazard Mater* 2013; 262: 17–25.
52. Taboada E, Angurell I, and Llorca J. Dynamic photocatalytic hydrogen production from ethanol–water mixtures in an optical fiber honeycomb reactor loaded with Au/TiO_2. *J Catal* 2014; 309: 460–7.
53. Tao Y, Wu CY, and Mazyck DW. Removal of methanol from pulp and paper mills using combined activated carbon adsorption and photocatalytic regeneration. *Chemosphere* 2006; 65: 35–42.
54. Dela Cruz N, Romero V, Dantas RF, Marco P, Bayarri B, Giménez J, and Esplugas S. o-Nitrobenzaldehyde actinometry in the presence of suspended TiO_2 for photocatalytic reactors. *Catal Today* 2013; 209: 209–14.
55. Shamim N and Sharma Virender K (Eds.). Sustainable Nanotechnology and the Environment: Advances and Achievements. ACS Symposium Series 2013, American Chemical Society.
56. Hayes RE and Kolaczkowski ST. Introduction to Catalytic Combustion. London: Gordon and Breach, 1998.
57. Hayes RE and Mmbaga J. *Introduction to Chemical Reactor Analysis.* Boca Raton, FL: CRC Press, 2012.
58. Pabst W and Gregorova E. Characterization of particles and particle systems. *Inst Chem Tech* 2007, Prague.
59. Fogler HS. Elements of Chemical Reaction Engineering. Englewood Cliffs, NJ: Prentice-Hall Inc., 1999.
60. Korologos CA, Philippopoulos CJ, and Poulopoulos SG. The effect of water presence on the photocatalytic oxidation of benzene, toluene, ethylbenzene and m-xylene in the gas-phase. *Atmos Environ* 2011; 45: 7089–95.
61. Tang F and Yang X. A "deactivation" kinetic model for predicting the performance of photocatalytic degradation of indoor toluene, o-xylene, and benzene. *Build Environ* 2012; 56: 329–34.

section three

Operation and monitoring

chapter twelve

Clean room technology—General guidelines

Matts Ramstorp

Contents

Abstract

Clean rooms are used to create an environment good enough for the thing and/or items handled within. Such a room is built and used in a way so it is easily cleaned and easy to keep clean during the desired time of usage. However, a clean room is not a room that is just built as a clean room; it also needs proper handling as well as monitoring to comply with the quality demands stated. This chapter deals with clean room operations as well as monitoring in order to reach the desired cleanliness for the processes taking place.

12.1 Introduction

In the first chapter of this book we discussed what a clean room is, what makes a clean room clean, and what differences there are in standards, norms, good manufacturing practices (GMP), etc.[1] In this chapter on general guidelines, we are following up on the previous chapter in order to look closer at how to operate a clean room and, not least, how to monitor it for compliance. As in the former chapter we are going to take a closer look at what the differences are in the GMPs used around the world, with special focus on clean rooms in the in vitro fertilization (IVF) area.

12.2 Clean room operations

Clean room operations can be summarized as all the different general activities that take place in a clean room and/or the airlocks leading to the room.[2,3] These activities include the way personnel move from an uncontrolled environment and further into a clean room. The same goes for all the material that is needed inside a clean room during work, as well as all the things that are brought out of the room after work has been finished. Another aspect included in operations relates to cleaning and disinfection, which must be mentioned at this early stage as one of the most contaminating operations normally performed in a clean room.

12.2.1 Entering a clean room—Not a walk in the park!

The general procedures when going to work in a clean room start long before you come to the first airlock. In some cases, there are demands on the personnel working in the clean rooms that they must abide by certain rules, even when at home. This might concern smoking, personal hygiene, the use of hair products, cosmetics, jewelry, etc.

Every operation must have detailed and written instructions and rules for how these situations must be handled. Personnel must not only read these, they must also understand the rules and most of all accept them!

In this part of the chapter we will deal with the following:

- Clean room garments
- Cleaning and disinfection of a clean room
- Personal responsibility before and when entering a clean room

12.2.2 Clean room garments

The garments used in clean rooms are highly specialized ones, which act like filters in order to create a barrier between the person wearing the garment and the outside surrounding environment.[4] The textile material used in producing such a garment often consists of stringently woven 100% polyester microfilament, resulting in a good air and water vapor permeability with good filtration efficiency for particles generated by the wearer. Different clean room classes or grades use different types of garments. As a general rule, one can state that the cleaner the clean room, the higher the degree of coverage of the personnel working in the clean room. In practice, this means that in a lower classification clean room, such as a Grade D clean room, according to the EU GMP, Appendix 1 of Volume 4, the garment normally comprises trousers and a T-shirt underneath a jacket or frock, together with special shoes or overshoes and hair cover.[5] The GMP does not state anything concerning the material in Grade D, but in practice blended cotton/polyester or 100% polyester is used.

When we come to clean rooms with a higher degree of cleanliness, for example, Grade B and Grade C, the EU GMP states that the material in practice should shed virtually no particles from the garment.

12.2.2.1 Clean room garment according to the EU GMP

The EU states recommendations of clean room garments as follows[5]:

Grade D: Hair and, where relevant, beard should be covered. A general protective suit and appropriate shoes or overshoes should be worn. Appropriate measures should be taken to avoid any contamination from outside the clean area.

Grade C: Hair and, where relevant, beard and moustache should be covered. A single or two-piece trouser suit, gathered at the wrists and with high neck and appropriate shoes or overshoes should be worn. They should shed virtually no fibers or particulate matter.

Grade A/B: Headgear should totally enclose hair and, where relevant, beard and moustache; it should be tucked into the neck of the suit; a facemask should be worn to prevent the shedding of droplets. Appropriate sterilized, non-powdered rubber or plastic gloves and sterilized or disinfected footwear should be worn. Trouser legs should be tucked into the footwear and garment sleeves into the gloves. The protective clothing should shed virtually no fibers or particulate matter and retain particles shed by the body.

12.2.2.2 General behavior when dressing for the clean room

When going into a clean room all personnel must be fully aware of all the rules and regulations that must be followed before as well as while entering the different airlocks and finally entering the clean room itself. The airlocks are normally used as changing and preparation rooms in order to fully comply with the demands stated. These activities may differ from operation to operation, but normally they consist of some type of hand washing process followed by a gowning process.

In some operations, the personnel remove all private clothing except for underwear. In other operations, the personnel are allowed to wear some parts of their private clothing underneath the clean room garment. The introduction of private clothing underneath the clean room garment is something that is worth considering. In many cases, the private parts of our clothing are uncontrolled, meaning that we do not really know where these clothes have been, and what the wearer has been doing and exposed the clothes to.

Many operations therefore do not allow anything private underneath the clean room garments other than private underwear, and instead supply the personnel with specially designed and clean room acceptable undergarments, in 100% polyester. These clean room undergarments not only supply better control in regard to what is brought into the clean room, but also act as pre-filters before the coverall is used. Many different studies have been made on this pre-filtration action, and the results from one of them are shown in Figure 12.1.[6]

Figure 12.1 shows the difference between using a coverall alone and a coverall that was studied together with clean room undergarments. This test is not based on humans in a body box, but instead performed in a test bench where particles similar to human skin particles are forced through pieces of textile, and particles in the air stream are counted before as well as afterward. In summary, private clothing must be minimized underneath clean room garments. The use of specially designed clean room undergarments has a decreasing effect on the particle dispersion from personnel in clean rooms.

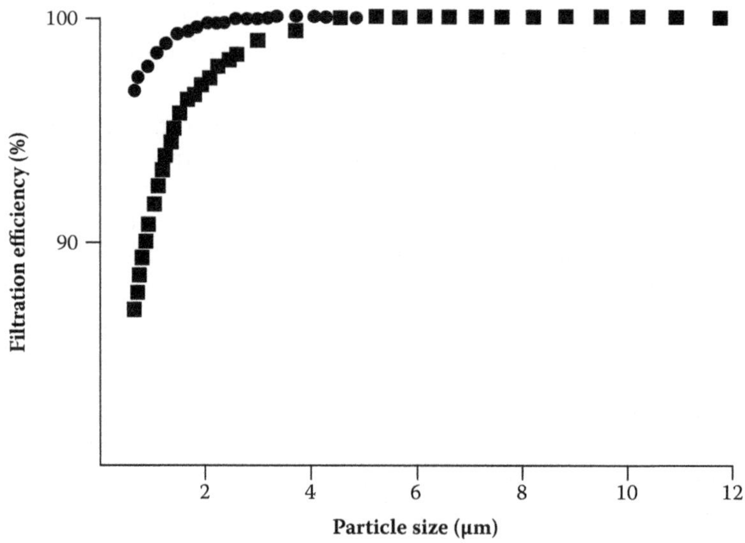

Figure 12.1 The difference in filtration efficiency between a coverall alone as compared to a coverall together with specially designed undergarment in polyester: Coverall alone (■) and combined coverall and undergarment (●).

12.2.3 Cleaning and disinfection of clean rooms

A clean room must be thoroughly cleaned on a regular basis. However, the cleaning process itself turns out to be one of the most contaminating activities in clean rooms. This means that if cleaning is performed and materials and equipment are stationed in the clean room, materials and equipment must often be protected in order not to be contaminated. The best rule of practice is to remove cleaning materials and equipment as much as possible after cleaning.

In the ISO 14644-5 standard with the title "Operations," some aspects on cleaning are given.[2] In all this, there is a way to divide the various surfaces within clean rooms in accordance with their different criticalities. There is also a helpful way to divide the various cleaning techniques available depending on the desired end result. The various methods are divided into

- Gross cleaning
- Intermediate cleaning
- Precision cleaning

Further to this, each of these different cleaning methods is also given a size limit for what is to be removed by each of them. Gross cleaning is intended to remove particles with a particle size of ≥50 μm. This particle size is the visibility limit for the naked human eye without any optical aid and in normal daylight, which in practice means that the gross cleaning result is by the naked human eye visibly clean. Intermediate cleaning concerns particles in the size range of 10 μm–50 μm. Finally, precision cleaning is used in order to remove or destroy particles with a particles size of ≤10 μm.

One important aspect of these cleaning methods is that all of them must be used one after another if precision cleaning is to be performed. This means that it is not effective enough to disinfect a surface, that is, to perform a precision cleaning, if the surface has not been gross cleaned followed by intermediate cleaning.

12.2.3.1 Cleaning technique

There are different types of cleaning techniques that might be used in clean rooms.[4] It is of great importance to demonstrate that the chosen technique fulfills the following:

- Should be able to release and/or dissolve the contaminant from the surface
- Should be able to be collected in something that is moveable
- Removed from the clean room alternative away from a critical area in the clean room

The cleaning process can be divided into:

- Dry methods
- Damp methods

Dry methods include vacuum cleaning, dry moping, dry wiping, and adhesive methods. It is worth noting that vacuum cleaning has low efficiency with smaller particles, albeit it being highly efficient (100% efficiency) to remove particles of ≥100 μm. Particles sized <100 μm will be released to a smaller extent as is shown in Figure 12.2.

Vacuuming can be performed in a clean room for removing larger contaminants, but needs to be in the form of a central system or a special type of clean room vacuum cleaner.

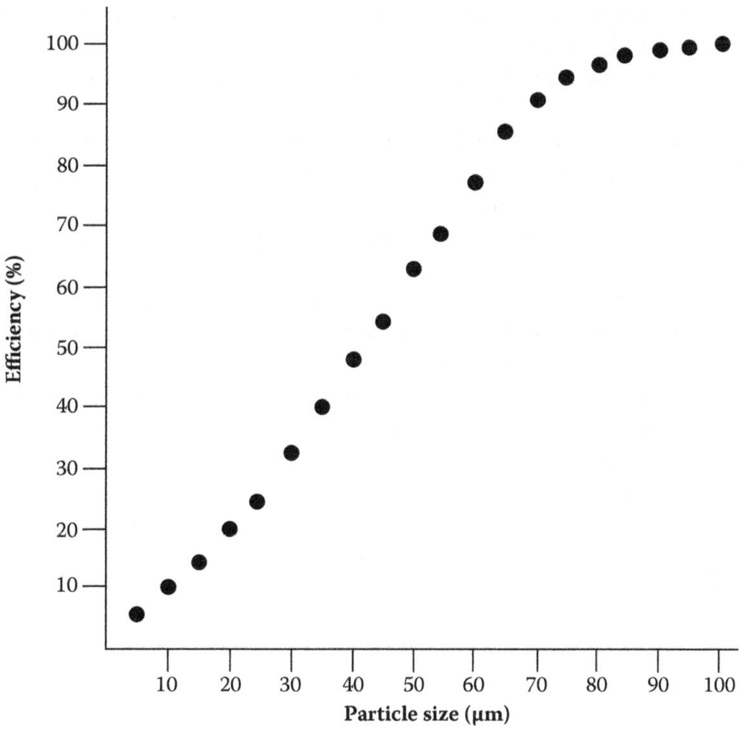

Figure 12.2 Schematic illustration of the overall efficiency of a vacuum cleaner to remove contaminants from surfaces as a function of particle size.

Such a vacuum cleaner is available at quite a high cost, but some of them are even possible to autoclave.

The most common cleaning procedure is performed by using mops and cloths that have been dampened with a liquid to facilitate the removal of contaminants. Traditionally the cleaning liquid consists of a water base with chemical compounds that help in the cleaning process. When choosing a cleaning liquid, it is important to consider that the agent:

- Is effective in removing (dissolving) the contaminants
- Is inert to the surface treated
- Is not drying too fast
- Is not hazardous to the personnel
- Is not leaving chemical residues on the surfaces
- Is free from particles

The demands from the list above cannot always be fulfilled, but one should have in mind that a cleaning liquid is needed in order to produce a clean surface and therefore not result in a surface that has been contaminated with something else after cleaning.

12.2.3.2 *How is a cleaning process performed?*

The biggest problems associated with cleaning processes in clean rooms are

- A surface can look clean although it can be extremely contaminated.
- We clean at home as well as in clean rooms with the same types of techniques, but normally in a different way.
- It is quite hard to clean a surface that from the beginning looks clean.

This means that quite a lot of effort must be put into training the personnel dealing with cleaning and, furthermore, to have good methods to study and analyze if the surface is clean enough after cleaning is performed.

Looking at how to clean a clean room, the following principles are of vital importance:

- Always clean a clean room from the cleanest part of the room and work toward the more contaminated part. Since a clean room is often more contaminated at the entrance, that is, at the area where you enter the clean room from the airlock, you should always start cleaning at the other end of the room and work your way out toward the airlock.
- When cleaning walls, the part of the floor nearest the wall is normally more contaminated compared to the part of the wall closest to the ceiling. Therefore, you dry a wall by beginning at the top and working your way down toward the floor. Always work in parallel streaks when mopping and drying with cloths. These parallel strokes should also be overlapping. Never use circular movements because these movements have a tendency to disperse contaminants from one point of a surface to another.

12.2.3.3 *Analyzing a cleaning process*

Studying and analyzing a cleaning process turns out to be a heavy task. When it comes to studying the microbiological cleanliness, contact plates together with swabs are quite good. However, when it comes to analyzing particles of nonmicrobiological heredity, there is a problem. Some standards have specified the following:

- Darkening of a cloth or a textile glove
- Collection with glued tape
- Collection with a magnet
- Bright white light
- Ultraviolet light
- Microscope

All the tests mentioned in the list above are unfortunately not quantitative, that is, you do not get a figure describing the cleanliness. There are, however, other test techniques available, but normally they are too expensive.

12.2.4 *Monitoring clean rooms*

Since clean rooms and clean zones are built and used in order to create a clean surrounding background for the material to be handled, it is of huge importance to measure and monitor the cleanliness to see if it is in compliance with the demands.

Measuring cleanliness is also important for the person working in the clean room because nearly all contaminants in the form of particles are so small that they cannot be identified and therefore not seen by the naked human eye. This means that a clean room that looks clean when performing a visual inspection may not be clean enough for the intended use.

Monitoring of clean rooms can be divided into several parts:

- Measuring particles[7]
- Measuring microorganisms[8]
- Measuring volatile solvents[9]
- Measuring humidity
- Measuring differential pressure

Of these parameters some measurements are performed in the air and some both in the surrounding air as well as on more or less critical surfaces.

Today we have access to analytical equipment that is capable of counting particles in the air, in gases, and in liquids as well as on surfaces. This equipment does not separate dead particles from living ones, that is, microorganisms. On the contrary, the equipment available for counting particles on surfaces is not widely used and is quite costly, so we have a problem when dealing with measurements of general particles on surfaces. On the other hand, traditional sampling methods of microorganisms are widely used for measuring microbiological cleanliness on surfaces. We will return to this later on in this chapter.

12.2.4.1 *Measuring particles*

In the following subsection we will focus on the measurement of particles in the surrounding air.[3,4] This parameter is also used for the classification of clean rooms (see Table 12.1) as discussed in Chapter 1. Particles in the air can be counted using three different techniques:

- Filter–microscope
- Optical particle counter
- Condensation nucleus counter

Table 12.1 Maximum number of particles per m³ in accordance with EU GMP, Appendix 1 of Volume 4 (2008)

	Maximum permitted number of particles/m³ equal to or larger			
Grade	At rest		Operational	
	0.5 µm	5 µm	0.5 µm	5 µm
A	3520	20	3520	20
B	3520	29	352,000	2900
C	352,000	2900	3,520,000	2900
D	3,520,000	29,000	Not defined	Not defined

12.2.4.1.1 Filter–microscope The technique called filter–microscope is from a practical point of view only used to count particles with a size ≥5 µm. The method utilizes a filter holder connected to a pump with a known flow rate. An efficient filter disc is placed inside the filter holder and the pump is started. The pump draws air from the surrounding environment inside the filter holder through the filter. After allowing a certain volume of air to pass through the filter, the sampling is stopped and the filter taken out of the holder and placed in a microscope. By looking at the particles collected on the filter in a microscope, larger particles can be counted.

This technique has one major advantage and that is that you get the opportunity to view the particles, and you can determine if they are round or, for example, fibers. You can see their color and by doing this you can, in some cases, be able to determine the source of the particles. Personally, I have used this technique to determine the overall particles in lower classification clean rooms, and have detected red fibers from T-shirts worn by operators by mistake.

12.2.4.1.2 Optical particle counter An optical particle counter, which normally is shorted to OPC, is the particle counter that nearly every clean room uses to determine the number of concentrated particles in the surrounding air. Figure 12.3 shows the schematic principle of such a counter. The OPC utilizes the fact that particles have the ability to

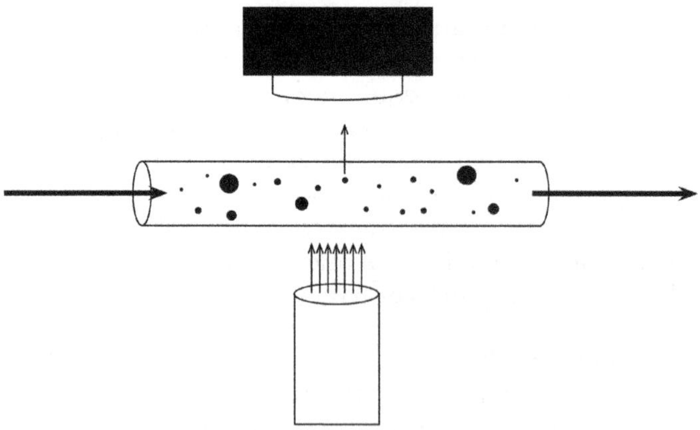

Figure 12.3 Schematic illustration of an optical particle counter (OPC). Air is drawn into the equipment by means of a pump and passes through a narrow glass tube. The glass tube is illuminated with a laser beam and particles in the air stream reflect the incoming air toward a sensor. The sensor cannot only count the number of reflections but also measures the intensity of the reflection and thereby indicates the size of the particle in the air.

reflect light when illuminated. All of us have probably seen particles floating in the air at home, especially when cleaning. If the sun shines through a window, many more particles can be observed, and when the sun is shaded many of the particles disappear. The observations above are all based on the fact that all particles reflect light, but only the ones that are large enough will be detected by our eyes.

The same principle applies for the OPC. As shown in Figure 12.3, air is drawn into the equipment by a pump. The air is then forced through a thin glass tube, which is illuminated by a laser beam. Particles that are large enough will reflect this incoming light and reflect it toward a sensor that counts the light flashes formed when particles pass through the glass tube. An OPC has the ability, in this way, to determine and count particles with a size ≥0.1 μm. The latter corresponds to the lowest particle size shown in the ISO 14644-1 clean room classification table.[1]

12.2.4.1.3 Condensation nucleus counter In some cases, especially in the microelectronics industry and in aerosol science, there is a need to measure and count particles with a size lower than 0.1 μm. However, the OPC mentioned above is not sensitive enough, but if smaller particles in the surrounding air are enlarged before entering an OPC, they can be determined and counted. Figure 12.4 shows the schematic principle of a condensation

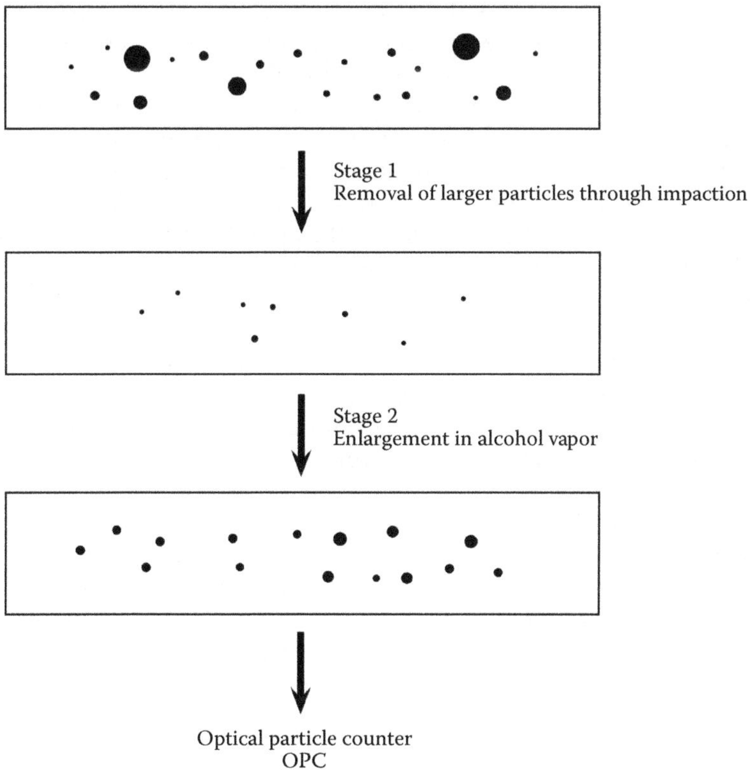

Figure 12.4 Schematic illustration of a condensation nucleus counter (CNC). The CNC contains exactly the same components as compared to the OPC, but with the addition of two separate parts. The first part will remove particles with a size greater than 0.1 μm and the air stream will thereafter continue to a part containing alcohol vapor. The vapor will condense on the small particles making them large in size and detectable by the sensor.

nucleus counter (CNC). In general, it resembles an OPC, but with the addition of two pretreatment parts. In the first one, particles larger than 0.1 μm are removed by impaction. In the second stage, all the smaller particles are allowed to come in contact with an alcohol vapor that will condense on the particles and thereby enlarge them. The size limit of a CNC is approximately 0.01 μm.

12.2.4.2 Measuring and monitoring microbiological contaminants

Microorganisms have been grown in laboratories in order to identify and use them to develop analytical tools as well as vaccines. This principle is also used when it comes to measuring cleanliness from a microbiological view, for example, in a clean room.

When working in a clean room with demands on microbiological cleanliness, we always try to make things worse for microorganisms so that they do not start to proliferate. When it comes to the determining and measuring microbiological contaminants in clean rooms, we work the other way around, that is, after a sample has been drawn or taken, the microorganisms in the sample are supplied with everything they need to prosper and reproduce to such a level that visible colonies can be observed and counted.

Microorganisms are quite like humans in their needs. Like humans, microorganisms need food and water, but are often satisfied with humidity and thrive in a certain temperature interval. In a clean room, we always try to make life for microorganisms as unpleasant as possible. We remove their food by cleaning, and we try to keep everything as dry as possible and in some cases also change the surrounding temperature (refrigeration and freezing) to a level that the microorganism does not like.

When it comes to measuring microbiological cleanliness, we work differently. After sampling we supply the organisms with food and moisture as well as the correct temperature for their reproduction. Two of the demands of microorganisms are supplied by the agar in which samples normally are taken, that is, food and water. After sampling the agar plates or tubes, depending on the sampling technique, they are placed in temperature-regulated incubators for as long as needed for the collected microorganisms to form, for our eyes, visible colonies.

12.2.4.2.1 Microbiological sampling of air The surrounding air of a clean room can be sampled in two ways, either by passive or active sampling. Passive sampling is sometimes referred to as settle plate sampling. Active sampling is carried out by collecting particles and eventual microorganisms from extracted air.

12.2.4.2.1.1 Passive air sampling of microorganisms in air Passive sampling is by far the easiest way of measuring microbiological cleanliness in the air. The only thing needed is an agar plate. An agar plate is a plastic holder into which a thin layer of agar has been cast. The entire plate is covered by a lid, including the agar, is that sterile.

This agar plate is placed on the sampling spot, the lid is removed, and the agar layer in the bottom of the plate is exposed to the surrounding air. Due to gravity as well as air movements caused by personnel, fans, etc., air and particles, including microorganisms, are deposited on the agar surface and after a predetermined exposure time, the lid is replaced and the entire plate is placed in an incubator with the correct incubation temperature.

After incubation the plates are removed and examined. Colonies of microorganisms on the agar surface are then counted and their number is what is called colony forming units (CFUs), which is a way to describe the microbiological cleanliness. The CFU concept is used because we cannot state what type of microorganisms have given rise to a certain colony and, furthermore, we cannot state if the colony on the agar plate aroused from one or several cells.

12.2.4.2.1.2 Active sampling of microorganisms in air Active sampling needs some type of equipment that can collect microorganisms from a certain volume of air. There are many different types of samplers available on the market, and in this context we will look into the general principle and some of the most commonly used equipment.

All equipment used in active air sampling of microorganisms is based on impaction. Extraction of particles from air by impaction is based on the fact that particles behave differently when blown toward an obstacle that air cannot pass through (Figure 12.5). Particles with different masses, which is correlated to their respective size, behave differently; smaller particles will follow the air as it deviates from the stream pattern, whereas large particles, due to their momentum, will continue toward the obstacle and finally collide with it.

Different equipment is available for measuring the impaction process. A few of them are cited here:

- Surface air sampler (SAS)
- Microbiological air sampler (MAS)
- Reuter centrifugal air sampler (RCS)
- Slit sampler

Surface air sampler

In an SAS the surrounding air is drawn into the equipment by an integral pump. The air is then allowed to blow down toward an agar plate placed underneath an inlet lid on the top, covered with many small precision-drilled holes (Figure 12.6). The

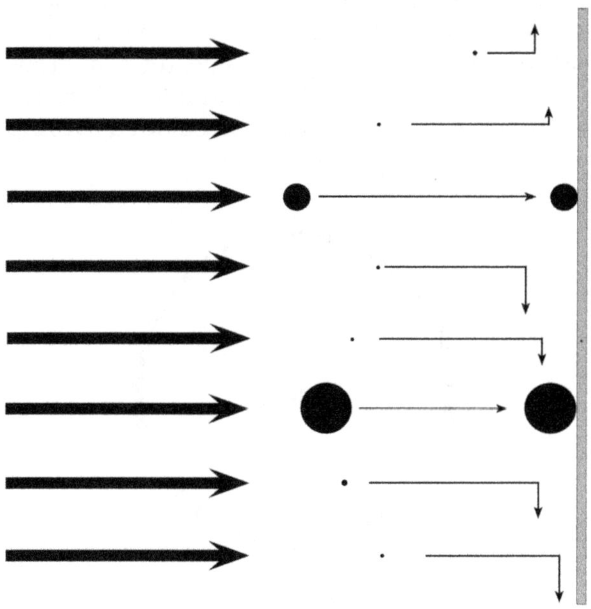

Figure 12.5 Schematic illustration of the principle of impaction utilized in much of the traditional equipment used for active sampling of microorganisms in air.

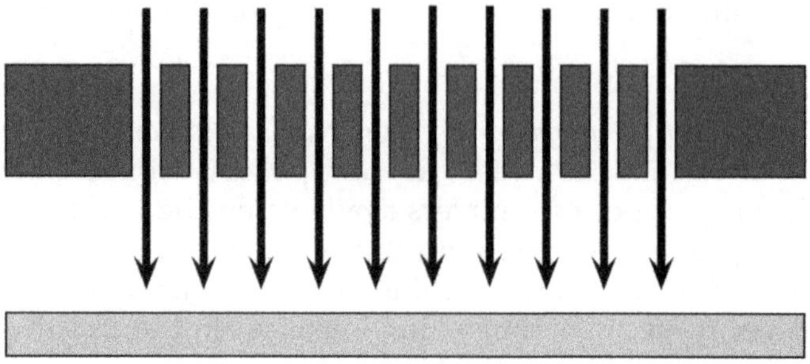

Figure 12.6 Schematic illustration of a surface air sampler (SAS) for active air sampling of microorganisms. The air is drawn into the equipment, by means of an internal fan, through a number of precision-drilled holes. The size of the holes gives the air stream a certain velocity, and microorganisms are collected on an agar plate situated directly underneath the holes.

smaller the holes, the higher the speed of air flow toward the agar plate and the higher the degree of collection of particles and microorganisms. However, the relation between the diameter of the holes in the top and the distance down to the agar plate is of vital importance when it comes to the collection of microorganisms that have the ability to reproduce. If the air speed is too high, many more microorganisms will be collected, but at the cost of decreased viability. After sampling the desired volume of air, the equipment is turned off, the perforated top is removed exposing the agar plate, the lid of the agar plate is replaced, and the plate is finally removed and placed in an incubator.

Reuter centrifugal sampler

This equipment does not have any precision-drilled holes where the air is introduced. Instead, it comprises a turbine wheel that draws air from the surroundings into the equipment and when entering the turbine the air is forced to change directions and will continue to a 90-degree angle, toward a rounded shell protecting the turbine blades. This shell is hollow and into it there is a plastic band; a strip containing small holes filled with agar can be fitted. During the action of an RCS

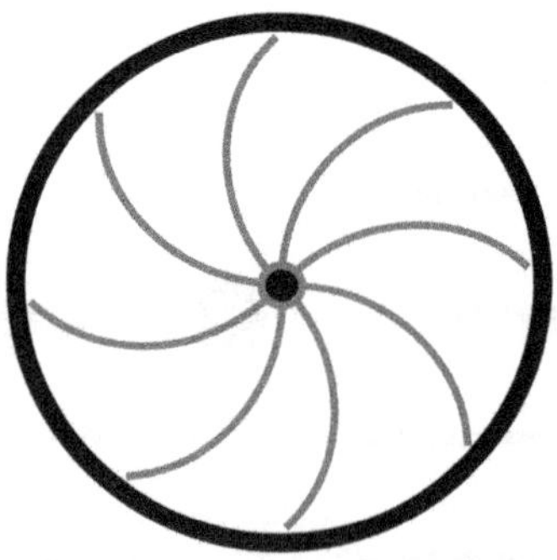

Figure 12.7 Schematic illustration of a reuter centrifugal sampler (RCS). The air is drawn into the equipment by means of a turbine. Once inside the equipment, the airflow changes direction and forces the air, together with microorganisms, toward an elastic plastic holder containing agar medium.

microorganism in the sampler, the air is forced from the outside and onto sterile agar on the strip (Figure 12.7).

Slit Sampler

A slit sampler is also called a slit to agar sampler. It is not equipped with either drilled holes or a visible turbine. Instead, the air is drawn into the equipment through a narrow slit that is placed over an agar plate in such a way that the slit only covers less than the radius of the plate (Figure 12.8). This means that only half of the agar plate is exposed to the air entering the equipment. The agar plate is subsequently placed on a holder that rotates, resulting in the collection of microorganisms on a time basis. The agar plate rotates with one revolution per 20 minutes, or more, depending on the supplier.

After sampling has been completed the equipment is opened, the lid of the agar plate is put back, and the agar plate is removed and incubated.

12.2.4.2.2 Analysis of microorganisms on surfaces It is not only the surrounding air that is of interest to those working in clean rooms and clean zones. We are also interested in the microbiological cleanliness of surfaces. The surfaces analyzed are floors, walls, benches, equipment, clean room clothing as well as the gloves of the operators.

The easiest way to perform a microbiological analysis on a surface is by using a contact plate. Such a plate is, compared to a traditional agar plate, overfilled to form a convex surface sticking out of the plastic plate, that is, it resembles an inkpad.

In the same way as a traditional agar plate, a contact plate is sterile and has a lid that has to be removed before sampling. When sampling, the lid is removed and the agar surface is pressed gently and thoroughly toward the surface, for as long as it is stated in the sampling instruction. The force by which the plate is pressed toward a surface and the contact times are extremely important for the number of microorganisms collected on the surface. After sampling the lid is replaced and the contact plate is incubated.

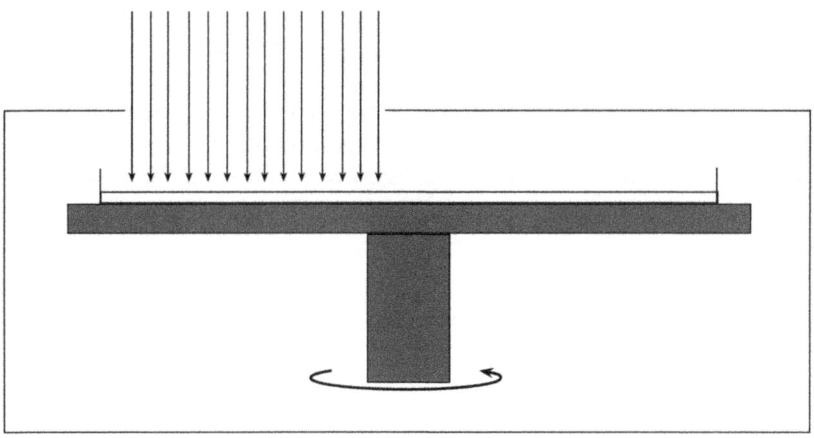

Figure 12.8 Schematic illustration of a slit sampler. A slit sampler consists of a thin slit through which the air is drawn into the equipment. The thin slit gives the air a certain velocity so that microorganisms can be captured on an agar plate situated below the slit. The agar plate is turning with a slow speed, making a slit sampler an active air sampler that measures microorganisms as CFUs per unit time.

Contact plates are used on all surfaces that are smooth and that have no larger crevices, holes, etc. They cannot be used in corners, and for this reason we instead use the swab technique. Swabbing is performed with a sterile pin equipped with some type of porous top that normally is dampened with a sterile liquid (saline, water, etc.). The swab is then used to collect microorganisms from the sampling spot. After sampling, the swab is placed in a test tube, either empty or filled with agar, and sent for further treatment. My experience tells me that contact plates are far better as compared to swabbing, and I normally recommend contact plates as much as possible.

12.2.5 Particle and microbiological limit values in clean rooms

Not only must equipment and methods be available for the detection and counting of particles as well as microorganisms, there is also a need for limit values in order to determine if the cleanliness level is good enough. Some operations have developed their own limit values for particles, as well as microorganisms, but most operations look to standards and norms that are presently used.

The European GMP, Appendix 1 of Volume 4 covers both particles as well as microorganisms, based on the CFU.[5] It comprises two tables. Table 12.1 shows maximum limits for four different clean room classes for particles per cubic meters of air, measured with an OPC, at two specified particles sizes, 0.5 μm and 5 μm, respectively.

Table 12.2 shows limit values for four different clean room classes based on the number of CFUs when measured with passive and active air sampling, surface sampling as well as sampling gloves on operators when working in Grade A and B, that is, when performing aseptic work.

Work is now in progress within the ISO to supplement the ISO standard in clean room classes based on particles, with a standard covering microbiological contaminants and their classification.

12.2.6 Modern technology

All the techniques discussed above are based on traditional microbiological methods. There are some shortcomings with these techniques; for example, the results from the tests are presented as CFUs and not as individual numbers of microorganisms. Another disadvantage is the time period from taking a microbiological sample until the numbers of CFUs are counted; in many cases, it takes at least one day but usually more. These two factors are some of the reasons for developing new methods to be able to get results on microbiological cleanliness faster.

Table 12.2 Maximum recommended number of CFU in accordance with EU GMP, Appendix 1 of Volume 4 (2008)

	Maximum number of viable organisms			
Grade	Air sample CFU/m³	Settling plate CFU/90 mm/4 h	Contact plate CFU/55 mm	Glove print CFU/5 fingers
A	<1	<1	<1	<1
B	10	5	5	5
C	100	50	25	–
D	200	100	50	–

The new methods are called rapid microbial methods (RMMs). All these new methods are based on the same principle as the OPC previously discussed for counting particles in the surrounding air. The RMM counts particles, but the wavelength of the laser light used has been chosen in such a way to excite certain biomolecules only existing in living cells. When the living cell is exposed to this light, in practice it will deliver a very low intensive light. This low intensive light is extremely hard to detect and measure, but with the aid of a special high-tech mirror acting as a dish it is possible to amplify and detect the signal.

RMMs can be used for analyzing gases and liquids as well as for surfaces; however, the surfaces to be analyzed must be swabbed and the collected microorganisms are suspended in water that is analyzed in an RMM.

When the RMM is totally accepted, all the limit values for microbiological contaminants must be updated, going from CFU to individual numbers of microorganisms.

12.2.7 Frequency of monitoring

After discussing the different techniques to measure cleanliness, the next question would be how often and how our clean rooms and clean zones should be sampled and monitored. The answer is quite simple: To measure is to get knowledge. New operations tend to sample much more frequently as compared to well-established operations. However, there are certain rules stated in the European GMP that are used within tissue banks. In the part of Annex 1 with the title "Clean Room and Clean Air Device Monitoring" the following is worth noting: "Clean rooms and clean air devices should be routinely monitored in operation and the monitoring locations should be based on a formal risk analysis study, together with the results obtained during the classification of the clean rooms and/or the clean zones."

It further states, "for Grade A zones, particle monitoring should be undertaken for the full duration of critical processing, including equipment assembly, except where justified by contaminants in the process, that would damage the particle counter or be a hazard, e.g., live organisms and radiological hazards. In such cases, monitoring during routine equipment setup operations should be undertaken prior to exposure to the risk. Monitoring during simulated operations should also be performed. Grade A zones should be monitored frequently and with suitable sample sizes that all interventions, transient events, and any system deterioration would be captured and alarms triggered if alert limits were exceeded. It is accepted that it may not always be possible to demonstrate low levels of ≥5.0 μm particles at the point of fill when filling is in progress, due to the generation of particles or droplets from the product itself."

Grade A zones are not the only zones covered. It is also recommended that a similar system is used for Grade B zones although the sample frequency may have decreased. The norm states, "The importance of the particle monitoring system should be determined by the efficiency of the segregation between the adjacent Grade A and B zones."

"The Grade B zone should be monitored at such a frequency and with suitable sample size that changes in levels of contaminants and system deterioration would be captured and an alarm triggered if limits were exceeded." When it comes to what type of system to be used, the norm states, "Airborne particle monitoring systems may consist of independent particle counters, a network of sequentially accessed sampling points connected by a manifold to a single particle counter or a combination of the two. The system selected must be appropriate for the particle size considered. Where remote sampling systems are used, the length of the tubing and the radii of any bends in the tubing must be considered in the context of particle losses in the tube."

"The selection of the monitoring system should take into account any risk presented by the materials used in the manufacturing operation, for example those involving live organisms or radiopharmaceuticals."

Thus far, only Grade A and Grade B have been discussed. Annex 1 also states recommendations for Grade C and Grade D. "The monitoring of Grade C and D areas in operation should be performed in accordance with the principles of quality risk management. The requirement and alert/action limits depend on the nature of the operations carried out, but the recommended cleanup period should be attained."

It is of vital importance to set alert and action limits. "Appropriate alert and action limits should be set for the results of particulate and microbiological monitoring. If these limits are exceeded, operating procedures should prescribe correct action."

12.2.8 *Humidity, temperature, and pressure*

Annex 1 states the following with regard to temperature and humidity: "Other characteristics such as temperature and relative humidity depend on the product and nature of the operations carried out. These parameters should not interfere with the defined cleanliness standard."

Not all operations control temperature and humidity, but every clean room uses controlled pressure. The use of pressure control in clean rooms is dependent on what type of protection is needed. The general principle states that if the clean room is used to protect the material handled or the handling process, the clean room is used with a positive pressure. This positive pressure will minimize the introduction of contaminants from the surroundings and together with the airlocks present they are a good barrier and protection.

On the other hand, if the material handled or the process itself is a danger to the operators and/or if the material might be dangerous and harmful for people outside of the clean room, the pressure situation will be reversed, that is, the clean room will have a negative pressure. A negative pressure will draw air into the room and thereby minimize the dispersion of dangerous materials outside of the room.

On some occasions there might be a need for both protection of the material handled and the personnel working in a clean room. On such occasions, the clean rooms must be designed and placed in such a way, together with different types of airlocks and differential pressure, that results in the correct and desired cleanliness.

Annex 1 states the following in regard to differential pressure: "A filtered air supply should maintain a positive pressure and an air flow relative to surrounding areas of a lower grade under all operational conditions and should flush the area effectively. Adjacent rooms of different grades should have a pressure differential of 10–15 Pascals (guidance values). Particular attention should be paid to the protection of the zone of greatest risk, that is, the immediate environment to which a product and cleaned components which contact the product are exposed."

References

1. Cleanrooms and Associated Controlled Environments—Part 1: Classification of Air Cleanliness, ISO 14644-1. International Organization of Standardization (ISO), Geneva Switzerland, 1999.
2. Cleanrooms and Associated Controlled Environments—Part 5: Operations. International Organization of Standardization (ISO), Geneva, Switzerland, 2005.
3. Ramstorp M. *Introduction to Contamination Control and Cleanroom Technology*. Wiley VCH Verlag GmbH, Weinheim, Germany, 2000.

4. Ramstorp M. Microbial contamination control in pharmaceutical manufacture. In: Saghee MR, Sandle T, and Tidswell EC (eds.). *Microbiology and Sterility Assurance in Pharmaceuticals and Medical Devices*. Business Horizons, New Delhi, India, 2010.
5. The Rules Governing Medical Products for Human and Veterinary Use, Volume 4, Annex 1 "Manufacture of Sterile Medicinal Products." The European Commission, Brussels, 2008.
6. Ramstorp M. Cleanroom clothing. In: Sandle T and Saghee MR (eds.). *Cleanroom Management in Pharmaceuticals and Healthcare*. Euromed Communications Ltd., Passfield, England, 2013.
7. Cleanrooms and Associated Controlled Environments—Part 3: Test Methods, ISO 14644-3. International Organization of Standardization (ISO), Geneva, Switzerland, 2005.
8. Cleanrooms and Associated Controlled Environments—Biocontamination Control—Part 1: General Principles and Methods, ISO 14698-1. International Organization of Standardization (ISO), Geneva, Switzerland, 2005.
9. Cleanrooms and Associated Controlled Environments—Part 8: Classification of Airborne Molecular Contaminants, ISO 14644-8. International Organization of Standardization (ISO), Geneva, Switzerland, 2013.

chapter thirteen

Just after construction and before the first IVF batch

Things to ponder

Lars Johansson

Contents

Abstract

The building of an ART clinic requires the input from a multidisciplinary task-force so it meets all demands from the legislation, owner and that guarantees the patients value for money. The latter will give the clinic a good reputation, increase the inflow of patients and generate an even higher income.

The clinic must proactively ensure that the couple's gametes and embryos are given an optimal chance to develop into top-quality embryos with high implantation and low miscarriage rates.

This chapter describes in detail the different steps needed for validating a newly built ART laboratory and the additional precautions that need to be implemented before any treatments can safely be undertaken.

13.1 *Introduction*

In order to construct and establish a high quality assisted reproductive technology (ART) clinic, a multidisciplinary skilled task force needs to be formed that guarantees that all aspects concerning the design and building of the clinic, selection of equipment and disposables as well as treatment procedures are taken into consideration. The clinic needs to be built in accordance to country-specific standards and legislations,[1] and perhaps also to international legislation if cross-border treatments[2] are also to be performed. In addition, the clinic must proactively prevent the exposure of oocytes and embryos to environmental embryotoxic pollutants from within the clinic (building materials, ventilation, laboratory furniture, light and gas source, disposables, detergents and cleaning agents, clothing materials and bio-burden of staff and therefore limit access), to ensure that the couple' gametes and embryos are given an optimal chance to develop into top-quality embryos with high implantation and low miscarriage rates.[3–10]

The classification of the clean room is carried out at three different stages in accordance with ISO-14644[11], namely, the installation stage, where the design, the facility, and the service support are validated. Has the facility been designed in accordance with the purpose, clean room standards, guidelines, and operational needs? If all requirements have been fulfilled for the installation stage, and after a thorough proper deep cleaning of the facility, all function-tested and pre-cleaned equipment are gradually introduced, via the anteroom, into the laboratory; this is the resting stage. During this stage, the settings of each instrument are adjusted to the specification for the media products, elevation of the clinic, and to the environment within the laboratory, so different requirements and threshold values are met. Each piece of equipment is also given a specific chronological identity and bar code, by which instrumental parameters (quality control [QC], services, and need of repairs) are registered. At the final validation, namely, the operational stage, the laboratory is validated while the staff is working.[4,11–17]

In addition, and before any treatment of patients can be undertaken, all staff categories must be educated and their competency tested in the operation of the area specific equipment (Technical Operational Procedures), treatment procedures (Standard Operational Procedures [SOPs]), quality control, how to enter patient specific data, and perform safety drills (first aid and fire).[18–19]

13.2 Installation stage: Validation of design, facility, and support services

Before the laboratory can be validated, the logistic layout, selection of building materials, and how support services are supplied to the laboratory must be commissioned (ventilation, delivery of correctly pressurized medical grade gases [gas station], uninterrupted power supplies [UPS], light and low current electricity [LAN]).

13.2.1 Logistic design, building materials, and support services

Most new ART laboratories are now built as clean rooms, which makes the validation more extensive. The layout, the selection of materials; finish of walls, ceilings, and floors; and all installations are controlled against the design and the expectations of the owners.[4] A logistic design facilitates and makes the work more efficient, and reduces the formation of particles and the spread of potential contaminations.

The laboratory surface finish should be very smooth, easy to clean, wear resistant, chemically resistant to cleaning detergents and disinfectants, preferably antibacterial, antistatic, and airtight, thus minimizing out-gassing and preventing the accumulation of hidden contaminations. Rounded corners of the floor and in the ceiling prevent the accumulation of contaminations and facilitate cleaning. Do not forget that the selected materials should preferably be fireproof. Ideally, the laboratory should be provided with fire detection and sprinkler systems. Fire and emergency escape routes should be clearly marked.

The most common floor foundation is concrete and on top of that a durable (epoxy paint, ceramic, vinyl, etc.), impervious, non-slippery, seamless, antistatic surface, resistant to wear and cleaning agents.[4] It is very important that the floor is conductive and earthed, since charged particles might adhere to and contaminate disposables and surfaces. Some floor adhesives are also very embryotoxic and must be given time for out-gassing. "Dust collectors," where the floor meets the wall, and silicone sealants for sealing of these joints, must be avoided. The walls and ceilings mostly consist of antibacterial nonparticle shedding material (coated steel partitions, epoxy painted or vinyl lined walls), which are easily cleaned. The ceilings are usually of walk-on steel panels since service staff need access to air conditioner and water ducts, gas pipelines, electric cables, and light fittings.

13.2.2 Ventilation system

Clean room laboratories can be divided into two categories, namely turbulently (non-unidirectional) and laminar flow (unidirectional) ventilated clean rooms. The turbulent ventilation system is the most commonly used ventilation for ART clean rooms, where high efficiency particulate air (HEPA), ultra low penetration air (ULPA), charcoal and volatile organic compound (VOC) prefiltered humidified and temperature controlled air enters the laboratory via several diffusers in the ceiling. The latest developed ventilation system for clean room ART is from Life-Aire, where the contaminants (total VOCs, aldehydes, biological spores) of the delivered processed air are all under the detection limits of the analyzing instruments.[4,12,20–22] The locations of the diffusers are adjusted to the location and function of sensitive equipment like incubators, ICSI workstations, and laminar air flow (LAF) benches, and to the procedures performed in the designated room.

The filtered air mixes with the laboratory air and removes airborne contaminations and pollutants from the facility, disposables, equipment, and staff, through air extractors located very close to the floor.[23–30] Low noise and vibration laminar flow benches and Class II cabinets further enhance the air quality within a restricted area where culture media products and disposables are handled and different specific ART procedures are performed. The pressure (30 Pascal, >20 air exchanges per hour) within the laboratory must be maintained while doors, hatches, and pass-through or air-showers are opened.

The clean room heating, ventilation, and air conditioning (HVAC) system is commissioned for:

1. Outer insulation, vibration and noise of the ventilation ducts, air duct and filter face velocity, filter integrities, UVC output and intensity, calibration of sensors, functioning of electrical back-up system
2. Temperature, humidity, room pressure and balancing pressure differences between rooms, air leakage test of doors, air-showers, hatches, and interlocks
3. Inlet air analyzed for particle count (e.g., 0.3 μm/cubic feet), total VOCs (TVOC in parts per billion [ppb]), aldehydes (μg/m^3), biological spores, and bacteria (colony forming units, cfu/m^3)

13.2.3 *Doors and pass-through hatches*

Clean room doors are mostly made of plastic covered wood or specially treated steel that is painted, and they should come with a small safety-viewing window. Avoid door handles because they minimize hand contamination and facilitates cleaning. Hang the doors so they are easily closed by the positive over-pressure within the clean room laboratory. The use of knee or foot pressure knobs, that regulates the opening of the laboratory door, facilitates the entry into the laboratory. All closed doors are checked for air leakage and there should be a positive air flow through the door of the laboratory when it is open, thus preventing contamination from entering the laboratory.[4]

The pass-through hatches are usually glazed and sealed with easy cleaning fittings. These hatches may be fitted with air showers and should only allow the opening of one side at a given time.

13.2.4 *Gas stations and pipelines*

The gas station delivers uninterrupted medical grade gas (CO_2, N_2, premixed gas) via an automatic switchover valve unit and argon welded stainless pipelines, which are connected to the wall or ceiling mounted pressure controlled reduction valves. The gas station, pipelines, and the reduction valves are function, leak, and pressure tested. In addition, the pipelines are controlled for correct labeling of type and quality of gas and the location and height of the reduction valves verified.

The reduction valves should be as close as possible to the location of the incubators since the shorter the nontoxic gas inert tubing is between the reduction valve outlet, the preclean gas inline charcoal, and potassium permanganate filter and the inlet of the incubator, the better.[31–33] All the connection points must also be leak tested. The 24-hour gas surveillance system functionality should also be tested.

13.2.5 *Lighting and other fixtures*

All indented yellow light fittings must be made out of top-quality components and checked for air leakage.[7,8] They are usually accessed via a false ceiling in order to change defect parts or lamps as well as to give access to terminal filters and gas and electrical fittings without contaminating the clean room.

13.2.6 *Electrical services*

The function of the UPS outlets should be controlled, their label and location verified so that sensitive equipment is connected to the correct outlet and directly inserted into the outlet without any extension cord. Also the local area network (LAN) power sockets, data and telephone systems, and security systems are evaluated. All outlets should be fitted so they reside within the wall, which prevents the collection of dust.

13.2.7 *Cryo-tank storage room*

The entry into the highly ventilated and low-oxygen alarmed cryo-tank storage room is via an air shower. This floor consists of anti-slippery aluminum, which prevents the destruction of the floor by overflowing liquid nitrogen.

The doors are checked for air leakage and the positive airflow through the air shower prevents contamination of the laboratory clean room.

13.2.8 *The rest of the facility*

13.2.8.1 *Anteroom*

The ventilation, lightings, fixtures, floors, walls, and ceilings are equipped with the same quality products as within the clean room laboratory. However, the overpressure is half of that in the clean room laboratory, thus preventing contaminations of the laboratory.

In the anteroom there are also ventilated storage cupboards for out-gassing of precleaned disposables before they are transferred, via the pass-through hatches, into the clean room laboratory.[9]

One ventilated cupboard is used for storing cleaning devices (telescope handles for mops, Dycem® mat squeegee, Ramrod distributor with switchable container), disposables (single use dry antibacterial microfiber mops, flat head mops for floors and walls, sterile antibacterial high absorbent wipes, irradiated sterile nonwoven and particle retention swabs), and detergents (Dygiene® for recharging of Dycem® mats, Oosafe® or FertiSafe®) for the laboratory and the anteroom.

The temperature, humidity, room pressure, and balancing pressure differences between the anteroom, ventilated cupboards, laboratory, and the change rooms are measured and corrected. All doors, air showers, hatches, and interlocks are leak and pressure tested.

As for the laboratory, the anteroom is analyzed for particle count, TVOCs, aldehydes, biological spores, and bacteria.

13.2.8.2 Change rooms

As for the rest of the facility, the change rooms are validated for logistic design and functionality after the installation of lockers, step-over metal barriers, hand wash facilities, dispensers containing hand-washing detergents (Oosafe, Alcogel, or other antibacterial soap solutions), clean room garments storage systems (gamma-irradiated, lint-free, antistatic coveralls with hoods [100% Polyester]), long powder-free nitrile gloves, footwear, face masks, washable color-coded autoclaved side vented and kick-off clogs, and just before the staff enter the anteroom they walk over a rechargeable sticky mat (Dycem® mats) and perhaps also need to go through an air shower.

When the design and the functionality of all rooms have been approved, they are deep cleaned with suitable detergents and allowed to fume (burn off). Then, the facility is retested for particle count, TVOCs, aldehydes, biological spores and bacteria, and the cleaned equipment, stainless steel furniture and chairs (polyurethane; easy clean) are introduced via the anteroom into the laboratory.

13.3 Resting stage

Once all equipment and furniture have been installed and the needed number of ventilated disposables has been introduced into the laboratory, the room temperature and the ventilation exchange rate are set to maximum to increase the release and elimination of VOCs—the so-called burn-off period.[4] During the burn-off period, the staff undertakes a comprehensive training program in clean room procedures and maintenance, education in technical and SOPs, and performs fire and safety drills. Each staff member shall also obtain a confidential staff job description, which includes a personal continuous educational program (PCD) and competency tests, which are updated on a regular basis and performed yearly.[4]

When the concentrations of VOCs are at an acceptable level, the room temperature is lowered, the air ventilation rates are set to normal values and all equipment is thoroughly calibrated to meet the expected threshold values for each parameter. The clean room is continuously monitored to ensure that all expected standards and quality controls are met, preferably via a wireless 24-hour surveillance QC program.

The facility is now commissioned during the resting stage and if all parameters are met, the facility will be validated while all staff is working in the laboratory—the operational stage.

13.4 Operational stage

Finally, an operational commission is performed while all staff is working in the laboratory. During this stage pre-incubated culture media are controlled for contaminations, which requires that staff are properly dressed (dress code), perform the daily QC routines, work and perform all procedures according to the clinics written SOPs, and all clean room routines are executed correctly.[18]

Whereas the concentrations of TVOCs (ppb), aldehydes (μg/m^3), biological spores, and bacteria (cfu/m^3) should be below the detection limits during the different developmental stages of the clinic, the highest concentration of particles (0.3 μm/ft^3) is measured at the operational stage.

13.5 Education

The clinic should educate all staff members in different techniques and procedures during the burn-off period, which varies between clinics before acceptable environmental values are reached. After this very thorough selection and investment in building materials, equipment, support services, and education of staff, it is of vital importance that the quality of the environment is maintained so that the couples are given an optimal treatment that generates excellent treatment outcomes and value for money invested. Therefore, all staff members must undergo a very comprehensive education program in standardization of all techniques and procedures and understanding the importance of constant quality improvements (QI) (see also TQM).[18]

Do not forget the effects of personnel bio-burden on the environment and the outcome. The dress code must be followed in all aspects and the staff must understand why jewelry, cell phones, long nails, nail polish, and scented products (cologne, perfume, deodorant, hairspray, facial foundation, body wash or powder, after shave, etc.) cannot be used. Smoking staff members should only work in the andrology or sperm preparation laboratory because tar particles within their breath and contaminations of skin and hair are released for a prolonged period of time after smoking.[34]

13.6 Calibration and quality control of purchased equipment

Equipment selection is based on evidence-based medicine for best outcome in human ARTs and on delivery the company should also perform the installation, educate the clinical staff, and calibrate the equipment. For the equipment to work satisfactorily, it is necessary to have a constant and stable environment within the laboratory that is not affected by outer seasonal variations, thus eliminating time-consuming recalibrations of equipment or troubleshooting when results are affected. The calibrations need to be performed with equipment that repeatedly gives reliable and accurate measurements within the expected threshold values. The frequency of measurements for a specific parameter (air, surfaces and liquids, temperatures, CO_2, O_2, pH, particle counts, humidity, etc.) and equipment is usually much higher during the start-up period because environmental factors affect their performance. This strategy will also increase the possibility of detecting malfunctioning equipment. It is therefore better if the equipment is purchased from local dealers since it simplifies communications and servicing.

13.6.1 Suggestions for equipment QC parameters and threshold values

Each piece of equipment is provided with a specific chronological identity and bar code, which is used to register all parameters (QC), services, yearly recertifications, reason for malfunctioning, and repairs.

13.6.1.1 Room temperature

The laboratory ambient temperature should be set at 22–24°C. The higher the temperatures, the higher sweat production, bacteria growth, and staff fatigue, which reduce their concentration and might lead to mistakes.

13.6.1.2 Workstations, laminar flow (LAF) benches, class II cabinets, and IVF chambers

The equipment is analyzed for the release of particles and bacteria, and the bench surface temperature and the heating of the light source are calibrated within the most frequently used culture dish, at a specific fan speed, with a surface temperature probe. The final temperature should be within 36.5–36.9°C for the best outcome, which also causes less damage to the most sensitive stage of the oocyte, namely, the meiotic spindle.[35]

If the workstation is also supplied with a premixed tri-gas mixture, the concentration of CO_2 is adjusted to the elevation of the clinic, and the pH measured and adjusted to the optimal values for the selected media products.

13.6.1.3 *Test-tube warmer and heat-blocks*

As for the workstations, the temperature of the heat blocks and test tube warmer is adjusted to the 36.5–36.9°C range, with a liquid temperature probe placed inside water prefilled and overnight prewarmed test tubes.

13.6.1.4 *Aspiration pump*

The optimal aspiration flow rate is set according to the instruction for the equipment. The flow rate is corrected if the clinic starts using another type of aspiration needle or different lengths of tubings between the aspiration needle and the test tube that collects the follicular fluid.

13.6.1.5 *Microinjector*

As for the surface of the workstations, the glass heat plate on the inverted microscope is also calibrated to 36.5–36.9°C, with a surface temperature probe in a flat ICSI dish.

The ICSI equipment should not be placed underneath a ventilation inlet, which may cause temperature fluctuation of the heat plate, release of small particles, vibrations of the injection pipettes, and which might increase the lysing rate of the injected oocytes.

13.6.1.6 *Incubators*

Make sure that the incubator inlet pressure is correct because it will otherwise affect its performance. There is also a need for an infrared (IR) sensor, which is not affected by humidity or temperature, which gives more stable culture conditions. Adjust the inflow of CO_2 to the elevation of the clinic and the media products. Large incubators, with a large door and shelves with pre-made holes, have a long recovery time (temperature, CO_2, pH, O_2, and humidity) of the culture conditions. Mini-incubators, of a much smaller volume, and direct warming of the dishes has a much quicker recovery of all parameters and generates embryos of higher quality and pregnancy rates.

The formation of condensation droplets on the inner glass doors of large incubators or within the gas tubing of mini-incubators is mostly due to defective temperature distribution within the incubator. The latter can depend on the location of the incubator.

Always reanalyze the pH when new gas cylinders are installed or when the clinic obtains new media batches. See that you obtain a signed analysis certificate for the content within each medical grade gas cylinder.[36–42]

Take the precaution of prerinsing the gas, with a charcoal-potassium permanganate filter, before it enters the incubator. The frequency of filter changes is dependent on the quality of the gas.

In order to obtain a low oxygen environment, some incubators have a built-in gas-mixer, of which the oxygen sensor is very sensitive and needs to be replaced yearly.[43–46]

13.6.1.7 *Slow freezers*

The accuracy of the temperature curve of each freezing program is controlled with an accurate temperature probe inserted into the carrier (straw, vial, ampoule, etc.) and at the exact height of the slow-freezer's temperature sensor. Compare the measure temperature curve with that for the provided program and adjust it if needed. Pay special attention to the seeding temperature is correct.

13.6.1.8 Medical refrigerators

The refrigerator comes with a built-in temperature probe that provides a written digital graph and alerts the staff if the temperature is not within the approved range.

13.6.1.9 Cryo storage tanks

The cryo tanks should be properly cleaned before being filled with sterile liquid nitrogen. Each cryo storage tank is connected to a low-level liquid nitrogen alarm and the cryo-room is supplied with a low oxygen alarm for the safety of the staff.

13.6.1.10 Alarm system

Room temperature, particle counts, and all equipment can also be connected to a 24-hour surveillance system, which graphically records the parameters and alarms if any of the parameters are outside the expected set threshold values.

13.6.1.11 Patient identification

The use of electronic witnessing of dishes with transparent barcoded labels prevents misidentification and errors, and increases traceability and automatic paperless traceability of labware and media batches.[4]

13.6.1.12 Disposables

Disposables for human ARTs are mostly mouse embryo assay (MEA), sperm survival or limulus amebocyte lysate (LAL) tested, and are usually nonpyrogenic. However, these disposables have not been tested for VOCs that are highly embryo toxic.[21] In fact, a recent study of human ART approved disposables were found to contain very high concentrations of embryotoxic VOCs. After one hour out-gassing in an LAF bench, most of the disposable VOC levels were below 0.1 ppm, whereas the impact on clinical outcome is seen already at the 2 ppb level.[9] It is therefore very important that all disposables are out-gassed for a prolonged period of time, in the ventilated cupboards in the anteroom, before they are transferred via the pass-through hatches into the clean room laboratory. Every batch of disposables, including the period and the couples it was used for, is documented in a logbook as well on the patient's individual treatment protocols.

Before disposables, and especially denudation and pipette tips, are used they are prerinsed directly with excess media, so that potential toxins from the manufacturing process are removed. Preferably a multi-pipette fitted with a prerinsed DNA, RNA, and pyrogenic free syringe (e.g., Eppendorf Biopur) is used for quick and safe dispensing of the culture media. Since the multi-pipette is only filled once, it reduces the risk for contamination of the vial or the flask, allowing quick reproducible pipetting of droplets from a sealed unit and preventing increase in osmolality and reducing the laboratory workload.[4]

Never use two-component syringes to aspirate culture media or to prepare culture media droplets for culture of embryos because the grease within the syringe contaminates and changes the properties of the media. Similar effects are also obtained if culture media are aliquot into disposables not approved for human ART (Patrick Quinn, personal communication).

13.6.1.13 Measurements of bacterial contamination

Before any treatments can start, the premises are thoroughly screened for bacterial contamination via air sampling, agar gel settle, or contact plates and swab tests. A higher frequency of analysis at the start-up of the laboratory identifies problems that need to be resolved before treatments can be started. Restricted laboratory access must be re-enforced since it prevents spreading of contamination.

13.7 Written standard operational procedures

Standard operational procedures (SOPs) can be of technical (equipment) or clinical type. The standardization improves the transparency and traceability of all actions performed, makes the processes and procedures more efficient, and improves services quality, which is beneficial for both customers and staff. The SOPs are upgraded yearly and the latest international technologies and benchmark processes and procedures are incorporated in a never-ending process. Each SOP track record and development must be saved.[18]

The staff's competency in the different techniques and procedures are tested yearly and saved in their personal file in a locked cabinet.

13.8 Total quality management

A total quality management (TQM) system, using domestic and international guidelines, should be implemented so that an optimal level of patient care and success rates can be maintained. TQM covers all aspects of ART, from facility and patient evaluations, treatment regimes, culture and embryo transfer techniques to the delivery of a healthy baby at a normal gestational time. There is a continuous improvement in procedures and incorporation of the latest developed techniques (quality improvements = QI) to optimize routines for the benefit of couples and staff. An experienced senior embryologist is appointed as quality manager (QM), who continuously controls that all parameters are within given threshold values, investigates and finds the reasons behind abnormal values and rectifies them.[4]

It is important to produce an organizational chart, which clearly shows the hierarchy, the line of communication, authority, and responsibility. This avoids many unnecessary misunderstandings and conflicts, and leads to more effective communication and interaction between different staff categories. Each staff member should have a detailed individual job description, which describes the required qualifications, health requirements, line of communication, responsibilities, and the yearly update of the job description, evaluation of performance, and competencies. All staff should be entitled to enjoy their work environment and develop their skills by attending continual medical education (CME). All certificates, competencies, health documents, job descriptions, and relevant papers are chronologically stored in a confidential personnel folder.[4]

All relevant data related to products and materials (batch number and expiry date), which come in contact with the patients' gametes or embryos during their treatment cycle, are recorded in the patients' files and a log book to allow traceability. Since all these data are also entered in a computer file, it is possible to quickly evaluate the effects of different materials or batch numbers on different steps in the procedure (fertilization, cleavage, implantation rate, pregnancy rate, etc.). The latter are called key performance indicators (KPIs) that are an important tool for auditing the clinic's performance over time, for detection of gradually declining results, performance of individual staff members, and areas of need for education. The indicators should be internationally defined and recognized, which reduces misinterpretations and facilitates internal as well as international communication and auditing. Unfortunately, many clinics only focus on the ultimate outcome, namely, pregnancy rates, which do not assess the overall quality of the ART program.[4,18]

13.9 Selection, preparation, and treatment of the first batch of patients

Before any treatment is performed, all equipment should have been properly calibrated and all parameters should be within the set threshold values. All staff should have also been properly trained in the different procedures and follow the written SOPs in detail.[47–53]

The first batch of patients is treated for free or for a lower fee since the clinic cannot, at this point of time, be sure of the outcome. The clinic should select couples with minor problems (anovulation woman combined with a normozoospermic man) since the expected outcome should be within normal ranges, facilitating interpretation of results and easier to find areas of concern. Perhaps the best option for these first cases is to perform 50% IVF and 50% ICSI to compare the outcomes and to avoid potential fertilization failures.

After each single treatment all staff should gather and go through routines and outcomes until all are satisfied (teamwork). Do we have any kind of contamination that affects the production of top quality embryos? Is all equipment optimally calibrated and generating acceptable results? Are there any areas of concern? Can we continue or should we stop? The questions are many and there are unfortunately multifactorial reasons for failures and equally many that lead to success. The routines should therefore be kept simple, effective, and the outcome should be easy to follow and interpret, if necessary. Remember to adjust the number of incubators to the number of treatments so optimal culture conditions and outcomes can be maintained.[4]

13.10 Final remarks

Despite the fact that TQM of an ART clinic is a never-ending effort, costly, time-consuming, and a lengthy process, the many positive outcomes that this leads to are highly beneficial for the clinic, staff, and especially the patients. There is no doubt that a standardization of the many processes within the clinic facilitates the communication between staff, patients, and other clinics. Remember that there are no shortcuts to perform a work of excellence and that all staff categories must be involved and committed.

References

1. ESHRE Report: Comparative Analysis of Medically Assisted Reproduction in the EU: Regulation and Technologies (SANCO/2008/C6/051), 2008.
2. ASRM Report: Cross-border reproductive care: A committee opinion. *Fertil Steril* 2013; 100: 645–50.
3. Zujovic L. IVF Culture systems: An overview. In: Varghese A, Sjoblom P, and Jayaprakasan K, eds. *A Practical Guide to Setting Up an IVF Lab, Embryo Culture Systems and Running the Unit.* Jaypee Brothers Medical Publishers (P) Ltd, New Delhi, 2013, pp. 31–44.
4. Johansson L. Establishment of an ART clinic: Location, construction and design. In: Varghese A, Sjoblom P, and Jayaprakasan, K, eds. *A Practical Guide to Setting Up an IVF Lab, Embryo Culture Systems and Running the Unit.* Jaypee Brothers Medical Publishers (P) Ltd, New Delhi, 2013, pp. 24–3017.

5. Nijs M, Franssen K, Cox A, Wissmann D, Ruis H, and Ombelet W. Reprotoxicity of intrauterine insemination and in vitro fertilization-embryo transfer disposables and products: A 4-year survey. *Fertil Steril* 2009; 92: 527–35.
6. Gardner DK and Lane M. Embryo Culture. In: Gardner D, Weismann A, Howles CM, and Shoham Z, eds. *Textbook of Assisted Reproductive Techniques. Laboratory and Clinical Perspectives.* Martin Dunitz Ltd, The Livery House, London, UK.
7. Ottesen LD, Hindkjaer J, and Ingerslev J. Light exposure of the ovum and pre-implantation embryo during ART procedures. *J Assist Reprod Gen* 2007; 24: 99–103.
8. Takenaka M, Horiuchi T, and Yanagimachi R. Effects of light on development of mammalian zygotes. *Proceedings of the National Academy of Sciences of the USA* 2007; 105: 14289–93.
9. Hua VK and Cooke S. Volatile Organic Compounds within the IVF Laboratory. FSA Australia, 2013.
10. Lierman S, De Sutter P, Dhont M et al. Double-quality control reveals high-level toxicity in gloves used for operator protection in assisted reproductive technology. *Fertil Steril* 2007; 88 (4 Suppl.): 1266–72.
11. www.iso.org.
12. Doshi A, Karunakaran S, Worrilow K et al. What makes an IVF laboratory successful? In: Varghese A, Sjoblom P, and Jayaprakasan K, eds. *A Practical Guide to Setting Up an IVF Lab, Embryo Culture Systems and Running the Unit.* Jaypee Brothers Medical Publishers (P) Ltd, New Delhi, 2013, pp. 13–23.
13. Esteves SC and Bento FC. Air quality in reproductive laboratories. In: Varghese A, Sjoblom P, and Jayaprakasan K, eds. *A Practical Guide to Setting Up an IVF Lab, Embryo Culture Systems and Running the Unit.* Jaypee Brothers Medical Publishers (P) Ltd, New Delhi, 2013, pp. 45–53.
14. Maalouf WE. Factors to consider when setting up a PGD laboratory. In: Varghese A, Sjoblom P, and Jayaprakasan K, eds. *A Practical Guide to Setting Up an IVF Lab, Embryo Culture Systems and Running the Unit,* Jaypee Brothers Medical Publishers (P) Ltd, New Delhi, 2013, pp. 61–68.
15. Tomlinson MJ and Harbottle SJ. Facilities and resources for the andrology service. In: Varghese A, Sjoblom P, and Jayaprakasan K, eds. *A Practical Guide to Setting Up an IVF Lab, Embryo Culture Systems and Running the Unit,* Jaypee Brothers Medical Publishers (P) Ltd, New Delhi, 2013, pp. 69–86.
16. Esteves SC and Bento FC. Implementation of air quality control in reproductive laboratories in full compliance with the Brazilian Cells and Germanitive Tissue Directive. *Reprod Biomed Online* 2013; 26: 9–21.
17. Esteves SC, Gomes AP, and Verza Jr S. Control of air pollution in assisted reproductive technology laboratory and adjacent areas improves embryo formation, cleavage and pregnancy rates and decreases abortion rates: Comparison between a class 100 (ISO 5) and a class 1.000 (ISO 6) cleanroom for micromanipulation and embryo culture. *Fertil Steril* 2004; 82(Suppl. 2): S259–60.
18. Mortimer S and Mortimer D. *Quality and Risk Management in the IVF Laboratory,* Cambridge University Press, Cambridge, England, 2015.
19. Hreinsson J. Quality management. In: Varghese A, Sjoblom P, and Jayaprakasan K, eds. *A Practical Guide to Setting Up an IVF Lab, Embryo Culture Systems and Running the Unit.* Jaypee Brothers Medical Publishers (P) Ltd, New Delhi, 2013, pp. 87–93.
20. Worrilow KC. The impact of UVC irradiation on clinical pregnancy rates in an ISO 5 cleanroom in vitro fertilization laboratory. *ASHRAE IAQ* 2009, 4–6.
21. Worrilow KC, Huynh HT, Bower JB et al. A retrospective analysis: Seasonal decline in implantation rates (IR) and its correlation with increased levels of volatile organic compounds (VOC). *Fertil Steril* 2002; 78 (Suppl 1): S39.
22. Forman M, Sparks ET, Degelos S et al. Statistically significant improvements in clinical outcomes using engineered molecular media and genomically modelled ultraviolet light for comprehensive control of ambient air (AA) quality. *ASRM* 2014; O–263.
23. Schimmel T, Gilligan A, Garrisi GJ et al. Removal of volatile organic compounds from incubators used for gamete and embryo culture. *Reprod Fertil* 1997; 68 (Suppl 1): S52–53.
24. Perin PM, Maluf M, Czeresnia CE et al. Impact of short-term preconceptional exposure to particulate air pollution on treatment outcome in couples undergoing in vitro fertilization and embryo transfer (IVF/ET). *J Assist Reprod Genet* 2010; 27: 371–82.

25. Cohen J, Gilligan A, Esposito W, Schimmel T, and Dale B. Ambient air and its potential effects on conception in vitro. *Hum Reprod* 1997; 12: 1742–9.
26. Boone WR, Johnson JE, Locke AJ, Crane M IV, and Price TM. Control of air quality in an assisted reproductive technology laboratory. *Fertil Steril* 1999; 71: 150–54.
27. Knaggs P, Birch D, Drury S et al. Full compliance with EU directive air quality standards does not compromise IVF outcomes. *Hum Reprod* 2007; 22 (Suppl.1): i164–65.
28. Hall J, Gilligan A, Schimmel T, Cecchi M, and Cohen J. The origin, effects and control of air pollution in laboratories used for human embryo culture. *Hum Reprod* 1998; 13 (Suppl 4): 146–55.
29. Khoudja RY, Xu Y, Li T, and Zhou C. Better IVF outcomes following improvements in laboratory air quality. *J Assist Reprod Genet* 2013; 30: 69–76.
30. Johansson L. Handling Gametes and embryos: Oocyte collection and embryo culture. In: Montag M, ed. *A Practical Guide to Selecting Gametes and Embryos*. CRC Press, Taylor & Francis Group, Boca Raton, FL, 2014, pp. 17–38.
31. Higdon H, Blackhurst D, and Boone W. Incubator management in an assisted reproductive technology laboratory. *Fertil Steril* 2008; 89: 703–10.
32. Rawcowsky C, Nureddin A, de los Santos MJ et al. Carbon-activated air filtration results in reduced spontaneous abortion rates following IVF. Proceedings of the 11th World Congress on In Vitro Fertilization and Human Reproductive Genetics, Sydney, Australia, 1999.
33. Mayer JF, Nehchiri F, Weedon VM et al. Prospective randomized crossover analysis of the impact of an incubator air filtration on IVF outcomes. *Fertil Steril* 1999; 72 (Suppl 1): S42.
34. Gerber A, V Hofen-Hohloch A, Schultze J et al. Tobacco smoke particles and indoor air quality (ToPIQ-II)—A modified study protocol and first results. *J Occup Med Toxicol* 2015; 10: 1–6.
35. Pickering SJ, Braude, PR, Johnson MH et al. Transient cooling to room temperature can cause irreversible disruption of the meiotic spindle in the human oocyte. *Fertil Steril* 2009; 54: 102–08.
36. Swain JE. Handling gametes and embryos: Quality control for culture conditions. In: Montag M, ed. *A Practical Guide to Selecting Gametes and Embryos*, CRC Press, Taylor & Francis Group, Boca Raton, FL, 2014, pp. 39–58.
37. Swain JE. Media composition: pH and buffers. In: Smith G, Swain JE, Pool TB, eds. *Embryo Culture Methods and Protocols*. Humana Press, Springer Science + Business Media, LLC, New York, 2012, pp. 161–75.
38. Will M, Clark N, and Swain J. Biological pH buffers in IVF: Help or hindrance to success. *J Assist Reprod Genet* 2011; 28: 711–24.
39. Phillips KP, Leveille MC, Claman P et al. Intracellular pH regulation in human preimplantation embryos. *Hum Reprod* 2000; 15: 896–904.
40. Swain JE. Optimizing the culture environment in the IVF laboratory: Impact of pH and buffer capacity on gamete and embryo quality. *Reprod Biomed Online* 2010; 21: 6–16.
41. Swain JE and Pool TB. New pH-buffering system for media utilized during gamete and embryo manipulations for assisted reproduction. *Reprod Biomed Online* 2009; 18: 799–810.
42. Pool TB. Optimizing pH in clinical embryology. *Clin Embryol* 2004; 7: 1–7.
43. Kovacic B and Vlaisavljevic V. Influence of atmospheric versus reduced oxygen concentrations on development of human blastocysts in vitro. A prospective study on sibling oocytes. *Reprod Biomed Online* 2008; 17: 229–36.
44. Waldenstrøm U, Engstrøm A, Hellberg D et al. Low-oxygen compared with high-oxygen atmosphere in blastocyst culture, a prospective randomized study. *Fertil Steril* 2009; 91: 2461–65.
45. Meintjes M, Chantilis SJ, Douglas JD et al. A controlled randomized trial evaluating the effect of lowered incubator oxygen tension on live births in a predominantly blastocyst transfer program. *Hum Reprod* 2009; 24: 300–7.
46. Catt J and Henman M. Toxic effects of oxygen on human embryo development. *Hum Reprod* 2000; 15 (Suppl 2): 199–206.
47. Morbeck DE, Khan Z, Barnidge DK et al. Washing mineral oil reduces contaminations and embryo toxicity. *Fertile Steril* 201; 94: 2747–52.
48. Otsuki J, Nagai Y, and Chiba K. Damage of embryo development caused by peroxidized mineral oil and its association with albumin in culture. *Fertil Steril* 2009; 91: 1745–49.
49. Wagner-Coughlin CM, Maravilla AE, Nikurs AR et al. Microdroplets under oil improves embryo quality even when an isolette is used. *Fertil Steril* 1994; 62 (Suppl 1): S177.

50. Swain JE, Cabrera L, Xu X et al. Microdrop preparation factors influence culture-media osmolality which can impair mouse embryo preimplantation development. *Reprod Biomed Online* 2012; 24: 142–47.
51. Ebner T, Shebl O, Moser M et al. Group culture of human zygotes is superior to individual culture in terms of blastulation, implantation and life birth. *Reprod Biomed Online* 2010; 21: 762–68.
52. Reed ML, Hamic A, Thompson DJ et al. Continuous uninterrupted single medium culture without medium renewal versus sequential media culture: A sibling embryo study. *Fertil Steril* 2009; 92: 1783–86.
53. Sepulveda S, Garcia J, Arriaga E et al. In vitro development and pregnancy outcomes for human embryos cultured in either a single medium or in a sequential media system. *Fertil Steril* 2009; 91: 1765–70.

chapter fourteen

Personnel practices in an IVF clean room facility

Martine Nijs and Greta Verheyen

Contents

Abstract

The in vitro fertilization (IVF) laboratory is the fundamental unit of the IVF center. Multiple IVF centers have demonstrated the feasibility of handling human gametes and culturing embryos in a clean room setting. Performing IVF in these controlled environments may optimize the outcomes. Better embryo quality, higher live birth rates, and lower miscarriage rates are being noted after switching to an IVF clean room facility. An IVF clean room has a "controlled" level of contamination of environmental pollutants such as dust particles, airborne microbes, aerosol particles, and chemical vapors. In order to maintain this low level of contamination, specific protocols for working and maintenance are to be installed, and they differ substantially from working in the traditional IVF laboratory. This chapter gives an overview of practices for personnel working in an IVF clean room environment.

14.1 What is an IVF clean room?

The IVF laboratory is the fundamental unit of the IVF center. Multiple IVF centers have demonstrated the feasibility of handling human gametes and culturing embryos in a clean room setting and even suggested that performing IVF in this controlled environment may optimize the outcomes. Better embryo quality, higher live birth rates, and lower miscarriage rates are being noted after the switch to a clean room IVF facility.[1–3]

An IVF clean room is a controlled environment where gametes, embryos, and reproductive tissues are collected, processed, and cultured. It is a room in which the concentration of airborne particles is controlled to specified limits.

The International Organization for Standardization (ISO) has set standards for environmental management. Standard 14644-Part 1 is the standard that classifies air cleanliness and it defines a clean room as "a room in which the concentration of airborne particles is controlled, and is constructed and used in a manner so as to minimize the introduction, generation and retention of particles inside the room and in which other relevant parameters, like temperature, humidity, lighting and air pressure are controlled as necessary." Moreover, a clean room is an environment with a low level of environmental pollutants such as dust, airborne microbes, aerosol particles, and chemical vapors.

A clean room therefore has a "controlled" level of contamination that is specified by the number of particles per cubic meter per specified particle size. In order to get and maintain this low level of contamination, specific protocols for working and maintenance are to be installed.[4,5]

First, strict IVF clean room conditions can be maintained by supplying the clean room with clean air that has been filtered with high efficiency filters under pressure. This will ensure that generated particles, bacteria, and chemicals cannot enter or are diluted and are removed. Second, a cascade of positive air pressure is created so that no "dirty" air can enter the clean room. Third, clean rooms are built with materials that should not generate/create particles and specific chemicals. Fourth, specific clothing should ensure that dust particles are not released and that staff members cannot disperse particles or microorganisms. And finally, all activities and procedures should be designed in such a way that the handling of gametes and embryos does not introduce, generate, or retain particles in the clean room.[4,5]

This chapter summarizes practices for personnel working in an IVF clean room environment. The instructions should be used as a guide to achieve IVF clean room specifications.

14.2 Dress code: What to wear and what not to wear in an IVF clean room facility

To minimize dispersion of particles in the IVF clean room, specific clean room clothing needs to be worn. Each person disperses up to 10^7 inert particles per minute (particles $\geq$ 0.5 μm) depending on the type of clothing worn. These particles originate from the skin, hair, mouth, and nose and from the clothing itself. Normally, some 40,000 skin cells are dispersed from human skin every hour. These skin cells carry flora; primarily those associated with human skin are Gram-positive cocci. Common bacterial genera include Micrococcus, Staphylococcus, Coryne bacterium, Bacillus, and fungi usually include Aspergillus and Penicillin.[6]

Clean room clothing is made from synthetic materials such as polyester or nylon. The fabrics should be woven so as to filter the particles generated from the skin or those from the clothing worn under the clean room clothing. Gore-Tex garments have shown to be very efficient and practical. Natural fabrics like cotton release a very high number of particles and must never be used in a clean room. Clean room fabrics should always be manufactured with conducting material woven into them in order to avoid static. Ideally a one piece zip-up overall with a hood that also covers the neck should be worn (Figure 14.1). Long sleeved coats combined with long trousers and cap covers are an alternative option. Shoe covers or dedicated shoes should be used. Beards should be covered when they are more than 3–4 mm long.

The clothing should be comfortable and of the correct size. Clean room clothing should be changed daily and washed and processed in a separate laundry facility. They should be inspected for holes, and folded and packed in specific clean bags. Non-woven fabrics such as Tyvek can be used for single use garments (e.g., visitors, builders, cleaners, etc.).

To avoid dispersion of contamination from mouth and nose (salts, microbes, hairs, etc.), facial masks can be worn over front of the nose and mouth. A typical example used in an IVF clean room is the surgical mask, a disposable non-woven mask with straps and loops.

Hands of personnel carry bacteria, oils, salts, DNAses and RNAses and hence can be a large source of contamination to the clean room and the culture system. Wearing gloves during the different laboratory procedures will not only protect staff members from contamination from the body fluids from the patients (follicular fluid, sperm sample, etc.) but will also prevent contamination to the culture system by staff hands. The choice of gloves

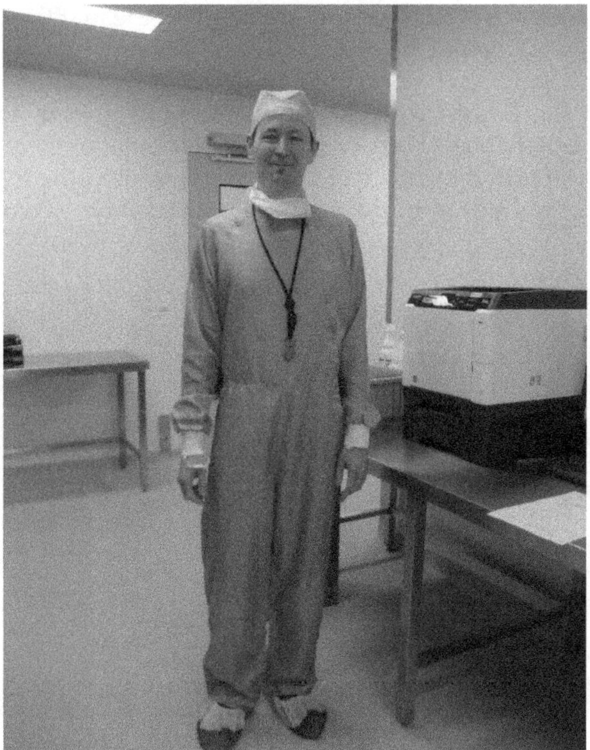

Figure 14.1 **(See color insert.)** Dress code for the IVF clean room: a one piece zip-up overall with long sleeves, a head cover, and shoe covers.

used during the handling of gametes and embryos is crucial because some gloves can carry toxicities that can be carried over into the IVF/ICSI culture system.[7]

Personal hygiene and cleanliness is essential for staff working in an IVF clean room setting. Staff are advised to not wear hair spray, artificial nails, nail varnish, deodorant, and perfumes. Released VOCs may be toxic to human gametes and embryos.[8,9] Fingernails and artificial nails are a main area of concern because they pose a hazard for infection. Watches, rings, and cell phones should be stored before changing into clean room garments.

14.3 Entrance to the IVF clean room facility by staff

A mistake often encountered in clean room facilities is the assumption that the dressing area is not part of the clean room. This area is the transition point from the "dirty" to the "clean" area, which means that the section (hatch) leading to the clean room should be at least as clean as the clean room itself. The design should segregate street/hospital clothes from clean room garments to minimize contaminates carry-over, particularly along the floor. It must be pointed out that clothing, such as overcoats, boots, and rubbers should be left as far from the room entrance as possible. The methods of entering into a clean room should guarantee that dust particles, bacteria, fungi, and viruses remain outside the clean room facility. In order to ensure this, personnel can move though three zones: a pre-changing zone, a changing zone, and an entrance zone.

In the pre-changing zone, street and/or hospital clothing should be removed. Watches and rings, wallets, and mobile phones are securely locked away. A hood, facemask, and if applicable a beard mask are put on; shoes are changed for the first time; and hands are thoroughly washed. Staff will then move to the changing room where they put on the proper clean room clothing. Clothing should be removed from its packing and put on without touching the floor. It should be inspected that garments are worn correctly, in front of a full-length mirror: check that hair is tucked in the hood, and that there are no gaps between clothing and hood. Staff will then move to the entrance zone using a "cross bench system" to change to clean room shoes or to put on a pair of overshoes (Figure 14.2). Staff should

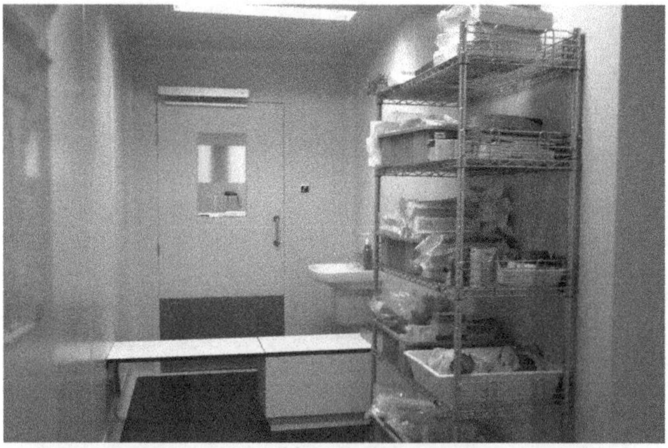

Figure 14.2 **(See color insert.)** Entrance room into IVF clean room facility using a cross bench. Staff should sit on the bench to remove their shoes, move the legs over the bench and put on the clean room shoes. Staff can stand up and move into the clean room by stepping on a sticky clean room mat. Hands should be disinfected after changing of shoes and before entrance into the IVF clean room facility.

sit on a bench, remove the shoes, move the legs over the bench, and put on the clean room shoes. Staff can stand up and move into the clean room by stepping on a sticky clean room mat. Hands should be disinfected after changing of shoes using a product that is safe for use in an IVF setting.[10] The cost of hand hygiene products should not be the primary factor for influencing a product selection. Staff suffering from respiratory or skin diseases should be advised not to work in the clean room until their health issues are solved.

Nothing should be allowed into the IVF clean room that is not required to support the work within the ART laboratory. Items that should be banned from entering into the IVF clean room include food, drinks, chewing gum, smoking materials, radios, mobile phones, towels, handkerchiefs, pencils and erasers, wallets, and purses to cite a few.

Clean room compatible documentation products should be used: clean room compatible paper and notebooks made from plastic fibers can enter the clean room. Some inks can be embryo toxic, so care should be taken when using printed labels or writing with ink pens. Pencils are not to be entered into the clean room.

Staff should be properly trained and instructed how to enter the clean room. Visitors should adhere to the same system for entrance into the clean room.

14.4 Entrance to the IVF clean room facility of materials and equipment

Equipment should evidently be first cleaned and disinfected before entrance into the clean room. Careful consideration should be taken when selecting cleaning products and decontaminating agents for use in human IVF centers as they may have a negative impact on the outcome of the fertility treatment.[10]

Materials and equipment can enter the clean room through a separate material airlock system or through a pass-through hatch. This airlock system or "sluice" works with a positive air pressure system that is lower than in the clean room and higher than outside. It often has interlocked doors, so only one door can open at a given time, in order to ensure that no particles enter the clean room. The pass-through hatch should also have an interlocked door system.

Materials and disposables used in the laboratories should be removed from their bulk packaging or cardboard boxes and placed into clean plastic boxes in the airlock before they are entered into the clean room. Not all materials used in ART are produced and packed for use in a clean room environment. Suppliers should be informed and simple changes to their production system will ensure the correct quality.

Staff bringing the materials or equipment into the material transfer room should leave this room. Air pressure in the material transfer room will be restored to the correct pressure, and staff from the clean room can now enter the material transfer room to collect the material.

The movement of materials between the inside and the outside of a clean room should be minimized. Each time a material is moved out of the clean room it can be contaminated, and hence contamination can be introduced into the clean room when backer-entering it into the laboratory.

14.5 Working in an IVF clean room environment: Basic principles

Within an IVF clean room, many rules must be followed in order to minimize contamination. Basically, movement of staff should be reduced to a minimum. In an IVF clean room setting, a sitting staff member produces 100,000 particles ≥ 0.5 μm per minute. A moving person sheds 1 million particles ≥ 0.5 μm per minute, and a walking person sheds over 5 million particles ≥ 0.5 μm per minute.[4] Quick movement of staff can disturb the unidirectional airflow in the IVF clean room and hence cause higher levels of contamination in the disrupted flow. It is suggested to walk slowly and avoid creating air turbulence.

Doors usually open inward into the laboratory and are held shut by the higher air pressure. Doors are opened and closed slowly and two adjoining doors are not opened at the same time. Doors should never be blocked in the opened position. When passing through the doors of an airlock, staff should ensure that the first door is locked before the second door is opened. Pass-through hatches used to pass items into the laboratory should be used in a similar way. Doors without handles will assist in preventing transfer of contamination of hands or gloves. Hand or foot sensors for opening of the clean room doors is advised (Figure 14.3).

IVF staff should anticipate the needs for each activity/handling and gather all necessary materials, tools, and supplies before performing the job. For example, cleaning solutions, wiping materials, petri dishes, pipettes and pipette holders, culture medium, and patient forms are assembled before and not during the work of preparing the culture dishes. Staff should not carry materials (like bottles or packs of petri dishes) against their bodies. Although they are wearing clean room garments, they are not contamination free. Fibers and particles can be transferred onto the materials, and hence enter into the tissue

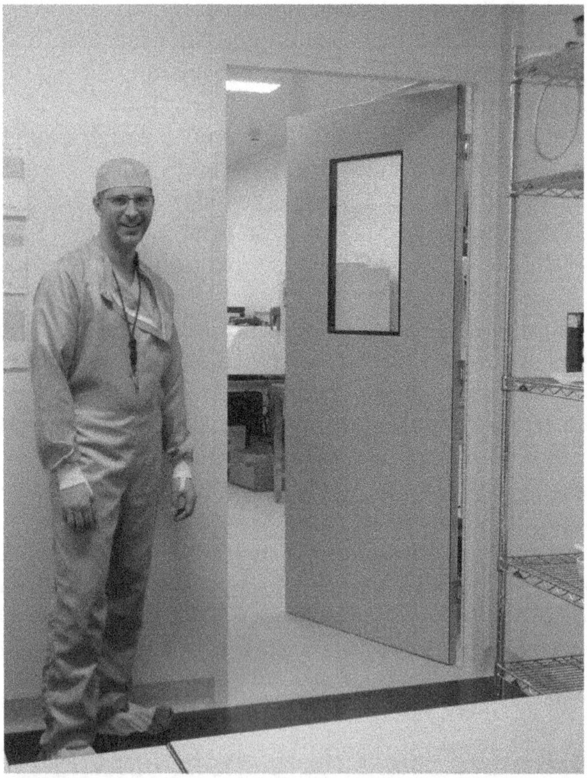

Figure 14.3 Doors without handles will assist in preventing transfer of contamination of hands or gloves. Hand or foot sensors for opening of the clean room doors is advised.

culture system. Plastic boxes are preferable to contain all the material needed for specific procedures or specific working stations.

Hands should not be put in the pockets, again to avoid spreading of particles and fibers when removing them from the pockets. Staff should try to avoid touching work surfaces. If personnel touch the mask or their garments, they will pick up particles and transfer them onto the surfaces. Hands grasped together in front of the body, in the style of a hospital surgeon, is the best way to prevent particle displacement.

Staff should not lean over the materials on the benches and flow cabinets, so they avoid fibers, particles, etc., to fall on or in the petri dishes, tubes, etc. IVF staff should not place themselves between the unidirectional flow of clean air and the materials in order to avoid a shower of particles deposited on the materials. IVF staff should not talk too much, cough, or sneeze, even when wearing a facemask because particles will be released from the mask. They must turn away the head from the benches or flow cabinets when doing so. Masks are replaced after sneezing or coughing.

All work is done under a tissue culture laminar flow cabinet. Standard aseptic working techniques will ensure that all cell culture procedures are performed in such a way that contamination from bacteria, fungi, and mycoplasma and cross-contamination are avoided. A movable glass panel or sash covers the face area of the tissue culture cabinet and acts as a physical barrier that helps to maintain a particulate-free environment and laminar air flow. Contamination by microorganisms may lead to subtle negative outcomes over time and may even be detrimental to embryo. For this reason, appropriate disinfection procedures and good personal hygiene are important factors in IVF clean rooms.[10]

Waste material should be collected into easily identified containers, one for glass pipettes and needles, one for bodily fluids, and one for overall waste. They should be removed frequently from the IVF clean room.

IVF staff must tidy up immediately when they are finished with each activity/handling and ensure that the clean room is properly cleaned.

14.6 Entrance and exit of samples into the clean room

14.6.1 Fresh semen samples

Semen preparation should be performed in a separate area or laboratory within the clean room, which is restricted to wet diagnosis and preparation of sperm samples. All tests that include fixation and staining of cells should be performed outside the clean room, to avoid spreading of the biocides in the air of the clean room.

Sperm samples are to be produced outside the clean room, but adjacent to it in a clean smoke-free area. Sperm containers are to be considered as contaminated on the outside surface because of handling of the container by the patient during production and the staff member on receipt. After correct identification check, sperm containers should be placed in a larger, clean container, hands are to be washed, and the container is to be transferred into the pass-through hatch of the andrology area. Staff in the andrology laboratory should never touch the sperm container itself but use a small sterile cotton cloth to open and close its lid, while holding the new clean container. Once opened, the sperm sample can be transferred into a correctly labeled sterile tube or container for further processing; the original sperm container can be discarded into the correct waste bin. Prepared semen samples can be left again in the wall mounted pass-through hatch (Figure 14.4).

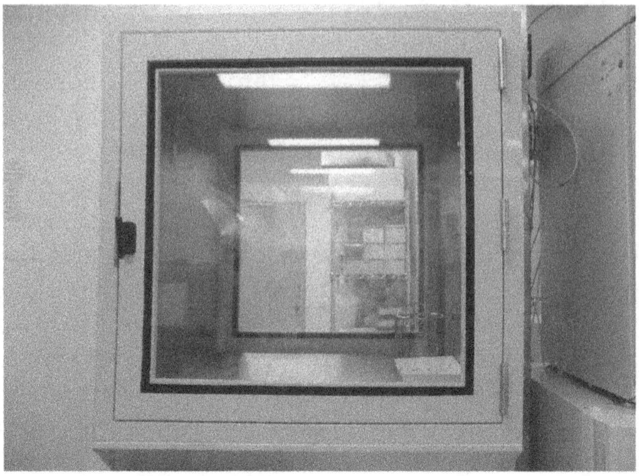

Figure 14.4 Wall mounted pass-through hatch for transfer of materials or samples (prepared semen samples, embryo transfer catheter, follicular fluid).

14.6.2 Follicular fluid

The oocyte retrieval room is located adjacent to the clean room. During oocyte retrieval, correctly labeled tubes with follicular fluid are collected in a sterile way and immediately transferred into a clean heated tube holder that is situated in the pass-through hatch between the oocyte collection room and the clean room. Staff in the IVF clean room will collect the tubes from this holder and transfer them into a new heated tube holder, and can start inspecting for oocytes.

14.6.3 Embryo transfer

A heated (37°C) pass-through hatch (Figure 14.4) is used for transfer of the embryo transfer catheter to the embryo transfer room that is located adjacent to the clean room. Staff in the embryo transfer room will notify laboratory staff when the embryo can be loaded into the embryo transfer catheter. After loading, the catheter is placed in a sterile packaging and transferred carefully into the heated hatch, for collection by trained staff in the embryo transfer room.

14.6.4 Cryopreserved materials

Cryopreserved samples like straws or vials with sperm cells, oocytes, or embryos have to enter the clean room as well for warming or thawing for further processing and culture. Samples are to be transferred from outside the clean room in a dry shipper or container with liquid nitrogen. The container is transferred by "outside" staff into the clean room via the material pass-through hatch or a room with a positive air pressure, but lower pressure than the clean room. Dry shippers or liquid nitrogen containers can only enter the clean room if properly cleaned; this can be done by the "outside" staff in the transfer room. Staff bringing the tank into the transfer room should leave the room. Air pressure in the material transfer room is restored to the correct pressure and staff from the clean room can now enter the transfer room to collect the dry shipper or container.

The exiting of cryopreserved samples is done in the same way of transfer through the material pass-through hatch or the material transfer room with positive air.

14.7 Cleaning and disinfecting

In a clean room, stringent and effective cleaning and decontamination protocols should be installed and followed carefully. Cleaning is the removal of contamination from the surfaces by physical means or by suitable agents. Disinfection is the process of reducing the number of microorganisms. Cleaning and disinfecting of walls, surfaces, benches, and the floor are essential in maintaining the standard clean room conditions. During the day, IVF staff should clean the working surface after each patient activity/handling. At the end of each day, a more thorough cleaning procedure for working surfaces and the floor is performed with the correct combination of products. A combination of different products should be used and in the correct order, ensuring cleaning actions, antibactericide as well as antisporicidal actions. A monthly rotation system should be installed in order to thoroughly clean cabinets, centrifuges, incubators, etc. At least once a year dedicated staff or a company should perform a complete deep cleaning of the clean room, including the walls and ceiling.

It is crucial that cleaning and decontamination products do not generate volatile organic compounds (VOCs) and that they are nonembryo toxic in order to avoid a negative impact on embryo development.[10] It should be ensured that appropriate bioassays have been applied to test their safety. Regular (three to four times a year) air quality and microbiological checks are to be planned in order to control the efficacy of the cleaning and decontamination protocols.

14.8 Exit from the IVF clean room facility by staff

When leaving the IVF clean room, the disposable garments should be discarded, and when re-entering, a new set of garments is to be used. If the same garments are to be used again on re-entry, they should be removed so that the outside of the garment is contaminated as little as possible.

14.9 Training of staff

Staff should be properly trained and instructed on how to dress, how to work in the IVF clean room, and how to clean. Auditing and retraining moments should be planned.

14.10 Conclusion

Working in an IVF clean room differs substantially from working in a traditional IVF laboratory because clean rooms have controlled levels of contamination of environmental pollutants such as dust particles, airborne microbes, aerosol particles, and chemical vapors. In order to maintain this low level of contamination, existing protocols for entrance, working, controlling, and maintenance need to be adapted or installed.

References

1. Boone WR, Johnson JE, Locke AJ, Crane MM 4th, and Price TM. Control of air quality in an assisted reproductive technology laboratory. *Fertil Steril* 1999; 71: 150–4.
2. Esteves SC and Bento FC. Implementation of air quality control in reproductive laboratories in full compliance with the Brazilian Cells and Germinative Tissue Directive. *Reprod Biomed Online* 2013; 26: 9–21.
3. Khoudja RY, Xu Y, Li T, and Zhou C. Better IVF outcomes following improvements in laboratory air quality. *J Assist Reprod Genet* 2013; 30: 69–76.

4. Whyte W. *Cleanroom Technology: Fundamentals of Design, Testing and Operation*. 2nd ed. John Wiley & Sons, Chichester, UK, 2010.
5. Whyte W. *Cleanroom Design*, John Wiley & Sons, Chichester, UK, 1999.
6. Sandle T. A review of cleanroom microflora: Types, trends, and patterns. *PDA J Pharm Sci Technol* 2011; 65: 392–403.
7. Nijs M, Franssen K, Cox A, Wissmann D, Ruis H, and Ombelet W. Reprotoxicity of intrauterine insemination and in vitro fertilization-embryo transfer disposables and products: A 4-year survey. *Fertil Steril* 2009; 92: 527–35.
8. Cohen J, Gilligan A, Esposito W, Schimmel T, and Dale B. Ambient air and its potential effects on conception in vitro. *Hum Reprod* 1997; 12: 1742–9.
9. Hall J, Gilligan A, Schimmel T, Cecchi M, and Cohen J. The origin, effects and control of air pollution in laboratories used for human embryo culture. *Hum Reprod* 1998; 13 (Suppl 4): 146–55.
10. Verheyen G, Sas S, Souffreau R et al. Toxicity testing of decontaminating agents and cleaning products used in human IVF laboratories. 30th Annual Meeting ESHRE, Munich, Germany, Abstract O72, ESHRE 2014.

chapter fifteen

Maintaining a clean in vitro fertilization laboratory

Sangita Jindal and Charlene A. Alouf

Contents

Abstract

IVF laboratories have been designed to provide optimal growth conditions for gametes in culture. Regardless of the environmental "hardware" in place, there are a number of "software" best practices that each laboratory can employ to ensure an optimal environment. Suboptimal laboratory environments expose human gametes and embryos to contamination and stress. Bacteria can cause degeneration of embryos, while fungus can retard embryonic development. All of these factors can impact embryo quality leading to lower pregnancy and live birth rates. Recently, epigenetic impairment due to stressful lab conditions has been described, providing yet another compelling reason to maintain a clean environment. Strategies for maintaining a clean IVF laboratory include development and review of protocols, quality assurance of reagents and equipment, quality control of the laboratory environment, and implementing simple checklists for proper maintenance. Each of these strategies can be customized for the end user, providing meaningful methods for optimizing culture conditions for oocytes, sperm, and embryos.

15.1 Introduction

Imagine the most sophisticated IVF laboratory in the world, engineered by experts and outfitted with the most up-to-date equipment. Now imagine that same laboratory being run by staff that is not committed to preserving a clean environment, and who do not follow a few practical guidelines for laboratory maintenance. Over time, the laboratory staff begins to notice that the number of expanded blastocysts has decreased, and pregnancy rates are dropping by a percentage point or two. Though there is no single cause they can pinpoint, the staff knows that something is not optimized in the engine that powers the IVF process.

The fact remains that regardless of the environmental "hardware" in place, the laboratory environment must be maintained as cleanly as possible in order to provide optimal growing conditions for the oocytes, sperm, and embryos. This involves containing or even eliminating possible sources of contamination to promote successful embryonic development and patient outcomes.

What classes of contaminants and stressors exist in and around IVF laboratories? The main toxicants measured in the air are low molecular weight aldehydes, air pollutants, and ozone.[1] Plastic ware and equipment may introduce chemical pollutants through off-gassing, and paper products may introduce particulate matter. Oocytes retrieved through the vaginal wall, and sperm delivered to the lab as semen, may be sources of bacteria, fungi, and viruses. Similarly, laboratory personnel are a common source of bacteria.

Given these and other potential sources of contamination, the task of maintaining a clean IVF laboratory requires a concerted and organized effort. In addition to standard protocols and excellent communication between team players,[2] a number of strategies are recommended to establish best practices for maintaining a clean environment. These include review of protocols, establishing checklists, maintaining quality assurance (QA) of reagents and equipment, and maintaining quality control (QC) of the lab environment. Each strategy can be customized for the end user, providing best practices for optimizing culture conditions for oocytes, sperm, and embryos.

15.2 Sources and types of contamination

15.2.1 Air

In recent years, the impact of air quality on IVF laboratory outcomes has been measured, quantified, and documented.[1–4] The four most potent air pollutants are

- Volatile organic compounds (VOCs)
- Small inorganic molecules such as nitrous oxide and carbon monoxide
- Substances derived from building materials such as aldehydes from flooring adhesives
- Other compounds such as aerosols, propellants, and heavy metals

These pollutants are introduced into the IVF laboratory most often by overuse of alcohol to wipe clean lab surfaces, thereby generating VOCs, off-gassing laboratory equipment, off-gassing laboratory supplies, anesthesia gasses, and refrigerants. Particulate matter may be introduced into laboratory air by paper and cardboard. Air also contains biological pollutants such as bacteria, fungi, and viruses.

15.2.2 *Physical plant and staff*

The IVF laboratory itself—which includes the floors, walls, ceilings, countertops, and heated surfaces—can be a major source of pollutants. A 2008 study demonstrated the challenge of maintaining a sterile controlled environment in a positive air flow operating room.[5] Forty-five sterile trays were opened using a sterile technique and were exposed for four hours. Bacterial culture specimens were obtained immediately after opening and every 30 minutes thereafter during the study period. Group 1 consisted of 15 trays that were opened and left uncovered in a locked operating room. Group 2 was identical to Group 1 with the addition of single-person traffic flowing in and out of the operating room from a non-sterile corridor every 10 minutes. Group 3 included 15 trays that were opened, immediately covered with a sterile surgical towel, and then left uncovered in a locked operating room.

The bacterial contamination rates recorded for the uncovered trays were 4% at 30 minutes, 15% at one hour, 22% at two hours, 26% at three hours, and 30% at four hours. There was no difference in contamination rate ($p = 0.69$) between the uncovered trays in the room with traffic and those in the room without traffic. The covered trays were not contaminated during the testing period. The survival time for those trays was significantly longer ($p = 0.03$) and the contamination rate was significantly lower ($p = 0.02$) than those for the uncovered trays. The authors concluded that culture positivity for bacteria correlated directly with the duration of exposure of the uncovered operating room trays.[5]

Foot traffic in and out of the laboratory is a significant source of pollutants into the laboratory environment. It has been estimated that humans shed roughly 1 billion skin cells daily[6], with each square centimeter of skin per human hand having a concentration of between 10^2 and 10^7 bacteria.[7,8] Desquamated human skin cells are an important contributor to particles in indoor air, and there is strong evidence that bacteria is associated with these skin cells.[6] Skin shedding may influence indoor air concentrations both through skin cells and their fragments directly becoming airborne, and also by deposition of cells onto floors and other surfaces followed by fragmentation and resuspension. Dust consists largely of skin cells and their accompanying bacteria.[9] Hospodsky et al. demonstrated that human occupancy produces a marked concentration increase of respirable particulate matter and bacterial genomes, and bacteria from human skin and from other environmental sources significantly contribute to indoor air bacterial populations.[9] The most common skin flora are *Staphylococcus epidermides, Staphylococcus aureus, Acinetobacter, Klebsiella,* and other enterobacters like *E. coli.*

Based on these and other published studies, it seems clear that many typical operations in an IVF laboratory can contribute to a suboptimal environment. Unpacking cardboard boxes, setting up gas tanks in or near the laboratory, and moving staff and sterile-wrapped plastic supplies in and out of a controlled environment such as an IVF laboratory can generate dust, dirt, and contaminants.

15.2.3 *Culture conditions*

Culture media and reagents may also be possible sources of contamination. A mineral or paraffin oil overlay employed during embryo culture provides temperature, pH, and osmolar stability. However, it has been demonstrated that oil may contain mold, zinc, or peroxides that cause sublethal cellular damage.[10–12] Depending on the storage conditions, peroxides may be generated which significantly and negatively impact blastocyst development. Therefore, it may be beneficial to wash oil with a protein-free medium in order to remove toxins.[13]

Chemical and biological toxins may be present or may be introduced by improper culture techniques. Water pans and baths and culture medium are strong aqueous sinks for many toxins; additionally, oil overlays are sinks for nonaqueous toxins.[14]

Most commercial suppliers of medium, medium supplements, or disposable plastic ware must adhere to stringent sterility requirements that greatly reduce the risk of contaminant transmission into the laboratory. Nonetheless, improper storage of IVF supplies or damage during packaging or storage could inadvertently result in contamination. Improper handling of any sterile device, such as allowing the outer wrap of a pipette to touch the sterile pipette, could result in the contamination of the culture medium. Attention must be paid to sterilization methods as some can produce residual toxicants. For example, a catheter should not be sterilized with ethylene oxide, as this could have deleterious effects on embryos.

All items from manufacturers and clinics should be sterilized properly in order to avoid the introduction of contaminants. Proper procedures for autoclaves and dry sterilizers must be followed, including regular monitoring of the effectiveness of these sterilizers using biological methods. Even the products of dead microorganisms (the lipopolysaccharide membrane of Gram-negative bacteria) can result in the destruction of embryos. For this reason, most fluids and contact materials are tested for endotoxins and must pass specific quality-control standards.

15.2.4 The patients

A source of contamination in the IVF laboratory that can best be controlled is the female patient who undergoes transvaginal oocyte retrieval, and the male patient who provides the seminal ejaculate. All biological fluids should be handled using standard precautions.

There are three major classifications of microbial contaminants that come from the female patient: fungi, bacteria, and viruses. The most common fungal contaminants in tissue cultures are *Aspergillus* (aerobic mold) and *C. albicans* (yeast). Common bacterial contaminants include *E. coli, mycoplasma, Staphylococcus,* and Gram-positive rods. Both bacteria and fungi have been identified in IVF cultures.[11,15,16] While bacterial contamination often results in the demise of the embryo, fungal contamination identified in the early stages seems not to harm the embryo. In a study by Ben-Chetrit et al., seven cases of fungal contamination resulted in pregnancies in all of the seven cases.[17] Embryos were merely washed free of the fungi and were then transferred. It may be that when fungi cause harm, it is either via depletion of energy substrates or a buildup of harmful metabolites. It appears that as long as the medium is replaced and fungal contaminants are removed, the embryos continue to grow.

Pelzer et al. examined the follicular fluid of 263 women undergoing oocyte retrieval for the presence of bacteria. They found bacteria in the follicular fluid of all 263 women. Seventy-one percent of the time these organisms were also cultured from the vagina, suggesting a vaginal source for the presence in the follicular fluid. This raises the question of whether some of these organisms might be introduced into the reproductive tract during follicular aspirations or even during embryo transfers. Some studies indicate that these contaminants can also result in lowered pregnancy rates when found in the vagina or uterus at the time of embryo transfer. Regardless of the source, follicular fluid is not sterile and could be one major source of contamination in the laboratory.[15]

In the semen, the prevalence of bacteriospermia has been well-documented,[18,19] and may range from 10 to 100%.[20] Microbial contamination of the semen sample collected for IVF could be of great importance as the natural defense mechanisms are compromised. Although centrifugation through gradient columns will reduce the microbial load of contaminated semen, it will not necessarily reduce it to zero, especially if the microbes bind to the sperm.[20] Bacteria in the sperm fraction can be contained by prophylactic treatment of the male with antibiotics or by sperm preparation in antibiotic-rich medium, which effectively eliminates 95% of organisms.[20] Apart from the herpes virus in semen, the presence of viruses has been less well documented. One study found that 83% of their study group (n = 172 men) had a herpes virus.[21] This included human herpes virus 6 (HHV6), Epstein-Barr virus (EBV), and cytomegalovirus (CMV). It appears that most semen is not sterile and likely contains bacteria and/or viruses.

15.3 Adopting a clean room philosophy

Given the numerous potential sources for and types of contamination described here and elsewhere, the challenge we face is to identify the best embryo-friendly practices for maintaining a clean IVF laboratory.

15.3.1 Testing

Most tests for IVF laboratory cleanliness are indirect. Unlike in-patient hospital stays and post-surgery assessments that measure length of stay, readmission rates, and outcome, culture conditions can only be tested by bioassay, which indirectly reflects the cleanliness of the environment. The mouse embryo assay (MEA) is widely used, though it has well-documented limitations.[22] Both the MEA and sperm bioassays measure chemical and biological contamination of the culture system.[10] Contaminants such as endotoxins, which are commonly found in purified water systems, may be specifically tested. Assessing embryo quality at discrete time points within the culturing process can be a useful way to measure the quality of the laboratory operations. Some feel that the quality of embryos derived from donor oocytes provides a "control" group for assessing optimal laboratory conditions.

15.3.2 Metrics

There are several studies that show a direct relationship between clean laboratory air and IVF cycle outcomes.[4,23–25] In a study of over 7400 women undergoing IVF, increases in nitrogen dioxide (NO_2) concentration both at the patient's home and at the IVF laboratory were significantly associated with a lower chance of pregnancy and live birth during all phases of the IVF cycle from medication start to pregnancy test (odds ratio [OR] 0.76, 95% confidence interval [CI] 0.66–0.86, per 0.01 ppm increase). After modeling for interactions of NO_2 and ozone at the IVF laboratory, NO_2 remained negatively and significantly associated with live births (OR 0.86, 95% CI 0.78–0.96).[4]

Several studies describe significantly improved IVF outcome measures after laboratories have been retrofitted with air filtration controls. In 2007, Merton et al. reported improved pregnancy rates ($p = 0.043$) for both fresh (46.3% vs. 41.0%) and frozen/thawed embryos (40.8% vs. 35.6%) following the transfer of in vitro–produced bovine embryos.[26] Improved implantation and clinical pregnancy rates and reduced no-transfer rates were seen by Dickey et al., following retrofitting of the air purification system in their human IVF laboratory.[23] In 2013, after retrofitting had been performed, Khoudja et al. saw significant improvements in fertilization rates (83.7% vs. 70.1%), embryo cleavage rates (97.35% vs. 90.8%), day 5 blastocyst formation rates (51.1% vs. 41.7%), and pregnancy/implantation rates (54.6%/34.4% vs. 40.6%/26.4%).[25] Finally, a study by Esteves and Bento compared outcomes between 255 couples treated at a conventional facility from the same practice before implementation of clean rooms and 2060 couples treated in the clean room facilities. No major fluctuations were observed in the clean room validation measurements over the study period. Live birth rates increased (35.6% vs. 25.8%; $p = 0.02$) and miscarriage rates decreased (28.7% vs. 20.0%; $p = 0.04$) in the first three months after clean room implementation.[24]

Recently, epigenetics and assisted reproductive technologies (ARTs) have been linked, specifically the exposure of early cleavage stage embryos to in vitro culture conditions in an IVF laboratory. ARTs involve several steps that subject the gametes and early developing embryos to environmental stressors, and this is the primary reason for an increased interest in the putative link between these techniques and epigenetic imprinting disorders. Although animal studies support such a link between ARTs and imprinting disorders via altered methylation patterns, data in humans are inconsistent.[27] Current ART protocols frequently employ prolonged in vitro culturing until the blastocyst stage before an embryo transfer, which results in higher pregnancy rates, higher implantation rates, and reduced multiple gestations. Extended exposure to and/or use of different types of culture medium during early embryo development potentially influences the process of remethylation.[27]

15.4 Strategies for keeping the laboratory clean

15.4.1 Best practices

The complexity of an IVF laboratory must be taken into account when assessing nonconformances. In the past 10 years, routine laboratory procedures during an IVF cycle, including documentation and record keeping, have gotten more complicated and involved. The American Society for Reproductive Medicine (ASRM) has recommended that clinics employ at least two embryologists per 150 cycles to maintain a safe environment.[28] In a recent updated version, the ratio between staffing and number of cycles was not included, but it remains true that the strict quality control (QC) and quality assurance (QA) required to maintain a clean IVF laboratory are easier with adequate laboratory staffing that minimizes the risk of shortcuts.[29]

Both ASRM and the European Society of Human Reproduction and Embryology (ESHRE) have published best practices guidelines for IVF laboratories. These guidelines are revised as needed as the field advances and innovations are introduced.[29,30] The guidelines address such topics as laboratory staffing, embryologist certification, laboratory design, policies and procedures, equipment, and safety measures. They are useful as a reference and foundation for creating end-user QA and quality management (QM) programs that monitor critical indicators of patient care and create an environment that provides consistent optimal culture conditions.

QC includes all activities or operational techniques within a process, and addresses both tangible elements (personnel, instruments, equipment, and supplies) and intangible elements (techniques, protocols, documentation, and record-keeping).[32,33] The main goal of QC is to evaluate the effectiveness of policies and procedures, identify and correct problems, assure the accuracy and precision of procedures, and monitor the performance and competency of the laboratory staff.[33]

QA provides a systematic monitoring of the testing process in order to help identify problems, errors, or improvements that may have occurred.[30,32] Results should be evaluated on a regular basis, indicators should be objective and relevant, and adequate thresholds should be established. Critical levels of laboratory performance for each indicator should be defined. While these indicators evaluate the entire process in the lab, they also indirectly reflect the ability to provide optimal culture conditions that are predicated on maintaining a clean IVF laboratory.

Assessing QA in an IVF laboratory presents certain difficulties: the final anticipated outcome is an ongoing pregnancy, which entails numerous components that are beyond the control of the laboratory. Therefore, common QM systems that apply a process approach and are directed to the end product of the process cannot readily be implemented in IVF laboratories.[31–34] The following indicators, however, can be regularly reviewed, analyzed, and discussed: rates of normally fertilized eggs, cleavage rates, rates of embryos of good quality, proportion of patients with failed fertilization, ongoing clinical pregnancy rates (fresh and frozen/thawed transfers), and implantation rates.[30,33]

Unfortunately, identifying a true decline in performance often occurs several weeks later when pregnancy rates decline, delaying the implementation of corrective action. Therefore, it is essential to establish minimal risk strategies in the form of a strict discipline of routines and procedures ensuring QC and QA. Attention to quality is a dynamic exercise, to be clearly defined and documented with general policies and delegation of responsibilities, carried out with continuous monitoring.[31–34]

15.4.2 Controlling the laboratory environment

15.4.2.1 Air

Two of the most common contaminants in laboratory air are VOCs and bio-pollutants. Therefore, the lab should have a dedicated and specialized air handling system (positive pressure, higher filtration, and higher frequency of air exchanges) and climate controls (temperature and humidity). The air handling system should function according to set parameters. Periodic testing for VOCs in the laboratory air should be implemented.

Air filtration systems should ideally be installed at the time of laboratory construction. Less ideally, laboratories may be retrofitted and/or floor units containing fans and an air filter may be placed in the lab. Most modern-day laboratories have installed into their air systems some or all of these air filters: high efficiency particulate air (HEPA), carbon, and/or potassium permanganate.[24] Additionally, the following modifications may be made to the environment in order to help control air contamination:

a. Frequent hand washing and glove changes between patients.
b. Use high-quality distilled water in the lab. This is high-purity, non-pyrogenic, endotoxin- and MEA-tested commercially available water for embryo culture. This should be used to clean surfaces and to dilute cleansers as described below.
c. Equip IVF laboratories with laminar flow hoods. These confined workspaces with stable vertical unidirectional flow (laminar) provide protection against contamination of items in the hood. Laminar flow hoods have HEPA filters and should be turned on at full (high) fan speed each morning 10 minutes prior to beginning embryology tasks in order to recirculate the air through the filter. One of the problems with any hood is that the insertion of items like a microscope into the airflow can result in contaminating that air. Further, these hoods are difficult to properly sterilize due to the volatiles used for sterilization.

d. Reduce the use of 70% ethyl alcohol (ethanol) when cleaning surfaces. The level of alcohol measured varies from laboratory to laboratory.[1] Alcohol used to wipe down surfaces becomes airborne, introducing VOCs into the laboratory air, which can deposit into the incubator humidifying water pans and open culture dishes. Make 70% ethanol with distilled water, apply to a lint-free wipe (e.g., gauze) and clean surfaces such as door handles. This can be followed directly with a distilled water wipe.
e. Clean laboratory surfaces regularly with distilled water and decontaminate with peroxide. Only distilled water should be used routinely with a lint-free wipe to clean surfaces of hoods, counters, and heating stages. For decontamination of surfaces including the hood between oocyte retrievals and after the last retrieval, use 6% hydrogen peroxide on a lint-free wipe followed by a rinse with distilled water.
f. Change water pans bi-monthly. In order to reduce the chance of water pan contamination and to maintain appropriate humidity levels, water pans should be replaced twice a month with new sterilized pans filled with prewarmed distilled water. Pans should be rinsed with the same water and allowed to off-gas in the hood prior to use. While changing the water pans, also wipe down the internal surfaces of the incubators with distilled water and a lint-free sterile wipe.
g. Clean incubators one or two times per year. Using a lint-free sterile wipe, all incubator doors, shelves, seals, walls, and handles should be wiped down with 6% hydrogen peroxide (30% hydrogen peroxide diluted with distilled water) followed by a generous rinse with distilled water. Apply the peroxide with a sterile wipe, so as not to bathe the incubator with it. Elbow grease is the key to successful cleaning, not a high volume of reagent.
h. Annual cleaning/decontamination. Once per year it is beneficial to give the incubators a more thorough decontamination during a period of non-use. A dilute solution of bezalkonium chloride (1:2000 dilution of the stock purchased solution [50%] dilute with distilled water) should be applied sparingly with a sterile lint-free wipe to all surfaces and shelves. Elbow grease is the key to successful decontamination. Rinse twice with distilled water and dry with a sterile wipe.
i. Biennial decontamination. If access to a large autoclave is available, the autoclavable components of the incubators should be disassembled and sent for autoclaving every two years. Once returned to the laboratory, remove components from the sterile packaging, and wipe all components with distilled water and a sterile lint-free wipe. If central sterilizing or autoclaving is not available, then perform the annual decontamination procedure using the working dilution (1:2000) of benzalkonium chloride on all surfaces of the disassembled incubator as described above.
j. Clean laboratory floors and procedure rooms with 7X cleaner or 3% hydrogen peroxide. 7X is a low-VOC cleaner diluted 1:7 with distilled water. Alternatively, commercially available 3% hydrogen peroxide can be applied to a large lint-free wipe to clean the floors. Follow with a rinse using distilled water.

15.4.2.2 *Physical plant and staff*

The following modifications should be made to the laboratory environment in order to help control the physical plant and the laboratory staff:

a. Ensure that the IVF laboratory is a protected and secure space. It should be protected from potentially toxic chemicals such as cleaning supplies, detergents, fragrances, and fumes as much as possible.

b. Restrict access to the laboratory and procedure room. Service technicians and other authorized visitors should always be accompanied.
c. Require embryologists and other authorized personnel to always wear scrubs, mask, and head and shoe covers.
d. Place sticky mats or tacky mats directly outside the laboratory door to capture dirt and dust from footwear as people are entering the laboratory.
e. Urge embryologists to wash their hands and exposed arms with biological soap (e.g., soap containing 4% chlorohexidine gluconate) and tap water each time they enter the lab. The MSDS of the biological soap should be reviewed and only soap without known hazardous ingredients should be used. Not all soaps have been evaluated for reproductive toxicity, unfortunately.
f. Insist that embryologists be attentive to sterile techniques. Skin cells and bacteria can exfoliate while reaching over dishes and cause inadvertent contamination.
g. Confirm that no painting, renovation, or repair is being done around the laboratory.
h. Ensure that noise and vibration levels are acceptable.

15.4.2.3 Protocols and workflow

Laboratory protocols and workflow should be reviewed to ensure the efficiency of all laboratory and clinical procedures. Protocols should require attention to detail and to sterile technique at all times. Maintenance of a clean IVF laboratory requires optimization of the QC and QA protocols in particular. The following is a list of possible QC and QA protocols that may be used to create a personalized QM program:

a. Document all QC, QA, and any corrective action in order to provide transparency and accountability.
b. Create a program to reduce or eliminate hazardous materials such as mercury thermometers and sterilizing products that contain ethylene glycol, betadine, or are otherwise embryotoxic.
c. Schedule and monitor equipment QC and QA. Tolerance limits on equipment should be observed at all times in order to maintain optimal culture conditions. The physical condition of equipment should be monitored in order to avoid breakdown, overuse, or expiry that can introduce contaminants into the laboratory environment. For example, overuse of gas tanks below 400 psi can stir up contaminants from the bottom of the tank into the gas supply. In addition, incubator seals can break down from overheating, dust buildup can occur in equipment not routinely used, and degradation of tubing can introduce contaminants into the gas supply.
d. Regularly schedule equipment QA for laminar flow hoods, incubators, and microscopes to ensure proper operation and cleanliness. All equipment should undergo an electrical safety inspection annually.
e. Establish scheduled testing of the laboratory environment by bioassays such as the mouse embryo assay and the sperm survival assay. Both can be used to detect any possible chemical and biological contamination of the culture system and thereby indirectly contribute to the cleanliness of the laboratory environment.
f. Change and clean distilled water and 70% ethanol bottles monthly.
g. Test the air handling system at least annually for pressure and balancing.
h. Test the air filtration system at least annually for new filtration substrate.

15.4.2.4 Items allowed in the laboratory

The following modifications may be made in order to help control what enters the laboratory:

a. Movement into the laboratory should be restricted. Only staff that needs to be in the laboratory should be permitted to enter attired appropriately in scrubs, mask, and hat and shoe covers.
b. Supplies should be unpacked outside the laboratory area in order to not bring in cardboard and increase the air particulate count. Supplies that are sterile and wrapped in plastic should be stored in cabinets or drawers to minimize introduction of off-gassing compounds into the air.
c. All new equipment should be off-gassed prior to placement in the laboratory in order to minimize VOC content in the environment.
d. No hand sanitizer, which is high in alcohol and therefore VOC content, should be used in the laboratory.
e. Only biological soap and water should be used routinely to wash hands and arms prior to entering the laboratory. If a new cleaning product is introduced, it must be reviewed and approved prior to use.
f. Areas should be designated as "clean" and require glove use at all times. Areas should be designated as "dirty" where items such as paperwork, computer work, cell phone use, etc., occur. As we live in a society where cell phones go everywhere (we may send and receive texts from clinical staff members during the day), it should be wiped clean before entry into the laboratory and used only during restricted times. A cell phone or tablet that is used routinely outside of the laboratory is one of the most highly contaminated items we own.

15.4.2.5 What is removed from the laboratory

The following modifications may be made to the environment in order to help control what is removed from the laboratory:

a. Biological waste should be removed daily from the laboratory and after every retrieval, if possible. Wash hands after removing and installing new bags.
b. Regular waste should be removed as needed from the laboratory.
c. Biological fluids (semen, serum, follicular aspirates) are to be handled with standard precautions, including the wearing of nonpowdered gloves and masks, and within a laminar flow hood if possible. If a spill of a biological fluid occurs, the material should be wiped up with a lint-free wipe and the surface should be cleaned with 10% bleach or 6% hydrogen peroxide (first applied to the lint-free wipe and not sprayed onto the surface), followed by wiping with distilled water applied to a lint-free wipe. This way the biological material is neutralized by the bleach but the air in the laboratory has minimal introduction of VOCs due to the rinse with distilled water.
d. If there is any concern that a product is contaminating the laboratory environment, it should be removed from use, evaluated for toxicity by the vendor or by bioassay, and replaced with a tested product. If there has been a change in supplies (e.g., gloves, syringes, plastic ware, etc.), all new supplies should be tested by bioassay prior to use.

15.4.2.6 Create a culture among the staff

The most important way to ensure a clean laboratory environment is to create an atmosphere of discipline, effective communication, and general attention to detail among the staff. The laboratory should have clear and documented QC and QA programs that are implemented daily and officially reviewed annually by all staff. Regular staff meetings can help with clarifying protocols, setting goals, assigning responsibility, and fostering a team environment through open communication. Laboratory maintenance and cleanliness can be reviewed periodically with emphasis given as needed to areas in need of remediation.

15.4.3 Checklists

In *The Checklist Manifesto*, published in 2009, Dr. Atul Gawande describes the valuable and critical use of checklists in a number of professions.[35] Using his own research, he designed a study to apply checklists to medicine and specifically to surgery, the findings of which were published in the *New England Journal of Medicine*.[36] Dr. Gawande and the other authors concluded that implementation of the checklist was associated with concomitant reductions in the rates of death and complications among patients at least 16 years of age who were undergoing noncardiac surgery in a diverse group of hospitals.

There are valuable lessons to be learned here. Checklists, as Dr. Gawande demonstrates, provide a kind of cognitive net, catching mental errors of memory, attention, and thoroughness. They allow for tracking and for communication and can make the reliable management of maintaining a clean IVF lab a routine. Checklists supply a set of checks to ensure that routine but critical items are not overlooked. They also supply another set of checks to ensure that people talk and coordinate and accept responsibility while maintaining the power to manage nuances.

Good checklists are precise, efficient, and easy to use in the most difficult of situations. They are not meant to be comprehensive but instead provide a reminder of only the most critical and important steps in any given process. Above all, checklists are practical. When making a checklist, there are a number of key factors to consider.

First, define a clear "pause point" at which the checklist is supposed to be used. This might be the moment just before starting the work of the day, or conversely the moment before closing the lab for the night. A pause point should be repeated daily at the same time so that it becomes routine.

Second, decide if you want a DO–CONFIRM or READ–DO checklist. In a DO–CONFIRM checklist, team members perform ("do") their job from memory or experience. Then they pause to run the checklist and confirm that everything that was supposed to be done was indeed performed. With a READ–DO checklist, tasks are carried out as they are checked off. It is important to pick the type of checklist that makes the most sense for maintaining a clean IVF laboratory. The rule of thumb is five to nine items on the checklist with simple and exact wording that fits on one page and is free of clutter and unnecessary colors.

Just checking boxes is not the ultimate goal of a checklist; embracing a culture of teamwork and discipline is. The checklist is a reflection of our code of conduct as individuals and as a team working in an IVF laboratory: selflessness, an expectation of skill, an expectation of trustworthiness, and discipline.

An example of a possible DO–CONFIRM checklist for an IVF laboratory is shown in Table 15.1.

Table 15.1 Checklist for maintaining a clean IVF laboratory

Checklist Category	Example of Activity on Checklist
Hygiene	Did you start by washing your hands with soap and water?
Cleaning	Did you finish by wiping down surfaces with distilled water?
Air flow	Are the laminar flow hood fans on during the day?
Waste removal	Has the regular waste and biological waste been removed?
Protocols	Have detailed protocols for daily shutdown been followed?

15.4.4 Audits

Audits are part of a good QA and QM program. This is the review of the prescribed procedures, often in the form of checking the standard operating procedures and rearranging the procedures if required. A system that monitors the individual performance of team members with regular appraisal is also helpful in maintaining an optimal standard of results. Measurement and feedback are crucial elements in quality management, which means that assessments and audits, both internal and external, should be applied systematically and periodically. The result is increased transparency and traceability, which helps refine the best practices that a laboratory establishes to maintain a clean environment.[37]

15.5 Conclusion

Maintaining a clean IVF laboratory is the first and last step in providing optimal embryology for the patient. Many engineering controls are used in the design and construction to ensure that laboratory access and air quality are controlled. Quality control and quality assurance programs are established and utilized on an ongoing basis to ensure that best practices are being followed and that the measures of embryology success are appropriate. Finally, embryologists individually and collectively as a team must create a culture of discipline and attention to detail in order to maintain the laboratory daily. Simple checklists may be helpful in ensuring that important basic tasks are completed, thus enabling the embryologist to focus on the art and science of embryology.

References

1. Cohen J, Gilligan A, Esposito W, Schimmel T, and Dale B. Ambient air and its potential effects on conception in vitro. *Hum Reprod* 1997; 12: 1742–9.
2. Van Voorhis BJ, Thomas M, Surrey ES, and Sparks A. What do consistently high-performing in vitro fertilization programs in the U.S. do? *Fertil Steril* 2010; 94: 1346–9.
3. Hall J, Gilligan A, Schimmel T, Cecchi M, and Cohen J. The origin, effects and control of air pollution in laboratories used for human embryo culture. *Hum Reprod* 1998; 13 Suppl 4: 146–55.
4. Legro RS, Sauer MV, Mottla GL, Richter KS, Li X, Dodson WC et al. Effect of air quality on assisted human reproduction. *Hum Reprod* 2010; 25: 1317–24.
5. Dalstrom DJ, Venkatarayappa I, Manternach AL, Palcic MS, Heyse BA, and Prayson MJ. Time-dependent contamination of opened sterile operating-room trays. *J Bone Joint Surg Am* 2008; 90: 1022–5.
6. Milstone LM. Epidermal desquamation. *J Dermat Sci* 2004; 36: 131–40.
7. Leyden JJ, McGinley KJ, Nordstrom KM, and Webster GF. Skin microflora. *J Invest Dermat* 1987; 88: 65s–72s.
8. Ritter MA. Operating room environment. *Clin Orthop Res* 1999: 103–109.

9. Hospodsky D, Qian J, Nazaroff WW, Yamamoto N, Bibby K, Rismani-Yazdi H et al. Human occupancy as a source of indoor airborne bacteria. *PLoS One* 2012; 7: e34867.
10. Hughes PM, Morbeck DE, Hudson SB, Fredrickson JR, Walker DL, and Coddington CC. Peroxides in mineral oil used for in vitro fertilization: Defining limits of standard quality control assays. *J Assist Reprod Genet* 2010; 27: 87–92.
11. Kastrop PM, de Graaf-Miltenburg LA, Gutknecht DR, and Weima SM. Microbial contamination of embryo cultures in an ART laboratory: Sources and management. *Hum Reprod* 2007; 22: 2243–8.
12. Otsuki J, Nagai Y and Chiba K. Damage of embryo development caused by peroxidized mineral oil and its association with albumin in culture. *Fertil Steril* 2009; 91: 1745–9.
13. Morbeck DE, Khan Z, Barnidge DR, and Walker DL. Washing mineral oil reduces contaminants and embryotoxicity. *Fertil Steril* 2010; 94: 2747–52.
14. Miller KF, Goldberg JM, and Collins RL. Covering embryo cultures with mineral oil alters embryo growth by acting as a sink for an embryotoxic substance. *J Assist Reprod Genet* 1994; 11: 342–5.
15. Pelzer ES, Allan JA, Waterhouse MA, Ross T, Beagley KW, and Knox CL. Microorganisms within human follicular fluid: Effects on IVF. *PLoS One* 2013; 8: e59062.
16. Selman H, Mariani M, Barnocchi N, Mencacci A, Bistoni F, Arena S et al. Examination of bacterial contamination at the time of embryo transfer, and its impact on the IVF/pregnancy outcome. *J Assist Reprod Genet* 2007; 24: 395–9.
17. Ben-Chetrit A, Shen O, Haran E, Brooks B, Geva-Eldar T, and Margalioth EJ. Transfer of embryos from yeast-colonized dishes. *Fertil Steril* 1996; 66: 335–7.
18. Kiessling AA, Desmarais BM, Yin HZ, Loverde J, and Eyre RC. Detection and identification of bacterial DNA in semen. *Fertil Steril* 2008; 90: 1744–56.
19. Moretti E, Capitani S, Figura N, Pammolli A, Federico MG, Giannerini V et al. The presence of bacteria species in semen and sperm quality. *J Assist Reprod Genet* 2009; 26: 47–56.
20. Cottell E, Lennon B, McMorrow J, Barry-Kinsella C, and Harrison RF. Processing of semen in an antibiotic-rich culture medium to minimize microbial presence during in vitro fertilization. *Fertil Steril* 1997; 67: 98–103.
21. Neofytou E, Sourvinos G, Asmarianaki M, Spandidos DA, and Makrigiannakis A. Prevalence of human herpes virus types 1-7 in the semen of men attending an infertility clinic and correlation with semen parameters. *Fertil Steril* 2009; 91: 2487–94.
22. Gardner DK, Reed L, Linck D, Sheehan C, and Lane M. Quality control in human in vitro fertilization. *Semin Reprod Med* 2005; 23: 319–24.
23. Dickey RP, Wortham Jr JWE, Potts A, and Welch A. Effect of IVF laboratory air quality on pregnancy success. *Fertil Steril* 2010; 94 Suppl 4: S151.
24. Esteves SC and Bento FC. Implementation of air quality control in reproductive laboratories in full compliance with the Brazilian Cells and Germinative Tissue Directive. *Reprod Biomed Online* 2013; 26: 9–21.
25. Khoudja RY, Xu Y, Li T, and Zhou C. Better IVF outcomes following improvements in laboratory air quality. *J Assist Reprod Genet* 2013; 30: 69–76.
26. Merton JS, Vermeulen ZL, Otter T, Mullaart E, de Ruigh L, and Hasler JF. Carbon-activated gas filtration during in vitro culture increased pregnancy rate following transfer of in vitro-produced bovine embryos. *Theriogenology* 2007; 67: 1233–8.
27. Iliadou AN, Janson PC, and Cnattingius S. Epigenetics and assisted reproductive technology. *J Int Med* 2011; 270: 414–20.
28. Practice Committee of American Society for Reproductive Medicine and Practice Committee of Society for Assisted Reproductive Technology. Revised guidelines for human embryology and andrology laboratories. *Fertil Steril* 2008; 90: S45–59.
29. Practice Committee of the American Society for Reproductive Medicine; Practice Committee of the Society for Assisted Reproductive Technology; Practice Committee of the Society of Reproductive Biologists and Technologists. Recommended practices for the management of embryology, andrology, and endocrinology laboratories: A committee opinion. *Fertil Steril* 2014; 102(4): 960–3.

30. Magli MC, Van den Abbeel E, Lundin K, Royere D, Van der Elst J, and Gianaroli L. Revised guidelines for good practice in IVF laboratories. *Hum Reprod* 2008; 23: 1253–62.
31. Kastrop PM. Quality management in the ART laboratory. *Reproductive Biomedicine Online* 2003; 7: 691–694.
32. Esteves S and Agarwal A. Ensuring that reproductive laboratories provide high-quality services. In: Bento F, Esteves S, and Agarwal A (eds.). *Quality Management in ART Clinics*. Springer US 2013, pp. 129–46.
33. Esteves S and Agarwal A. Defining what reproductive laboratories do. In: Bento F, Esteves S, and Agarwal A (eds.). *Quality Management in ART Clinics*. Springer US 2013, pp. 75–8.
34. Esteves S and Agarwal A. Explaining how reproductive laboratories work. In: Bento F, Esteves S, and Agarwal A (eds.). *Quality Management in ART Clinics*. Springer US 2013, pp. 75–127.
35. Gawande A. *The Checklist Manifesto*, 2009. Picador, New York.
36. Haynes AB, Weiser TG, Berry WR, Lipsitz SR, Breizat AH, Dellinger EP et al. A surgical safety checklist to reduce morbidity and mortality in a global population. *N Engl J Med* 2009; 360: 491–9.
37. Bento F. How to get information. In: Bento F, Esteves S, and Agarwal A (eds.). *Quality Management in ART Clinics*. Springer US 2013, pp. 59–68.

chapter sixteen

Clean room certification in assisted reproductive technology clinics

Alcir Leal dos Santos

Contents

Abstract

This chapter provides health care professionals working in assisted reproductive technology (ART) units equipped with clean room facilities knowledge and guidance on the concepts and definitions concerning clean room testing and certification processes. The standards and procedures detailed in this chapter are the minimum requirements to be followed by certified firms when performing clean room testing and certification procedures.

16.1 Introduction

Clean rooms and related controlled environments provide contamination control for particles in air suspension thus ensuring that activities sensitive to contamination are carried out in a safe environment. Aerospace, pharmaceutical, operating theaters, and assisted reproductive techniques (ARTs) are among the activities that benefit from air contamination control.

When clean room installations are completed, there is a need to prepare for certification with the purpose of validating clean room design and operational conditions. Invariably, at this stage, air flow balancing and differential pressure adjustments are paramount. Certification guarantees that facilities meet minimum requirements for a maximum concentration of specified-size airborne particles.

In this chapter, we will focus on the clean room certification process in accordance with the norm ISO 14.644 (Parts 1 to 3) issued by the International Organization for Standardization.[1–3] As for any testing, attention should be placed on specific operational requirements including a risk analysis of the installation concerned.

In some regions, including the European Union and Brazil, regulatory agencies enforce specific requirements regarding air quality control to in vitro fertilization (IVF) laboratories.[4] Under such regulations, testing and certification processes should be adapted to comply with both international and national standards tests. A detailed description of air quality control requirements as per Brazilian legislation is presented in Chapter 18.

16.2 Definitions

Airborne particle: Solid or liquid object, viable or nonviable, suspended in air.
Air cleanliness classification: A specified level of airborne particulate cleanliness applicable to a clean room or clean zone, expressed in terms of a cleanliness class, in accordance with a referenced standard.

Clean room certification according to occupational status:

As built: Defines a clean room fully built and operational, with all services connected and operational, but without equipment or personnel within the facility. This certification is most common because any failures at this stage can be immediately addressed and corrected by the clean room designers and builders.

At rest: Defines a clean room fully constructed and operational, with production equipment installed and operating (or operable), but with no personnel within the facility. This certification demonstrates compliance as per the design and requirements agreed between customer and supplier. Clean rooms that were modified also require "At Rest" certification.

Operational: Defines a clean room in normal operation, including equipment and personnel. This certification may occur after a partial—or full—complement of equipment is installed within the clean room. The intention is to demonstrate compliance with cleanliness standards. According to a Brazilian Cell and Tissue Directive[4] testing should be performed, whenever possible, with the facility operational. Exceptions apply when specific conditions prevent testing under operation, such as those related to the integrity of biological material; then simulation of routine activities should be done as close as possible to real conditions.

Clean room: A specially constructed room in which the air supply, air distribution, filtration of air supply, materials of construction, and operating procedures are regulated to control airborne particle concentrations to meet appropriate cleanliness levels and other relevant parameters (e.g., temperature, humidity, pressure, etc.) as defined by ISO 14644 or any other regulatory entity. Such environments are built and utilized to minimize the introduction, generation, and retention of particles.

Clean zone/clean area: A defined or dedicated space in which the concentration of airborne particles is controlled to specified limits or cleanliness levels and other relevant parameters (e.g., temperature, humidity, pressure) as defined by ISO 14644 or any other regulatory entity.

Contamination: The presence of any unwanted substance, material, or energy that adversely affects a product or procedure in a clean room.

Particle size: Diameter of the reference droplet that can generate an equivalent response to that of the particle being assessed by a measurement instrument.

Unidirectional air flow clean room: Controlled air flow through the entire cross section of a clean zone with a uniform velocity and approximately parallel air stream that is no greater than 14 degrees from plumb.

16.3 *Clean room certification process*

The certification process of a given clean room or clean zone consists in performing several tests, described henceforth, with the final goal of verifying compliance to meet the established acceptance criteria.

Only qualified and certified technicians or engineers who are duly graduated and formally registered in their respective boards should perform testing and certification. All test instruments should be calibrated to ensure precise and accurate readings. Precision relates to the ability of an instrument to produce repeatable readings under the same conditions. The accuracy of an instrument is the capability of that instrument to indicate the true value of a measured parameter.

16.3.1 *Tests*

This section provides an overview of clean room tests and their related procedures. Certification tests and procedures may vary from project to project. The choice of certification tests may be based on the cleanliness class level, type of clean room air flow, occupancy mode, and the product produced. As already mentioned, the scope of the clean room testing services should be based on international and national (if any) standards and contract document requirements agreed between the ART center and the certified firm.

The tests are related to airborne particulate cleanliness classes as required by ISO 14644 as well as particle and air movement. By performing these tests, the clean room will be correctly classified to the appropriate class level.

- HEPA filter integrity
- Airborne particle counting
- Air flow velocity and uniformity
- Clean room differential pressure
- Clean room recovery time (particle fallout rate)
- Filter saturation level

- Relative humidity and temperature of ambient air
- Lighting levels
- Noise levels
- Smoke test
- Air flow parallelism

16.3.2 How and why tests should be performed

16.3.2.1 HEPA filter integrity assessment

High efficiency particulate air (HEPA) filters are extended media, dry-type filters mounted in a rigid frame having a minimum particle-collection efficiency of 99.97% for 0.3 μm particulate at a rated air flow.

After installation, HEPA filters should be tested for leaks. This test is performed to confirm that HEPA filters are properly installed and operational. Test procedures include verification for any relevant leakage that might have occurred during installation, and that filters do not contain any defect such as puncture leakage, damaged filtration media, sealing and frame structure defects, and rack fixture.

HEPA filter integrity is evaluated by first injecting a known aerosol, usually dioctil phthalate (DOP) or poly alpha olefin (PAO) containing 0.3 μm particles in the upstream side of the filtration system. Subsequently, the aerosol concentration in a sample taken from the downstream side of the filtration system is compared with a similar measurement of

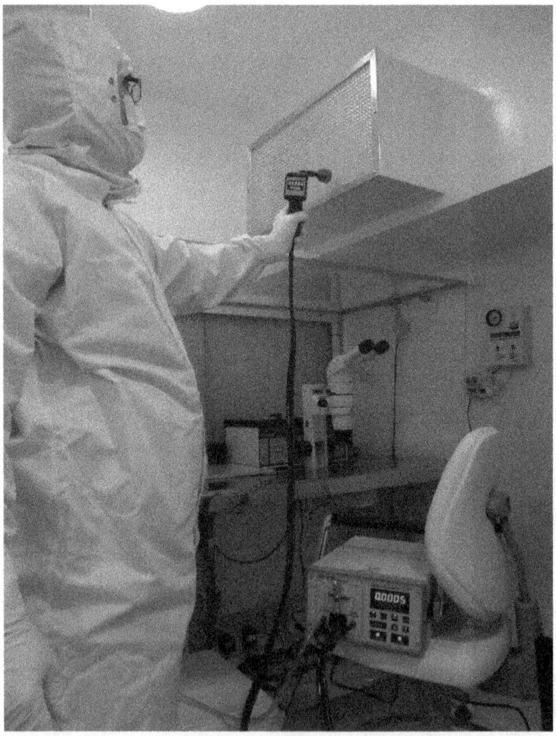

Figure 16.1 **(See color insert.)** In situ testing of HEPA filter installation. Photograph showing an engineer testing a HEPA terminal filter in the clean room IVF laboratory. (Courtesy of Androfert, Campinas, Brazil.)

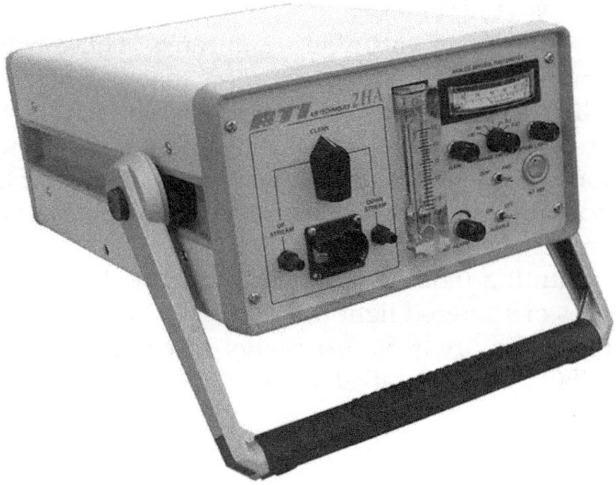

Figure 16.2 Aerosol photometer.

aerosol concentration in a sample taken from upstream side of the filtration system (Figure 16.1). Using a photometer, leaks are normally characterized by readings that are greater than 0.01% of the upstream challenge.

HEPA filter integrity assessment requires a photometer (Figure 16.2) and an aerosol generator (Figure 16.3).

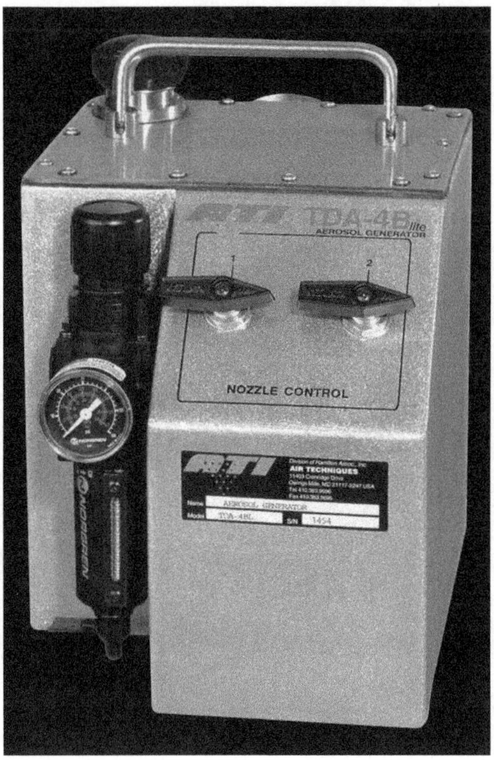

Figure 16.3 Aerosol generator.

16.3.2.2 *Airborne particle counting*

This test is performed to classify air cleanliness and consists of drawing a predefined volume of air from different points within the clean room to measure the number of particles of various sizes according to the ISO 14644-1 norm (Table 16.1). ISO 14644-1 establishes standard classes of air cleanliness for clean rooms and clean zones based on specified concentrations of airborne particulates. The number and location of measurement points should be in compliance with the aforesaid norm, but specific points can be monitored as per agreement between supplier and customer.

Airborne particle counting requires an electronic particle counter (Figure 16.4). The instrument counts pulses of scattered light from particles. The test probe is kept pointing upward during monitoring (Figure 16.5). Test results are compared with the specific allowable particle limits per ISO class as detailed in Table 16.1, and the clean room or clean area is classified accordingly.

Table 16.1 ISO classification (ISO 14.644-1) versus maximum particle concentration allowed

ISO classification	Maximum concentration limit of each particle size in m^3 per cleanliness class					
	0.1 μm	0.2 μm	0.3 μm	0.5 μm	1 μm	5 μm
1	10	2	–	–	–	–
2	100	24	10	4	–	–
3	1000	237	102	35	8	–
4	10,000	2370	1020	352	83	–
5	100,000	23,700	10,200	3520	832	29
6	1,000,000	237,000	102,000	35,200	8320	293
7	–	–	–	352,000	83,200	2930
8	–	–	–	3,520,000	832,000	29,300
9	–	–	–	35,200,000	8,320,000	293,000

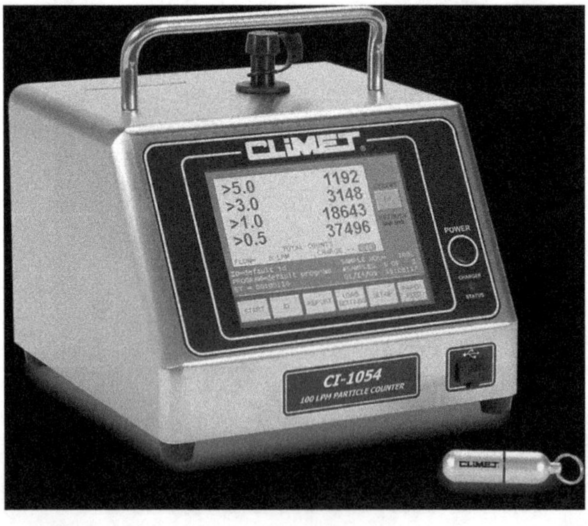

Figure 16.4 Particle counter.

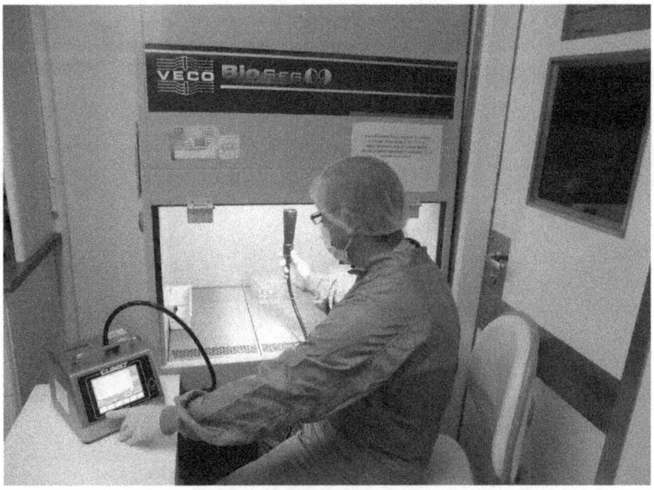

Figure 16.5 **(See color insert.)** Particle counting in Class II biosafety cabinet. (Courtesy of Androfert, Campinas, Brazil.)

16.3.2.3 Air flow velocity and volume

This test is performed to determine that the air flow velocity and volume of air supplied meet clean room design specifications. The data collected allow calculation of the total air volume injected, and is used to determine the number of air changes per hour. The latter represents the number of times the total air volume of a defined space is replaced in a given unit of time. This is obtained dividing the total volume of air supplied (or exhausted) in cubic meters (or cubic feet) per unit of time by clean room area.

Air flow velocity and volume assessments consist of reading the air speed and flow directly under the air diffuser in the clean area. Air flow volume is given in liters and velocity in liters per second (or cubit feet per second).

Air flow adjustments are carried out whenever necessary to ensure compliance with design specifications regarding the distribution of air among all areas served by the HVAC (heat, ventilation, and air conditioning) system.

The most commonly used instruments for measuring air flow velocity and volume assessments are the balometer and pitot tube (Figures 16.6 and 16.7), thermo-anemometer (Figures 16.8 through 16.10), and fan-anemometer (Figure 16.11).

16.3.2.4 Clean room differential pressure

Pressure is critical to the proper functioning of the clean room. If the pressure is too low, especially when a door is opened, contaminants can enter. If it is too high, energy is being wasted.

The test consists of determining the difference between pressures measured in different areas of interest, for instance, between a clean room and an adjacent room. An adequate pressure differential ensures that the air flow goes from the cleanest to the less clean room when doors and pass-throughs are opened. For instance, an ISO 7 clean room dumps air into an ISO 8 clean room.

The most commonly used instruments for measuring pressure differential include the manometer (Figure 16.12) and micro-manometer (Figures 16.13 and 16.14). The most commonly used unit of measurement is millimeters of water column.

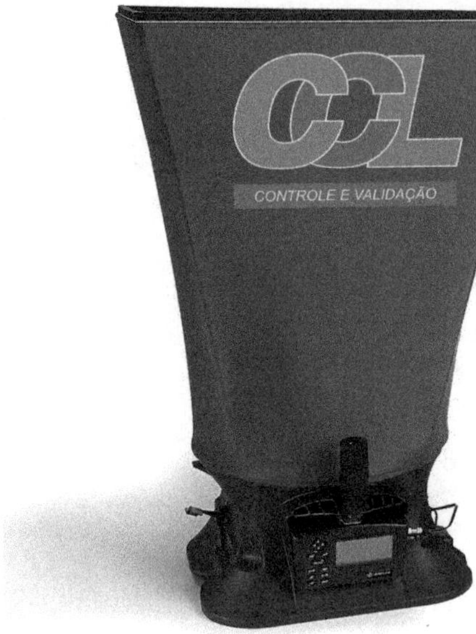

Figure 16.6 Balometer is an electronic flow meter custom designed to measure the air volume supplied by diffusers and grills.

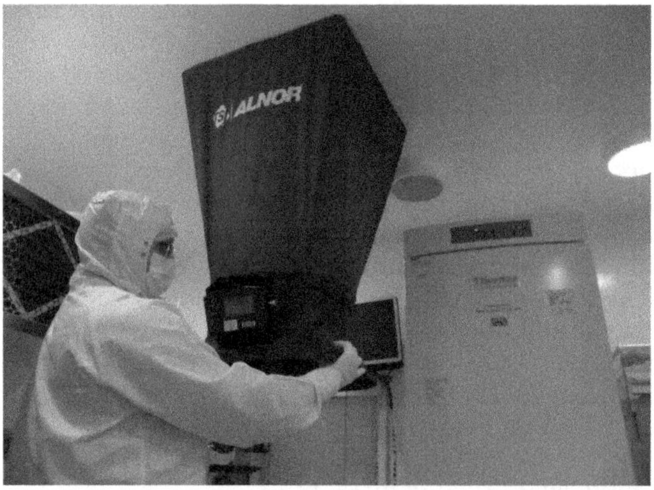

Figure 16.7 **(See color insert.)** Air flow volume and air speed assessment. Photograph showing an engineer testing an air diffuser with a balometer in the clean room IVF laboratory. (Courtesy of Androfert, Campinas, Brazil.)

16.3.2.5 *Clean room recovery time*

The recovery assessment test is performed to determine whether the installation is capable of returning to a specific cleanliness level within a finite time lapse after being briefly exposed to a generation of particles in air suspension, as a challenge to the system.

Testing consists of performing several particle counts within the clean area, ranking it according to the ISO classification (Table 16.1), then increasing the known air particle concentration and monitoring the readings until the room returns to its initial classification.

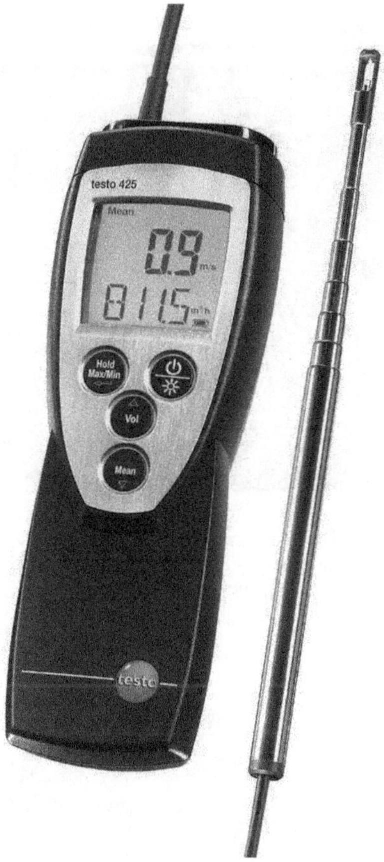

Figure 16.8 Thermo-anemometer.

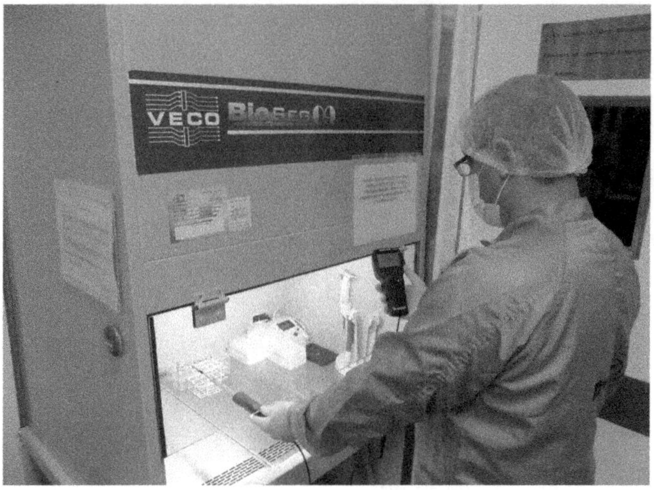

Figure 16.9 **(See color insert.)** Air flow volume and air speed assessment. Photograph showing a Class II biosafety cabinet being checked for air flow volume and speed with a thermo-anemometer. (Courtesy of Androfert, Campinas, Brazil.)

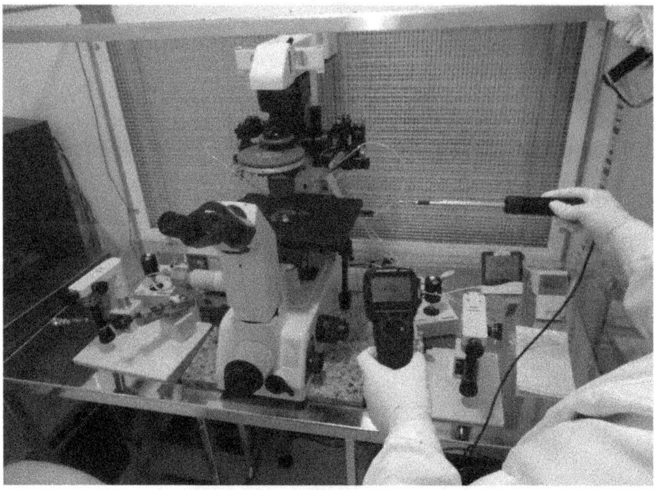

Figure 16.10 **(See color insert.)** Air flow volume and air speed assessment. Photograph illustrating an engineer checking air flow volume and air speed of an unidirectional air flow workstation with a thermo-anemometer. (Courtesy of Androfert, Campinas, Brazil.)

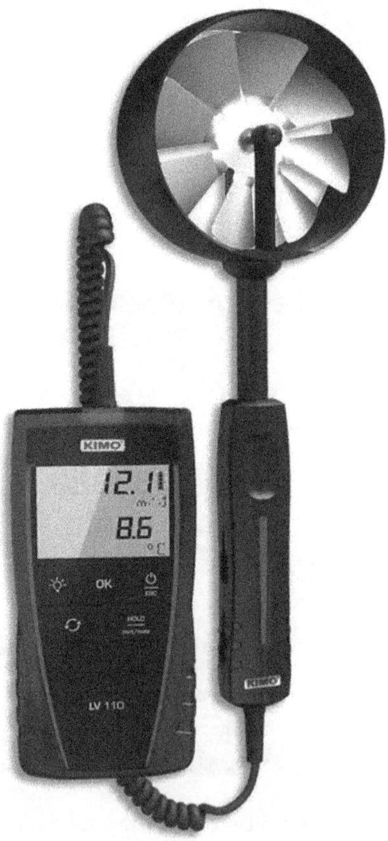

Figure 16.11 Fan-anemometer.

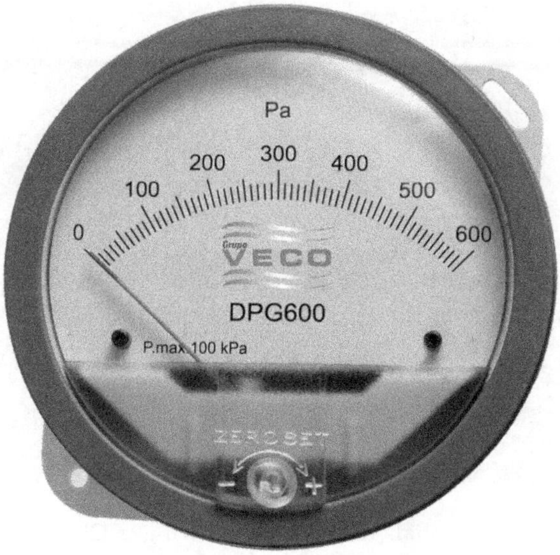

Figure 16.12 Manometer.

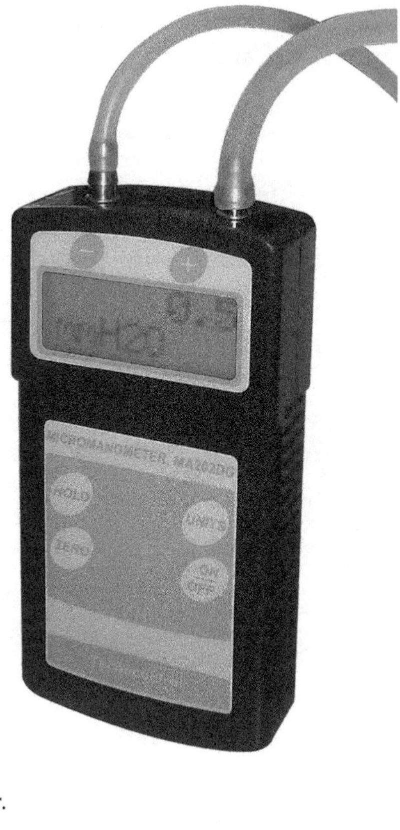

Figure 16.13 Micromanometer.

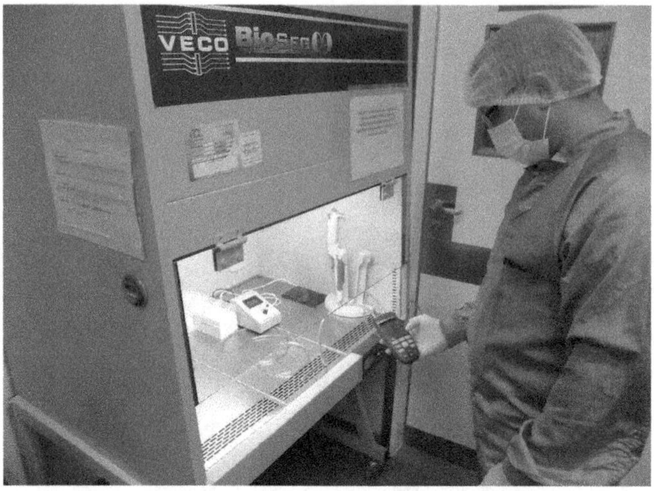

Figure 16.14 Air pressure differential. Photograph showing a Class II biosafety cabinet being checked with micromanometer. (Courtesy of Androfert, Campinas, Brazil.)

For instance, an ISO 7 room is ramped up to reach ISO 8, and at this point the particle generator is turned off and the stopwatch is started. The period of time required to return to the initial condition is recorded. The faster the recovery time, the better the capacity of the installed devices and the room design.

Clean room recovery time assessment requires an electronic particle counter (Figure 16.4), an aerosol generator (Figure 16.15), and a stopwatch (Figure 16.16). Figure 16.17 illustrates the recovery time test.

16.3.2.6 Filter saturation level

This test consists of determining the life span of the air filtration system, which provides an overview of all filters installed (pre-filter, fine dust, and HEPA filters). The procedure encompasses reading the pressure drop in the filtration system and comparing the results

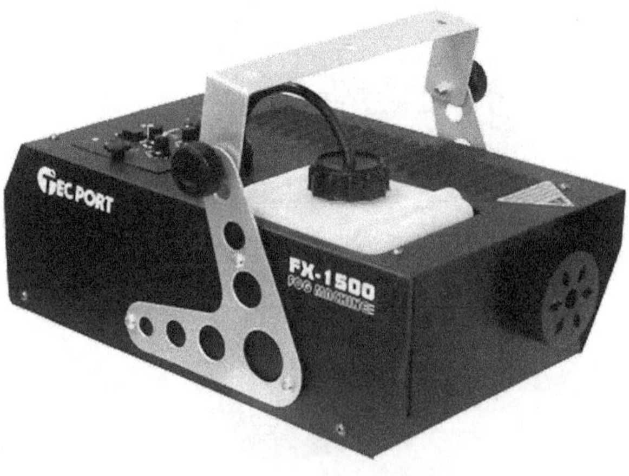

Figure 16.15 Aerosol generator.

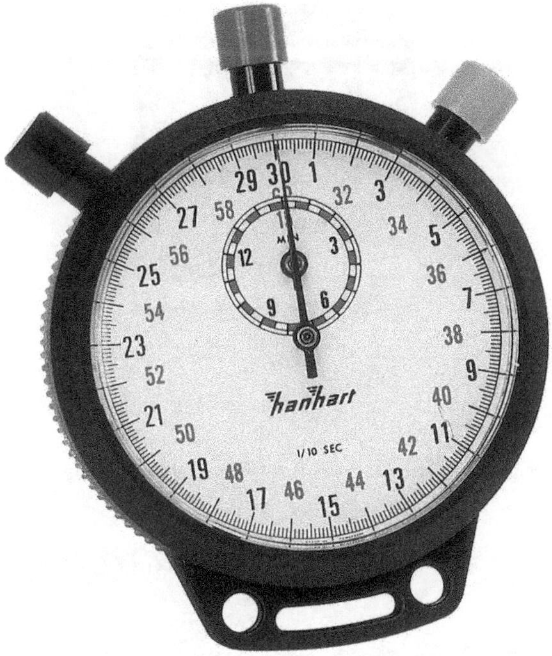

Figure 16.16 Stopwatch.

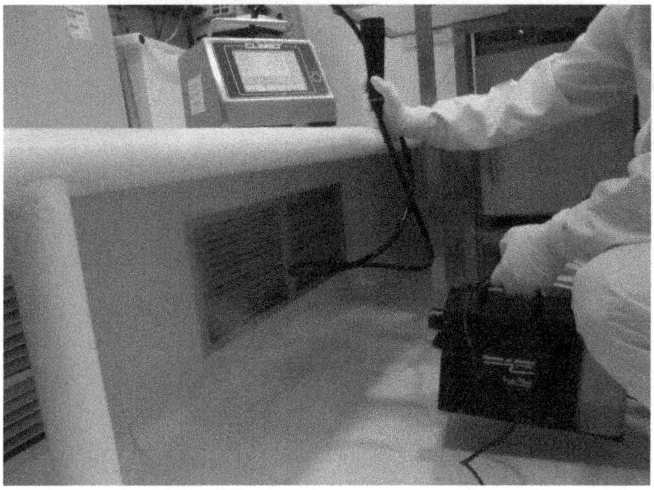

Figure 16.17 Clean room pressure differential testing. Photograph showing an engineer checking the recovery time in the clean room IVF laboratory. (Courtesy of Androfert, Campinas, Brazil.)

with pre-tested filter manufacturer's catalogue/datasheet. A high pressure drop is indicative of saturation, thus filter replacement will be recommended. Invariably, pressure drop is associated with reduction in air speed and flow, and as a consequence less air changes per hour.

Filter saturation level assessment requires the same instruments as listed in Section 16.3.2.4 (Figures 16.12 and 16.13).

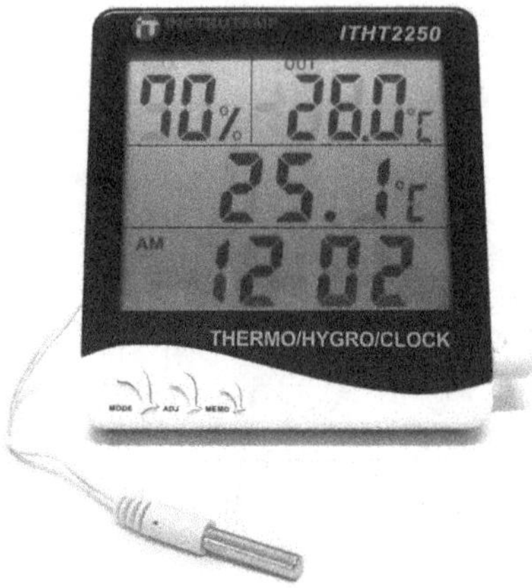

Figure 16.18 Thermo hygrometer equipped with a temperature probe.

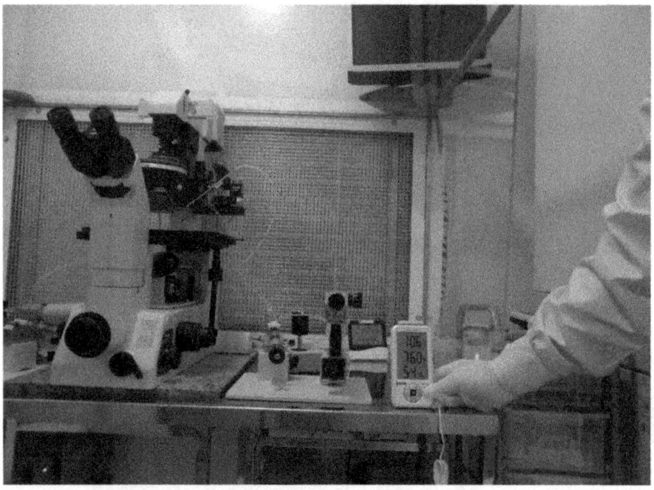

Figure 16.19 Ambient humidity and temperature measurement. Photograph showing an engineer using a thermo hygrometer to monitor air humidity and temperature in the clean room IVF laboratory. (Courtesy of Androfert, Campinas, Brazil.)

16.3.2.7 *Relative humidity and temperature of ambient air*

This test consists of determining the capacity of the HVAC system to maintain temperature and humidity levels within the pre-established limits according to design specifications.

Direct reading of percent humidity and temperature is performed in several points distributed throughout the clean area using a thermo hygrometer equipped with a temperature probe (Figures 16.18 and 16.19).

16.3.2.8 *Light intensity (luminance)*

This test consists of determining the luminance level inside the clean room or clean area. Luminance is a photometric measure of the luminous intensity per unit area of light travelling in a given direction. It describes the amount of light that either passes through or is

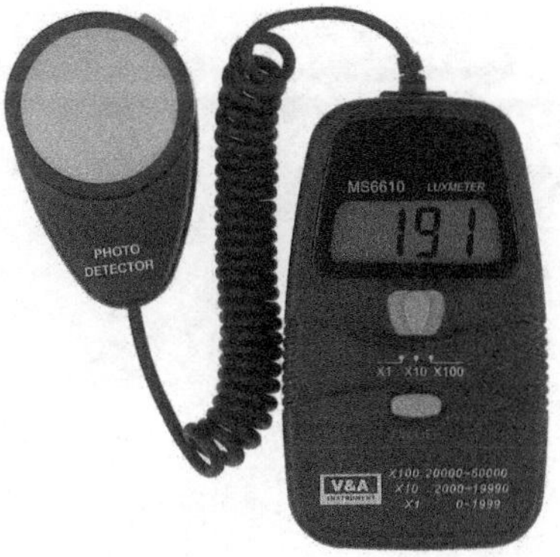

Figure 16.20 Light meter.

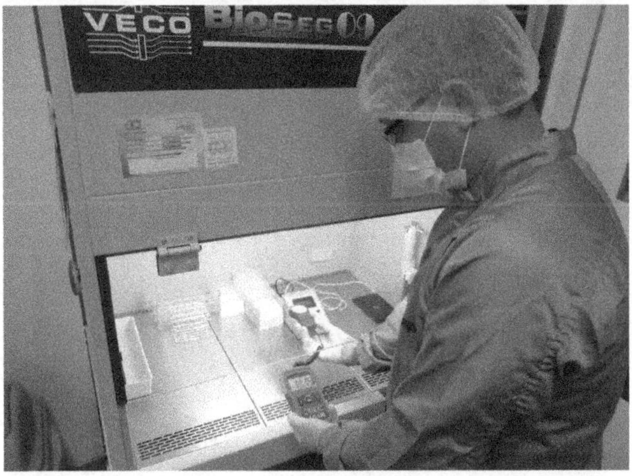

Figure 16.21 **(See color insert.)** Light intensity measurement. Photograph showing a Class II biosafety cabinet being checked with a light meter. (Courtesy of Androfert, Campinas, Brazil.)

emitted/reflected from a particular area and falls within a given solid angle. The SI unit for luminance is candela per square meter (cd/m^2).

The test consists of multiple readings of light intensity taken from several points distributed throughout the clean area using a light meter (Figures 16.20 and 16.21).

16.3.2.9 Noise levels

This test consists of determining the noise level inside the clean room/clean area in order to determine that employee noise exposure does not exceed maximum established limits.

The test consists of directly reading the noise level in several points distributed throughout the clean room/clean zone. The most commonly used instrument for measuring noise levels is the sound level meter (SLM). The SML consists of a microphone, an electronic circuit, and a readout display. The microphone detects the small air pressure variations associated with sound and changes them into electrical signals. These signals are processed and the results are expressed in decibels. The SML measures the noise level at one instant in every location of interest (Figures 16.22 and 16.23).

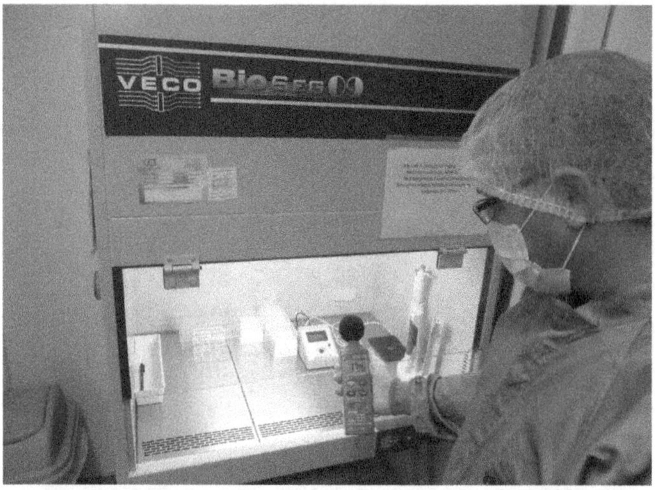

Figure 16.22 **(See color insert.)** Photograph showing a Class II biosafety cabinet being checked with a sound level meter. (Courtesy of Androfert, Campinas, Brazil.)

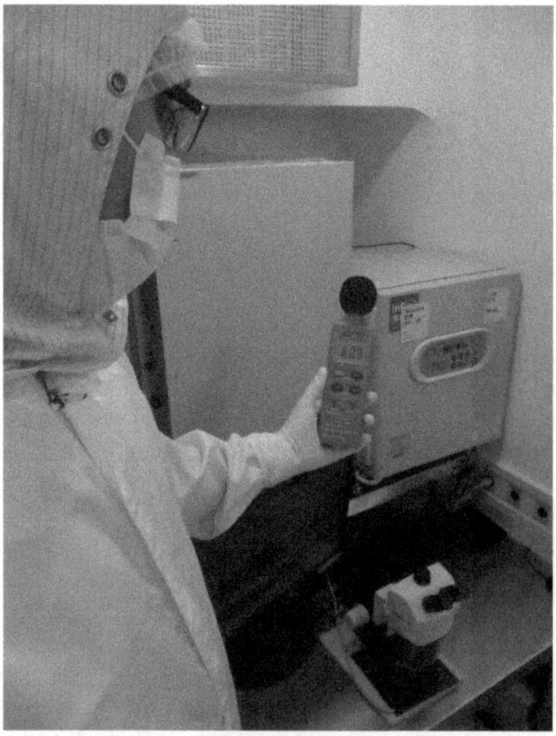

Figure 16.23 Sound level measurement. Photograph showing an engineer using a sound level meter to monitor noise level in the clean room IVF laboratory. (Courtesy of Androfert, Campinas, Brazil.)

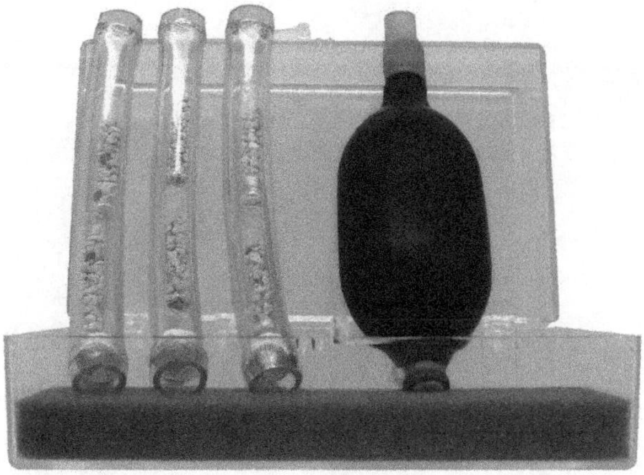

Figure 16.24 Small-volume smoke ampoules.

16.3.2.10 Smoke test

This test consists of visually inspecting the orientation and direction of the air flow inside the clean areas.

The smoke test is carried out by generating a large amount of smoke inside the clean area and confirming that smoke is drawn back to air return vents. It also serves the purpose of checking points with air reflow, design inconsistencies, or wrongful distribution of equipment and furniture within the clean room/clean area, including the micromanipulator, microscopes, the incubators, among others.

The smoke test can be filmed or photographed, and customers use this information for internal training procedures.

The most commonly used instruments in smoke testing include a large-volume smoke generation device (Figure 16.15), video recording, and a photographic camera.

16.3.2.11 Air flow parallelism

The purpose of the air flow parallelism test is to determine the parallelism of the air flow throughout the clean work area. It can also be used to demonstrate the effects of interposed equipment on air flow. Air should flow in a parallel stream to prevent the flow of outside air into the critical area.

The test consists of generating a small amount of visible vapor or smoke close to the airflow outlet immediately after the HEPA filter. Like the smoke test, the air flow parallelism test can be videotaped or photographed and be used for internal training purposes. The utilized instruments are a small-volume smoke ampoule (Figure 16.24), support, and video recorder, or a photographic camera. The angle of deflection should not be greater than 14° from center when measured 1 m away from the outlet (Figure 16.25).

16.4 Certification intervals

The recommended testing intervals range from 6–12 months. In ART Clinics equipped with clean rooms/clean areas, testing intervals of six months are suggested by CCL (Controle & Validação). CCL-Controle & Validação is a company specialized in testing and certification of clean rooms/clean areas, unidirectional air flow areas, and biosafety equipment in Brazil and South America. After the introduction of the Brazilian Tissue and Cell Directive, which

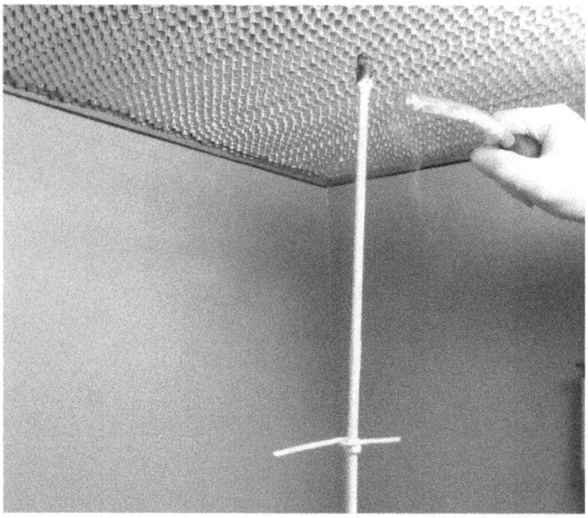

Figure 16.25 Photograph showing an engineer performing the air flow parallelism test inside a unidirectional air flow cabinet. (Courtesy of Androfert, Campinas, Brazil.)

requires air quality control in IVF laboratories and associated critical areas, CCL has been also devoted to testing and certification of IVF laboratories.

Our routine is to perform a complete set of testing once a year, named a "premium certification," intercalated by a less stringent one, named a "standard certification," every six months.

16.4.1 *Premium certification*

Tests included in the premium certification are as follows:

- HEPA filter integrity
- Airborne particle counting
- Air flow velocity and uniformity
- Clean room differential pressure
- Clean room recovery time (particle fallout rate)
- Filter saturation level
- Relative humidity and temperature of ambient air
- Lighting levels
- Noise levels
- Smoke test
- Air flow parallelism

16.4.2 *Standard certification*

Tests included in the standard certification are as follows:

- Airborne particle counting
- Air flow velocity and uniformity

- Clean room differential pressure
- Filter saturation level
- Relative humidity and temperature of ambient air

16.5 Reports

Upon testing completion, a report is generated with test results and clean room performance. The report includes a narrative synopsis of each test conducted and the occupational state.

It is our routine to include schematic diagrams of HVAC, filtration units, and measurement locations. The final report includes a list of all deficiencies (if any) and recommendations. Reports include all instrumentation and equipment used for testing, accompanied by copies of calibration certificates.

References

1. International Organization for Standardization, 1999. ISO NBR 14644-1:2005 on cleanrooms and associated controlled environments. Associação Brasileira de Normas Técnicas (ABNT), Brasilia, DF, Brasil.
2. International Organization for Standardization, 2000. ISO NBR 14644-2:2006 on cleanrooms and associated controlled environments—Part 2: Specifications for testing and monitoring to prove continued compliance with ISO 14644-1. Associação Brasileira de Normas Técnicas (ABNT), Brasilia, DF, Brasil.
3. International Organization for Standardization, 2005. ISO NBR 14644-3:2009 on cleanrooms and associated controlled environments—Part 3: Test methods. Associação Brasileira de Normas Técnicas (ABNT), Brasilia, DF, Brasil.
4. ANVISA. Brazilian National Agency for Sanitary Surveillance, 2006. Resolução no. 33 da Diretoria colegiada da Agência Nacional de Vigilância Sanitária (amended by RDC23 of May 27, 2011 on setting standards of quality and safety for the donation, procurement, testing, processing, preservation, storage and distribution of human tissues and cells). http://bvsms.saude.gov.br/bvs/saudelegis/anvisa/2011/res0023_27_05_2011.html (accessed August 8, 2015).

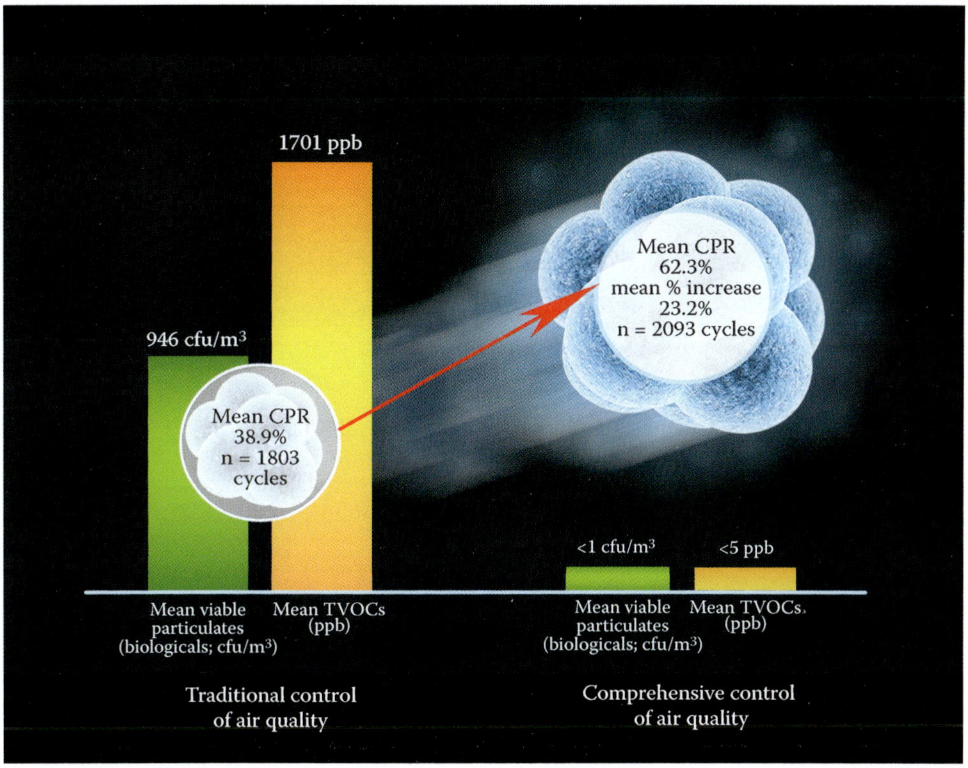

Figure 3.3 Statistically significant increase in clinical pregnancy rates (CPR) concomitant with comprehensive control of ambient air quality; viable particulates and total volatile organic compounds (TVOCs).

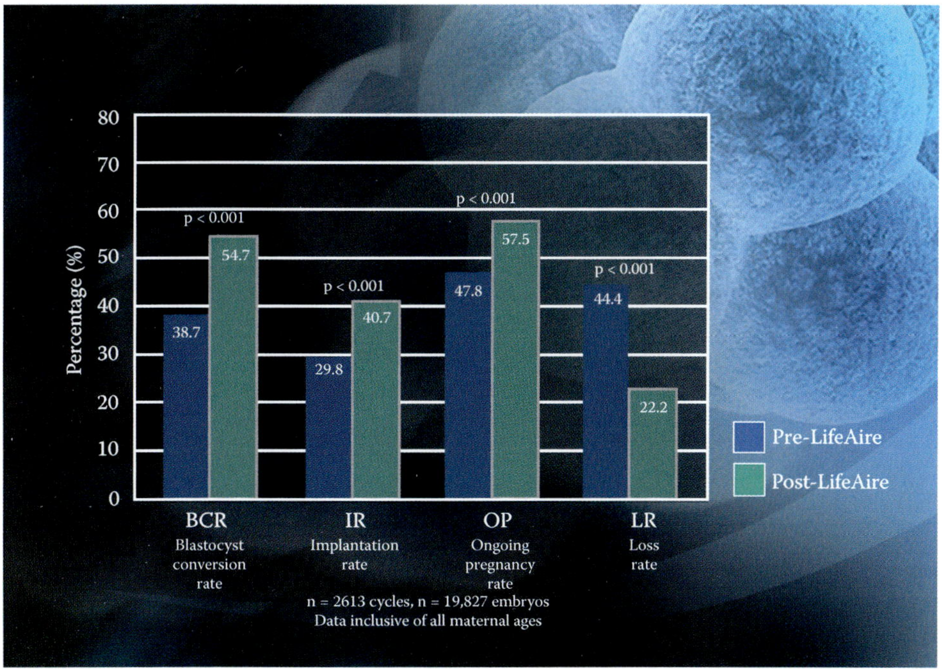

Figure 3.4 Statistically significant increase in BCR, IR, and OP rates and statistically significant decrease in LR with comprehensive control of ambient air quality—a multi-site study including 2613 non-donor patient cycles and 19,827 embryos. The data are inclusive of all maternal ages.

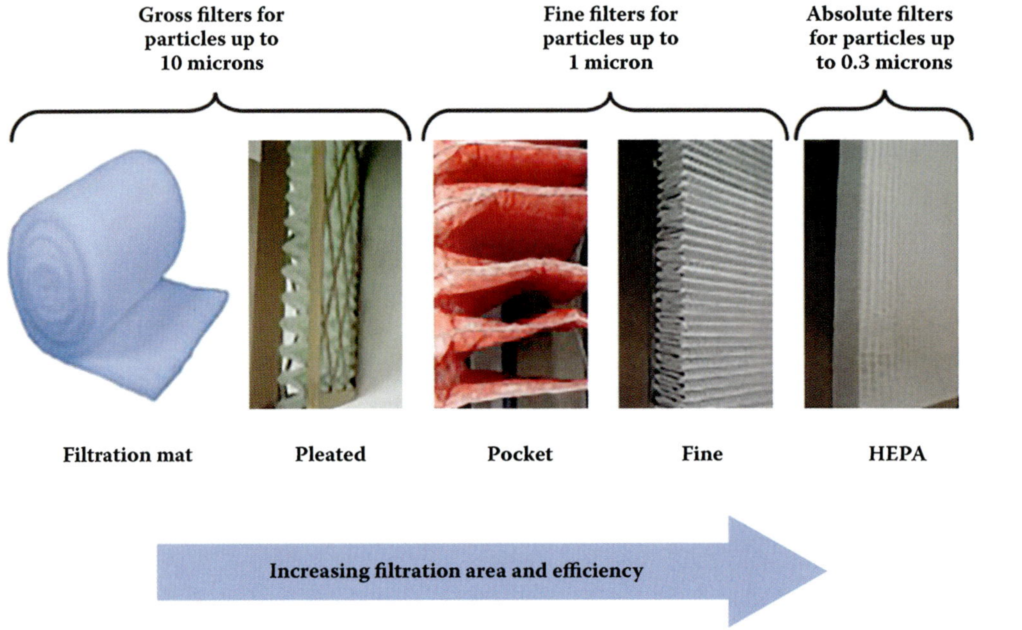

Figure 5.10 Particulate air filtration design for increased efficiency. Pre-filters and fine filters (less expensive) should be placed in series upstream the HEPA filter (more expensive).

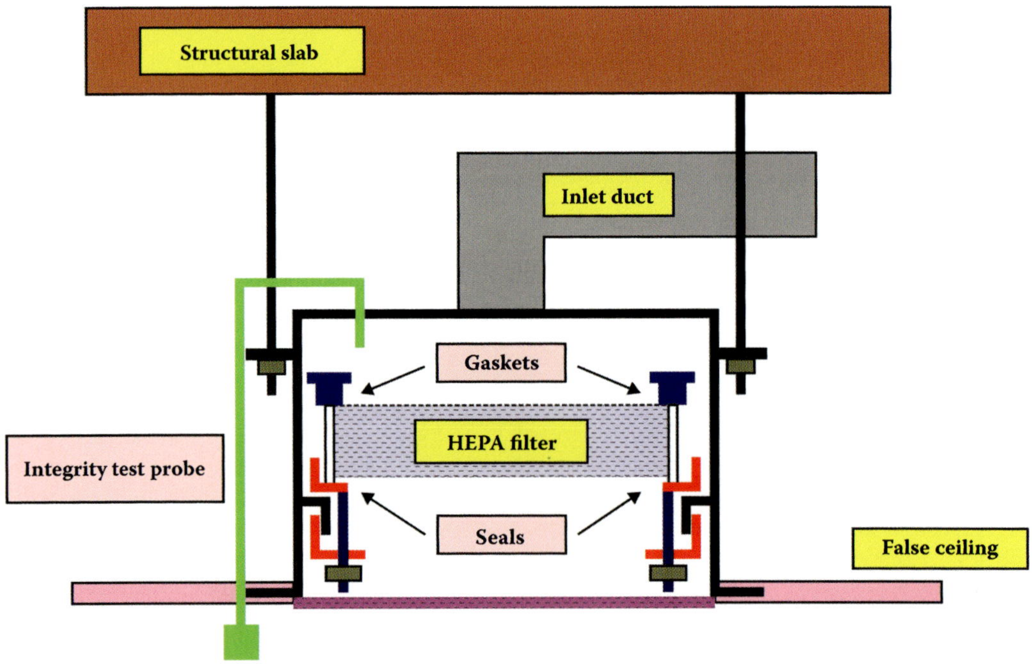

Figure 7.1 Example of HEPA filter installation.

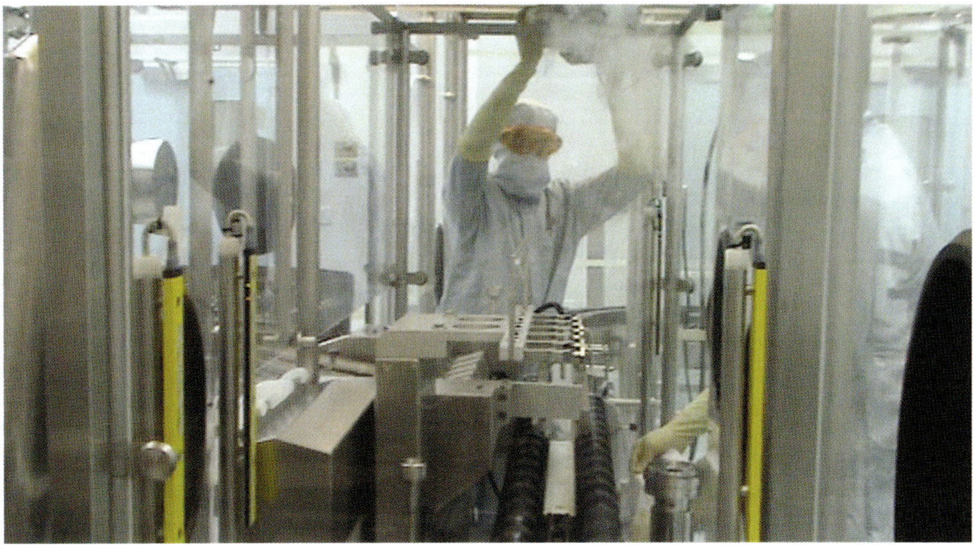

Figure 7.3 An example of turbulent airflow visualization.

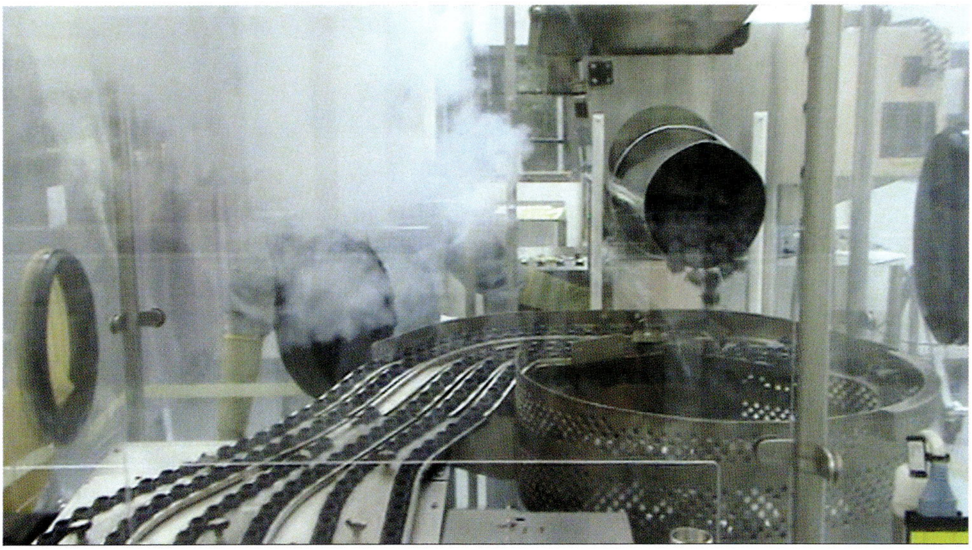

Figure 7.5 Illustration of air movement: UDAF unit (laminar flow) within a turbulent air flow clean room.

Gas	USA	International
Oxygen	Green	White
Carbon dioxide	Gray	Gray
Nitrous oxide	Blue	Blue
Helium	Brown	Brown
Nitrogen	Black	Black
Air	Yellow	White and black

Figure 9.1 Cylinder identification color code chart used for medical gases. In Europe, it is anticipated that the identification color codes will be standardized by 2025. The United States designations are as follows: (i) oxygen USP is a green background with white lettering or white background with green lettering; (ii) carbon dioxide USP is a gray background with black lettering or white lettering; (iii) nitrous oxide USP is a blue background with white lettering; (iv) helium USP is a brown background with white lettering; (v) nitrogen USP is a black background with white lettering; and (vi) air USP is a yellow background with black lettering.

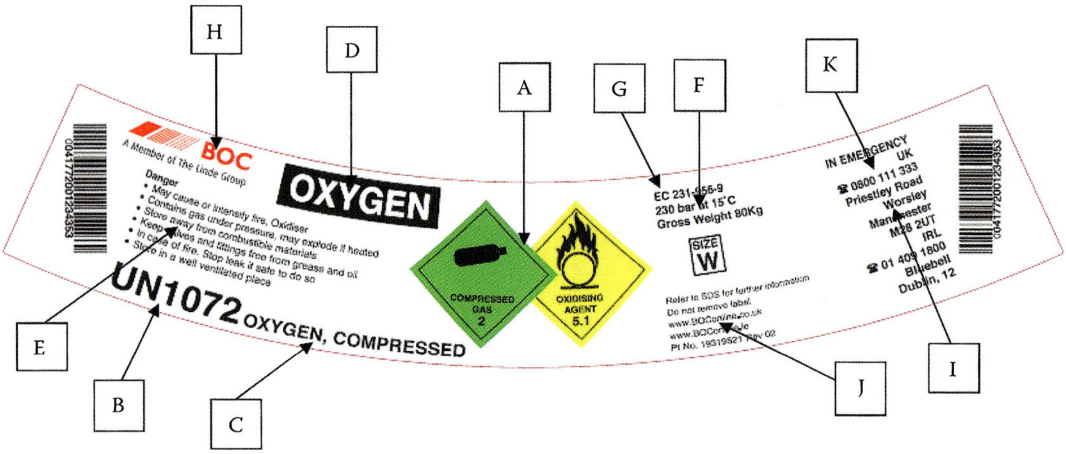

Figure 9.2 A typical label found on the neck of a compressed medical oxygen gas cylinder. The following information is required on a label: (A) a diamond hazard label, displaying the primary hazard with additional hazard labels displaying any subsidiary hazards. These labels will display the dangerous goods classification number. (B) The UN number, preceded by the letters UN. (C) The proper shipping name. (D) Product name (may be omitted if the proper shipping name is identical). (E) Signal word, hazard and precautionary statements. (F) Package size and pressure. (G) EC number, if applicable. (H) Company name. (I) Address of the gas company. (J) Additional company information. (K) A telephone number to call in an emergency. In addition, a bar code on the label identifies the cylinder and is used for inventory purposes and a yellow sticker indicating an oxidizing agent and can be harmful. (Courtesy of British Compressed Gases Association.)

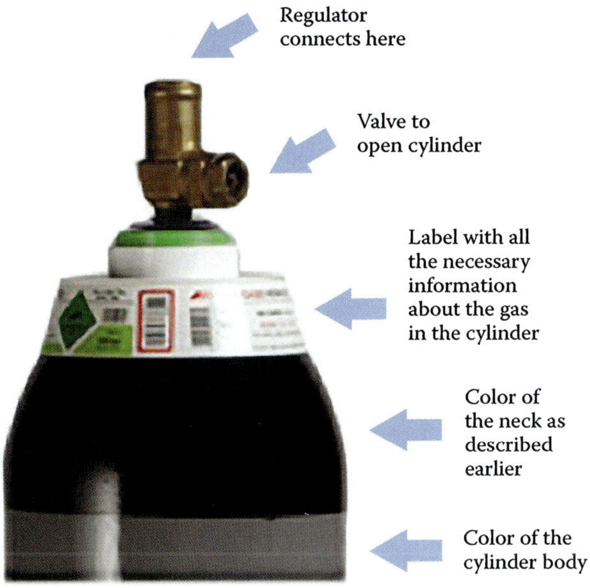

Figure 9.4 Nitrogen (oxygen free) 230 bar cylinder. Note the typical label that is attached to the neck of all certified medical gas cylinders. The cylinder identification color on the neck is different from that on the body. (Courtesy of BOC Health Care, UK.)

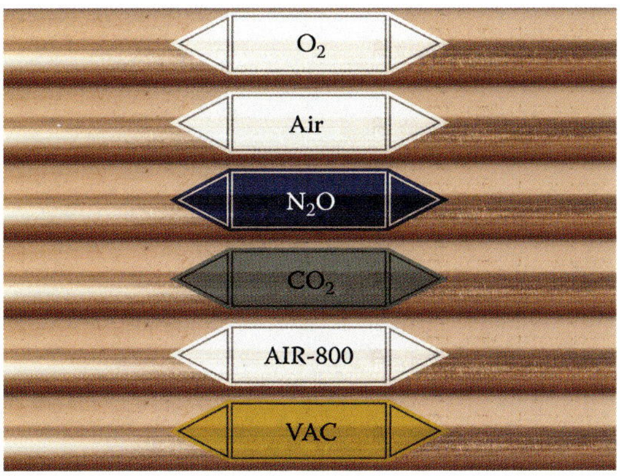

Figure 9.6 Labeling of each pipe of the medical gas pipelines system (MGPS). Although the color-coding may vary, the importance is to note that each pipe has a label.

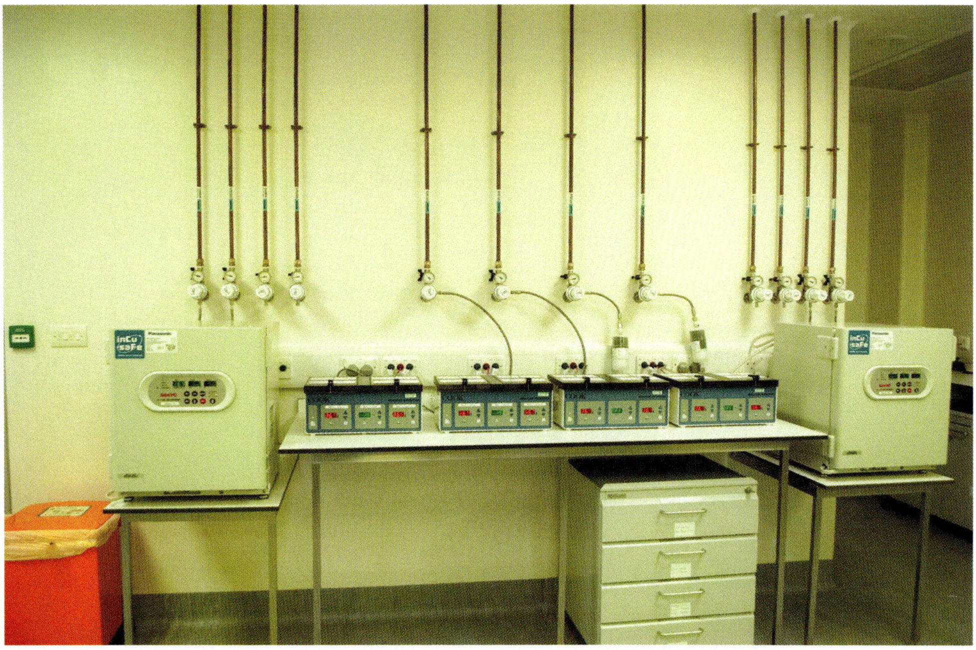

Figure 9.7 Individual gas pipe lines to IVF lab incubators. Each terminal can be connected to an inline filter to remove VOCs from gas bottles. (Courtesy of Magda Carvalho, Cambridge IVF, UK.)

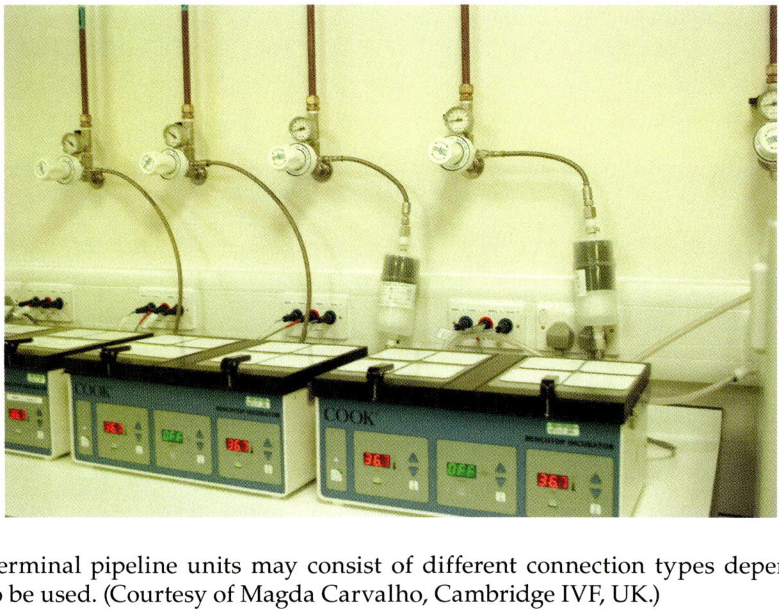

Figure 9.8 Terminal pipeline units may consist of different connection types depending on the equipment to be used. (Courtesy of Magda Carvalho, Cambridge IVF, UK.)

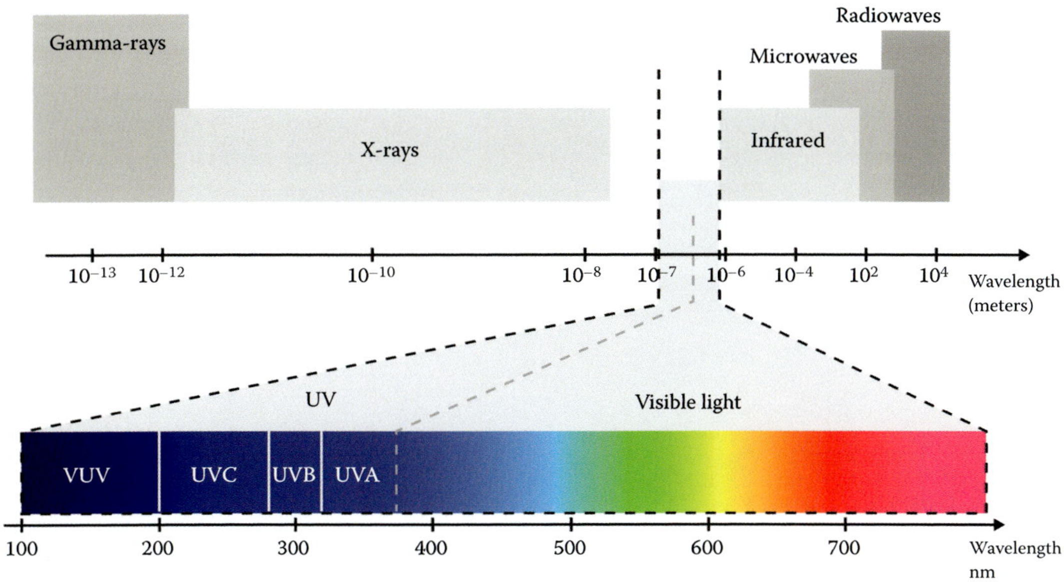

Figure 10.3 Light spectrum.

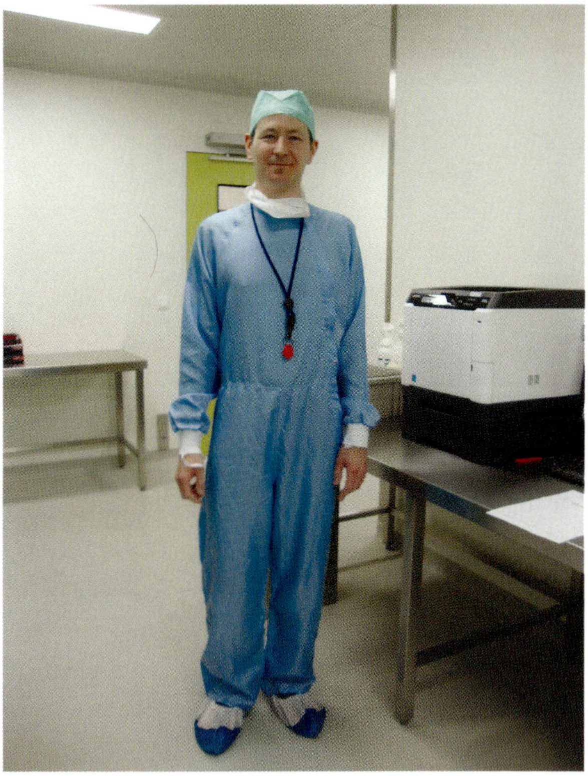

Figure 14.1 Dress code for the IVF clean room: a one piece zip-up overall with long sleeves, a head cover, and shoe covers.

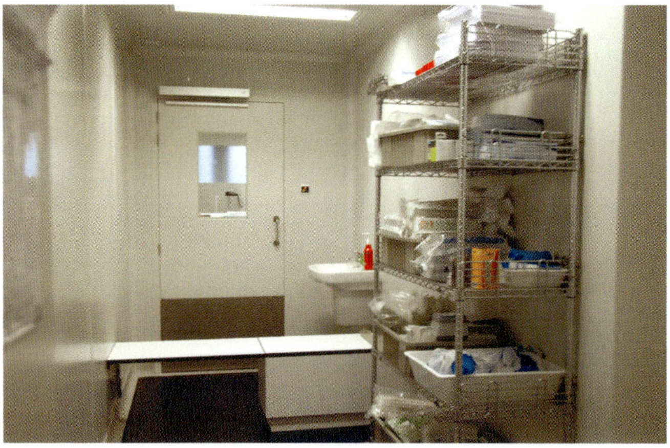

Figure 14.2 Entrance room into IVF clean room facility using a cross bench. Staff should sit on the bench to remove their shoes, move the legs over the bench and put on the clean room shoes. Staff can stand up and move into the clean room by stepping on a sticky clean room mat. Hands should be disinfected after changing of shoes and before entrance into the IVF clean room facility.

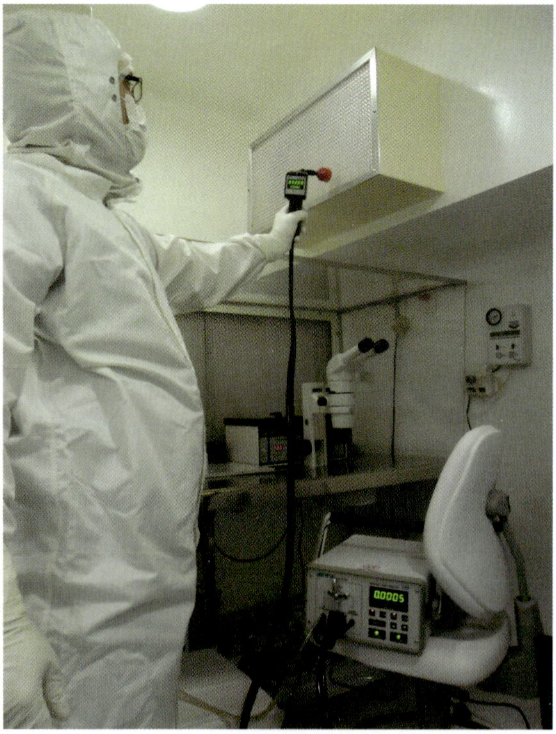

Figure 16.1 In situ testing of HEPA filter installation. Photograph showing an engineer testing a HEPA terminal filter in the clean room IVF laboratory. (Courtesy of Androfert, Campinas, Brazil.)

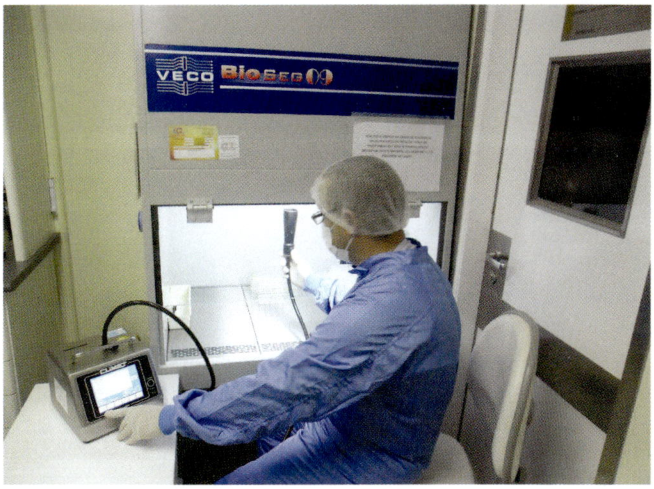

Figure 16.5 Particle counting in Class II biosafety cabinet. (Courtesy of Androfert, Campinas, Brazil.)

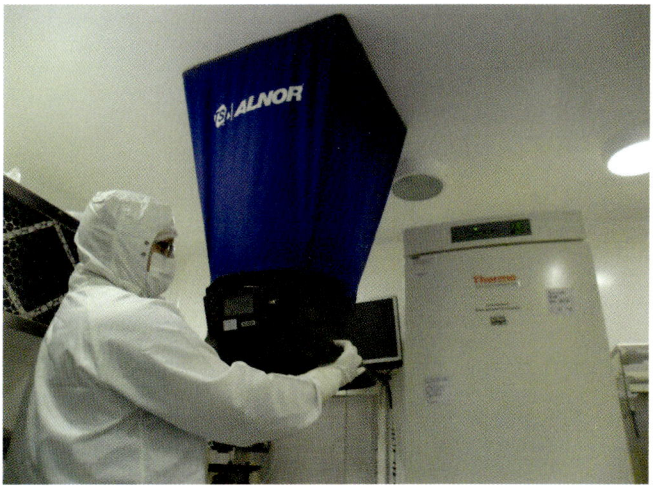

Figure 16.7 Air flow volume and air speed assessment. Photograph showing an engineer testing an air diffuser with a balometer in the clean room IVF laboratory. (Courtesy of Androfert, Campinas, Brazil.)

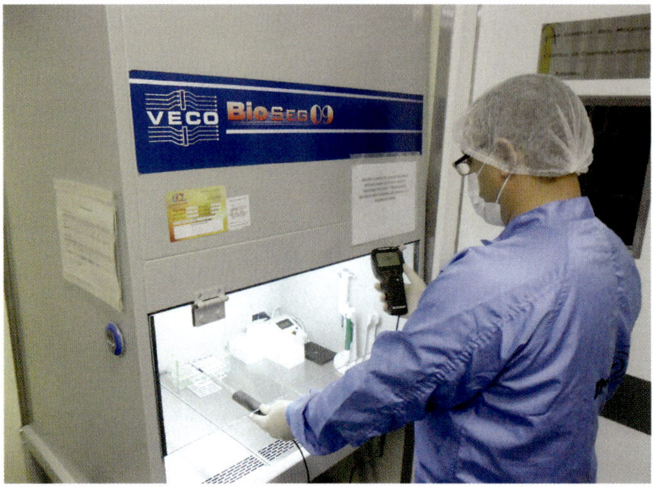

Figure 16.9 Air flow volume and air speed assessment. Photograph showing a Class II biosafety cabinet being checked for air flow volume and speed with a thermo-anemometer. (Courtesy of Androfert, Campinas, Brazil.)

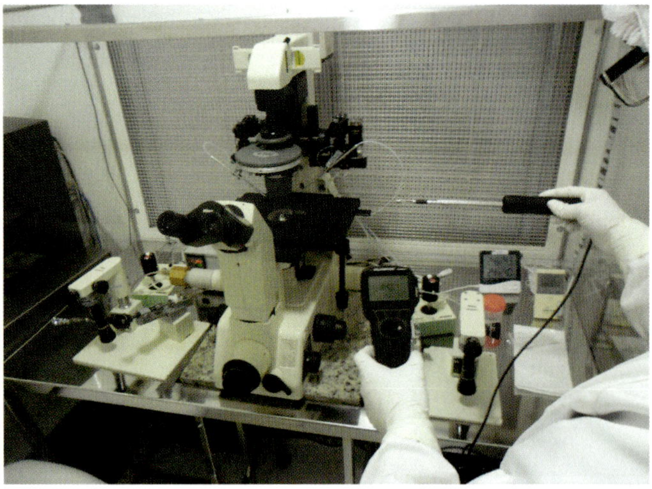

Figure 16.10 Air flow volume and air speed assessment. Photograph illustrating an engineer checking air flow volume and air speed of an unidirectional air flow workstation with a thermo-anemometer. (Courtesy of Androfert, Campinas, Brazil.)

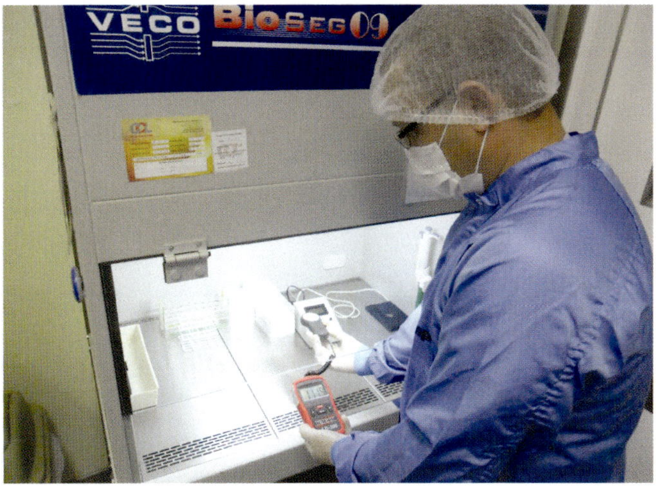

Figure 16.21 Light intensity measurement. Photograph showing a Class II biosafety cabinet being checked with a light meter. (Courtesy of Androfert, Campinas, Brazil.)

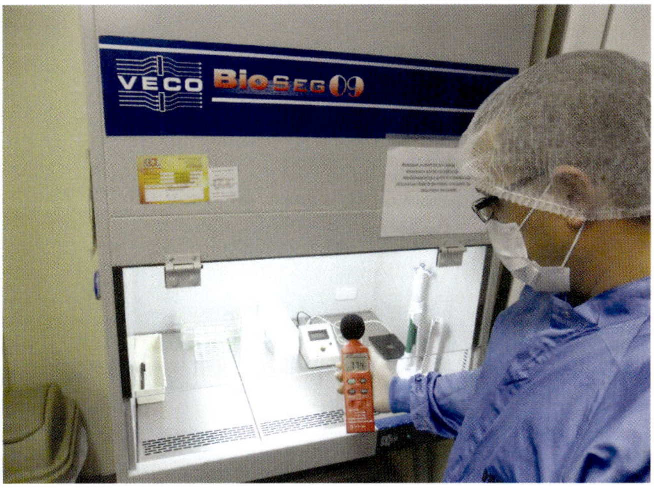

Figure 16.22 Photograph showing a Class II biosafety cabinet being checked with a sound level meter. (Courtesy of Androfert, Campinas, Brazil.)

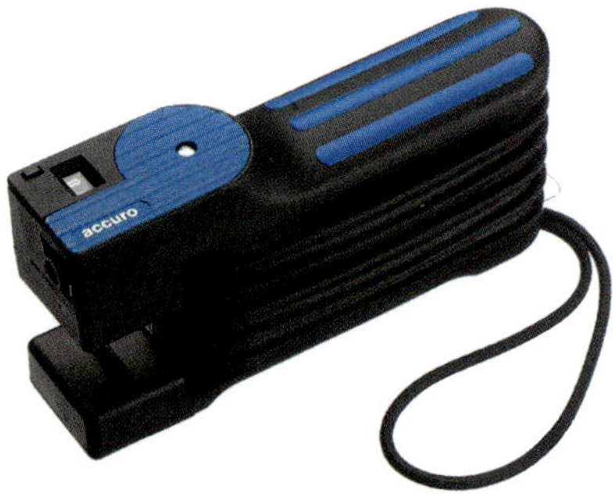

Figure 17.1 Hand pump for Tenax TA thermo desorption tube. (Drägerwerk AG & Co. KGaA, Lübeck, Germany.)

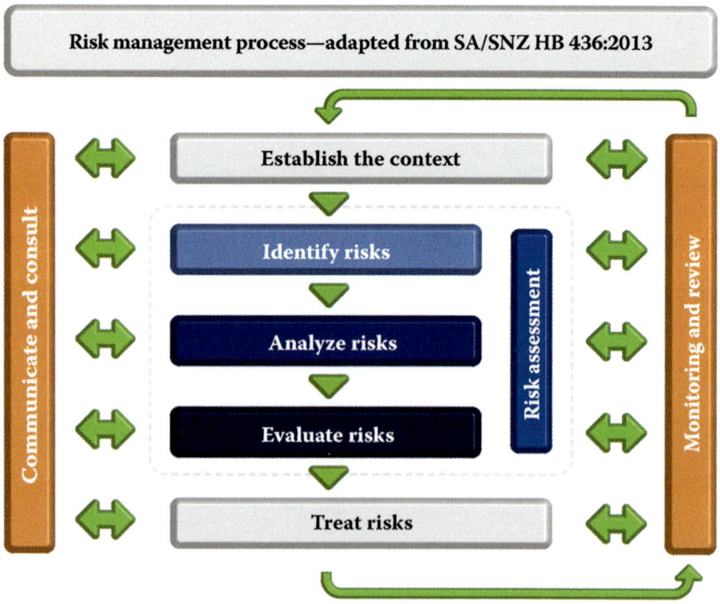

Figure 19.1 Risk management process.

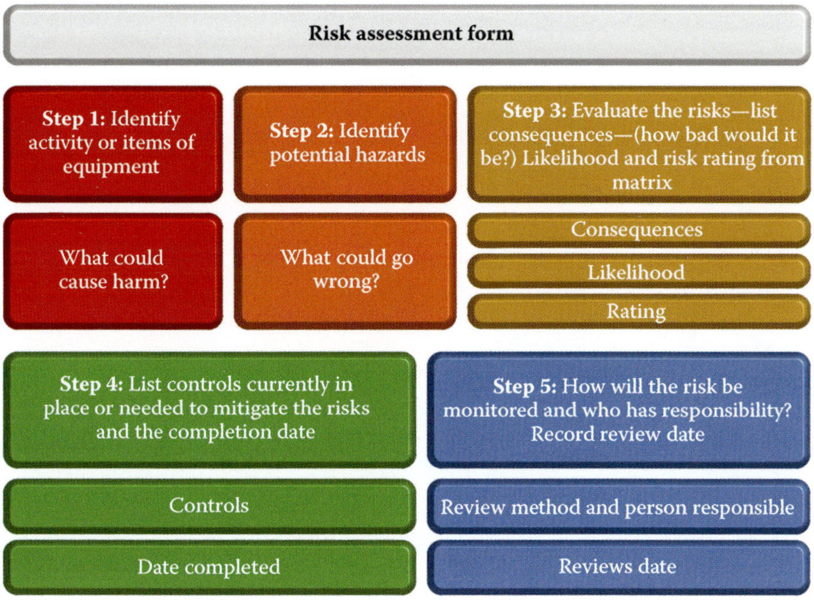

Figure 19.4 Example of risk assessment form.

Likelihood						
	Almost certain (5)	Medium (5)	High (10)	High (15)	Critical (20)	Critical (25)
	Likely (4)	Low (4)	Medium (8)	High (12)	High (16)	Critical (20)
	Possible (3)	Low (3)	Medium (6)	Medium (9)	High (12)	High (15)
	Unlikely (2)	Low (2)	Low (4)	Medium (6)	Medium (8)	High (10)
	Rare (1)	Low (1)	Low (2)	Low (3)	Low (4)	Medium (5)
		Insignificant (1)	*Minor (2)*	*Moderate (3)*	*Major (4)*	*Catastrophic (5)*
Severity						

Figure 19.5 Risk rating matrix.

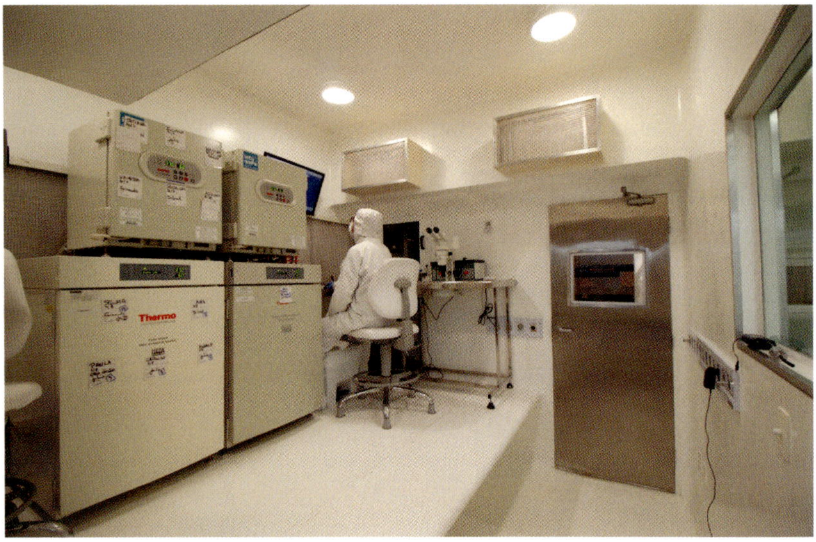

Figure 26.3 Overview of embryology laboratory suite.

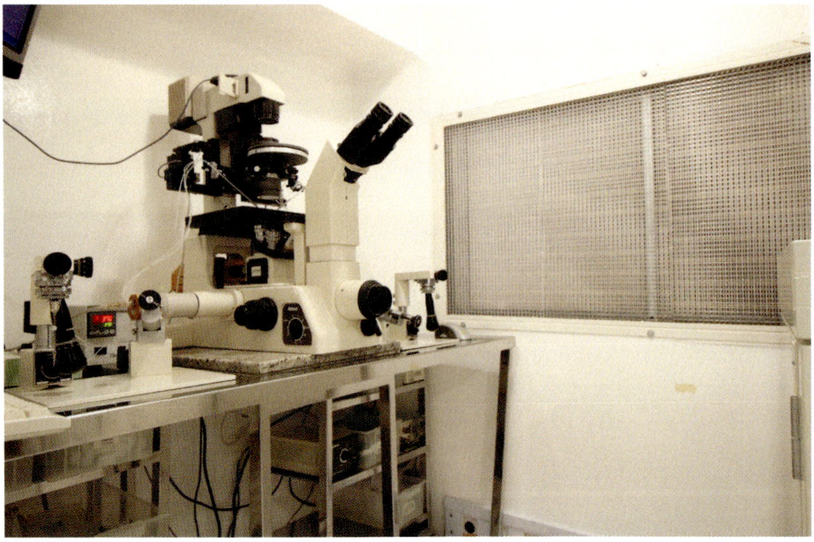

Figure 26.4 Overview of a workstation for micromanipulation of oocytes, sperm, and embryos. A wall-mounted frame with a terminal high efficiency particulate air (HEPA) filter supplies unidirectional airflow within the work area.

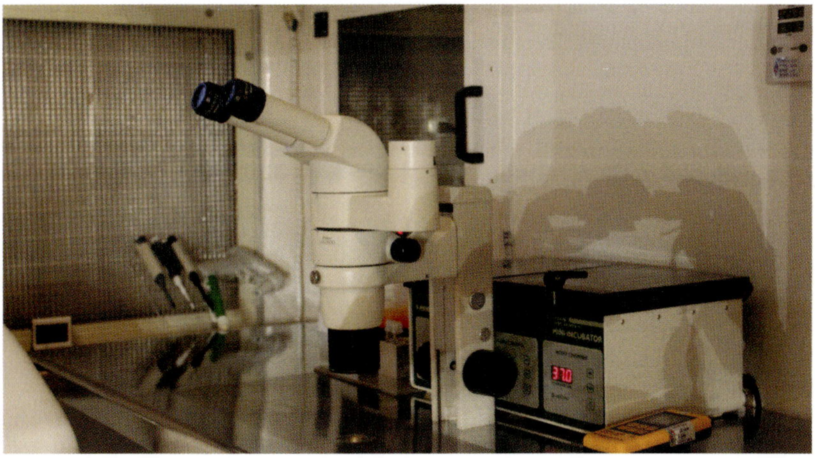

Figure 26.5 Overview of a workstation for handling oocytes and embryos. A wall-mounted frame with a terminal high efficiency particulate air (HEPA) filter supplies unidirectional airflow within the work area.

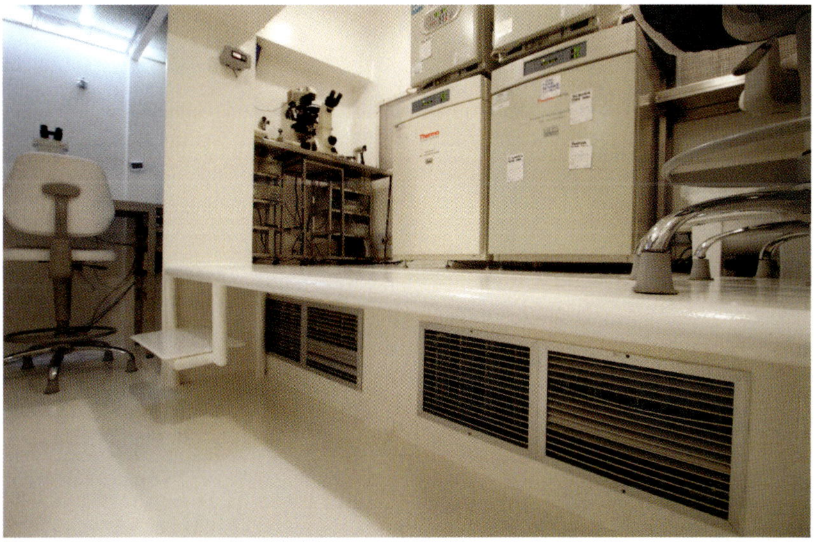

Figure 26.6 Overview of floor level return vents in the embryology laboratory suite.

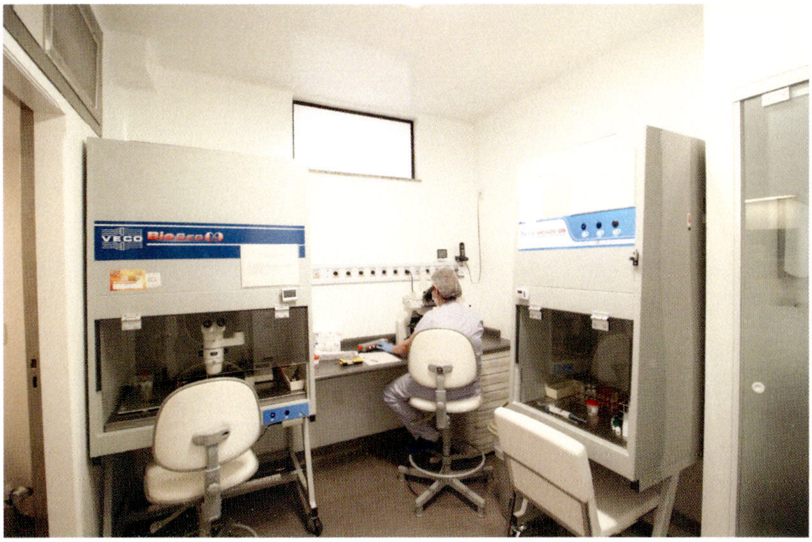

Figure 26.8 Overview of andrology laboratory suite.

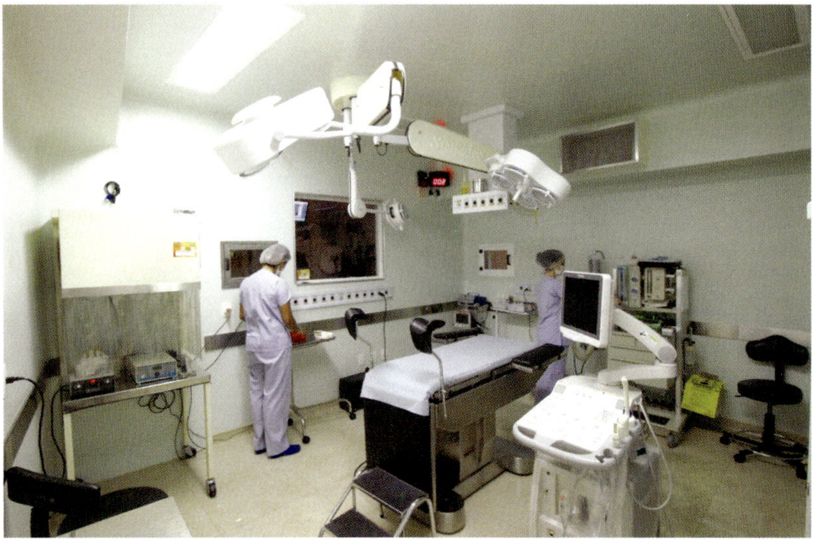

Figure 26.10 Overview of operating theater.

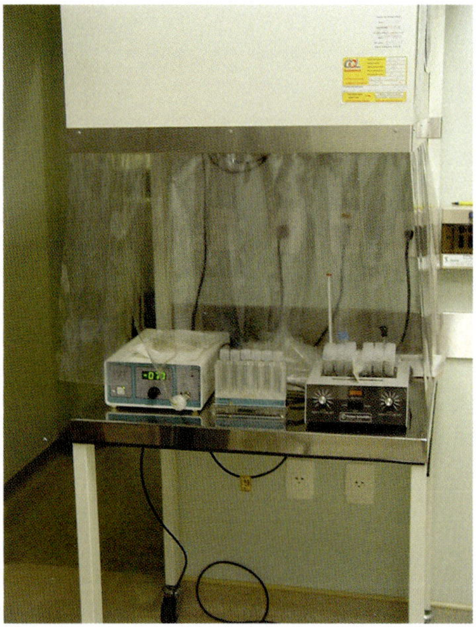

Figure 26.11 Cabinet in which tubes to collect follicular fluid are handled during oocyte pick-up. A ceiling-mounted high efficiency particulate air (HEPA) filtration system provides vertical unidirectional airflow to the work area.

chapter seventeen

Testing and monitoring: Volatile organic compounds and microbials

Benthe Brauer and Georg Griesinger

Contents

Abstract

The current state of the art dictates that IVF laboratories are systematically monitored for ambient conditions, such as air temperature, particle concentrations, and cleanliness. In this chapter, different methods and techniques for testing and monitoring volatile organic compounds and microbial contaminants are presented and discussed. As a final point, it should be noted that the threshold values for microbial contamination (e.g., defined by GMP guidelines) exist. In contrast, as yet little is known about the sources and concentrations of VOCs commonly present in IVF laboratories. It is known that VOCs may be emitted from various sources in the IVF laboratory setting. Some VOCs have been identified as potentially genotoxic or mutagenic in various contexts other than in-vitro fertilization. Exposure of human embryos in-vitro to VOCs may have harmful consequences on both the reproductive potential of the embryo as well as long-term child health. However, to date, no threshold values have been defined below which no adverse effects of individual VOCs or groups of VOCs can be expected. For the time being, VOC concentrations should therefore be kept at a minimum. Further research needs to urgently address the following issue: What VOCs at what concentrations may carry a risk of negatively impacting on human embryo health and developmental potential?

17.1 Introduction

It is reasonable to assume that chemical air contamination (CAC) frequently occurs in the context of assisted reproductive technology (ART) utilization; however, CACs have not yet received adequate recognition. Concerns about automotive and industrial emissions certainly exist to some degree among reproductive medicine health care providers, but reference values for air contents and gaseous emission limits have neither been consented nor routinely monitored. Herein, we intend to describe air sampling methods and assay systems, which can be applied to any laboratory or laboratory item. It should be noted that unfiltered outside air may, in many instances, be cleaner than high efficiency particulate air (HEPA) filtered laboratory air and in particular air obtained from the inside of incubators. The reason behind that phenomenon is most likely the accumulation of volatile organic compounds (VOCs) originating from spaces adjacent to the IVF laboratory or products used during the laboratory work, such as compressed CO_2, sterilized Petri dishes, and other materials or devices known to be sources of gaseous emissions. Specific groups of products such as anaesthetic gases, refrigerants, cleaning agents, hydrocarbons, and aromatic compounds such as benzene and toluene have been identified. The latter was shown to accumulate particularly in incubators.[1]

There are numerous indoor air pollutants that can spread throughout a building. They typically fall into three basic categories of biological, chemical, and particulate matter (i.e., "particles") origin.[2]

Biological. Relevant concentrations of bacteria, viruses, fungi, dust mites, animal dander, and pollen may result from inadequate maintenance and housekeeping, water spills, inadequate humidity control, condensation or water leaking into the building or from indoor piping.

Chemical. Sources of chemical pollutants (gases and vapors) include emissions from products used in the building (e.g., office equipment, furniture, wall and floor coverings, pesticides, and cleaning and consumer products); accidental spills of chemicals; products used during construction activities such as adhesives and paints, respectively, and exhaust gases such as carbon monoxide, formaldehyde, and nitrogen dioxide, respectively.

Particulate matter and aerosols (nonbiological). Such nonbiological particles are small enough to remain suspended in the air. Dust, dirt, or other substances may be drawn into the building from outside. Particles can also be produced by activities that occur inside buildings such as construction activities, printing, copying, and in the context of other utensil usage, for example, household equipment.

In this chapter, we provide an overview of the testing and monitoring of VOCs and microbial contamination. The measuring and monitoring of particulate matter and aerosols (nonbiological), which can be performed with commercially available particle counters, are not covered herein.

17.2 Testing and monitoring of volatile organic compounds

VOCs may be emitted from various sources in the IVF laboratory setting. Some VOCs have been identified as potentially genotoxic or mutagenic in contexts other than in vitro fertilization. Exposure of human embryos in vitro to VOCs may have harmful consequences on both the developmental potential of the embryo as well as long-term child health. However, as yet little is known about concentrations, sources, and potential deleterious consequences of VOCs commonly detected in IVF laboratories.

17.2.1 Sampling strategy

It should be kept in mind that the indoor air quality is static, that is, unaltered over a longer period of time, only in exceptional cases. The concentration in air of any substance typically fluctuates at all times and this fluctuation is influenced by the potency of emission from the source, the human activity, the room ventilation rate, the climatic conditions, and possible sorption or desorption on, for example, interior surfaces and furniture. Furthermore, the composition of the indoor air is likely to differ from one room to another.

These facts should affect the sampling strategy for indoor air surveys. Primarily it is necessary to identify the purpose and define when, where, how often, and for what duration the samples should be taken. Only after this has been clarified can the analysis of the indoor air components be planned. This requires a distinct strategy because there are different specific analytical methods for each respective VOC in indoor ambient air depending on their chemical origin. Thus far, an all-purpose strategy for the analysis of the whole range of VOCs, especially for VOCs in IVF laboratories, has not been engineered and described.

The ISO standard 16000 series "Indoor air" describes various methods that can be used for the measurement of VOC concentrations and can therefore also serve as an orientation for the design of a sampling strategy directed toward the substances that one wants to detect.[3] For example, the ISO 16000-6, Indoor air–Part 6, "Indoor air: Determination of volatile organic compounds in indoor and test chamber air by active sampling on Tenax TA® Sorbent, thermal desorption and gas chromatography using MS or MS-FID"[4] is a widely used standard method for VOCs between C_6 and C_{16}.

The determination of indoor air pollution usually runs in two phases:

1. Sampling should be performed on site with one device and the analysis is performed at a later stage in a laboratory, for example, using desorption tubes.
2. Sampling and analysis are carried out simultaneously on the site using direct-reading instruments, for example, using VOC probes from the Wolf Sense or Research Instruments companies.

Furthermore, two types of sampling must be distinguished by the duration of measurement: first, short-term sampling, which typically does not exceed one hour, and which provides an ad-hoc snapshot of the prevalence of specific VOCs and, second, longer-term sampling (several hours to several days), which aims at determining an average exposure over a longer time period.

17.2.2 Duration and time point of sampling

It is important to consider that the concentration of air pollutants is not constant over time, but—as stated earlier—varies temporally. If chemicals (e.g., detergents) are currently used in a room, typically outlier measurements can be expected. The relevance of results generated under such circumstances needs to be carefully considered. Further important parameters when deciding on the time to start as well as the duration of the sampling are, for example, the air exchange rate, the personnel activities, the type of room and the room temperature, as well as the relative humidity.

Activities like opening a window will disturb the previously established equilibrium status of the ambient air. With short-term sampling, it is therefore impossible to obtain representative results, when starting the measurement directly after ventilation or after detergent use. In most IVF laboratories, however, ventilation through windows is not allowed and therefore not a factor to be considered.

If the substance in question is emitted continuously, for example, by building materials or furniture, opening a window for ventilation or personnel moving in and out of the room, thereby opening and closing doors, may seriously affect short-term sampling results, as contaminants from outside or adjacent rooms may be introduced. For long-term sampling, the amount and frequency of ventilation should be documented and accounted for when interpreting the results.

If the emissions result from discontinuous sources, the point of the measurement and the duration of sampling will depend on the target of the investigation. It may fall within the period of peak concentration or cover the average load over a longer period. Eventually, even the person taking the sample or setting up the measurement device may introduce substances otherwise unrelated to the IVF laboratory air, like cigarette smoke or cosmetic/perfume odor.

If the building or the room is equipped with a ventilation and air conditioning system (heating, ventilation, and air conditioning; HVAC), further aspects should be considered. The HVAC system itself may be a source of adverse emissions (e.g., from sealing materials, from the humidification, or from dust) and may transfer contaminants from one room to another throughout the whole air-conditioned building—in particular if the HVAC system is operated with a high recirculation rate.

Ultimately, the intake port of air for the HVAC system may become a source of high levels of air contaminants, in particular if the air intake is near ground level, where, for example, exhaust fumes from vehicles may constitute a problem.

17.2.3 Sampling purpose

The most important points to be considered for a sampling strategy are

1. The biochemical interaction with the cells handled in the laboratory
2. The physical properties of the substances
3. The emission characteristics of the source
4. The detection limit of the analytical procedure
5. The overall objective of the measurement

The bio-chemical interaction of cells and contaminants of the highest concern is the potential genotoxicity. For substances with assumed acute effects on cells, a short-term sampling should be preferred, whereas for substances with long-term or cumulative effects a long-term sampling seems more appropriate. However, long-term sampling will not detect extreme peak concentrations. This may lead to false-negative measurement results.

The physical properties like fumes, dust, gases, and vapor as well as the chemical composition are factors that mandate the selection of the analytical instrumentation.

With regard to the emission characteristics, it seems to be clear that the detection of a temporary source is reasonably feasible only with a short-term measurement system. On the other hand, continuous sources seem to be best targeted by long-term measurements. The temporary peak concentration occurring during, for example, spraying of a slide fixer could only be detected by a short-term measuring system. In some cases, the nature of the emission characteristics of the suspected sources is initially unknown. A time-limited continuous recording of measured variables (e.g., sum of total carbon using a flame ionization detector [FID] or photo ionization detector [PID]) can provide valuable information to determine further procedures.

There is a wide range of analytical instrumentation and methods for the measurement of airborne substances available. The detection limits, range, specificity, and repeatability are factors to be considered when deciding on the survey strategy. The manufacturer normally provides these data, and in the literature one can find supporting data and indications for their applicability. Some methods deliver rapid results; some may take days, for example, absorption tubes.

The long-term sampling is usually used to determine the average exposure of the personnel to VOCs in the context of occupational safety and health issues, for example, issues originating from complaints concerning the "sick building syndrome (SBS)." Such results may in some cases be of use so that the objective of a survey can be narrowed to some degree, for example, to save on cost and time and limit the survey to short-term sampling of extreme situations (e.g., low air exchange rate, elevated temperature) in order to be able to estimate the maximum possible contamination impact. The conditions for use and the terms of use of the room during sampling should in any case be carefully documented in order to allow cross comparison between repetitive measurements or data from the literature.

In some cases, especially when only a few measurements are to be performed, a compromise is required and not all objectives (average exposure determination vs. peak-concentration determination) may be explored to a similar extent.

17.2.4 Location of measurement

In addition to the temporal fluctuation and accumulation of a given substance, the spatial distribution must be considered. Not only when, but also where to measure within a given setting may affect the results.

Regarding the location of sampling, one might have to measure in several different places, for example, in the middle of the room, to obtain a long-term value and at different places in the room for short-term values. It might even be worthwhile to elaborate a 3D picture of the room to optimize the measurements (e.g., to locate sampling points with the highest concentrations) and to document the results accordingly.

In buildings equipped with HVAC systems, measuring the supply and exhaust air can under certain circumstances be useful to analyze how the values are distributed around an average and thus to localize and rank the sources of air pollution.

Standard rules for occupational safety and health require that measurements are generally done in the center of the room. If this is not possible, the sampling device should not be closer than one meter away from the wall. Samples should be taken at a height about one to one and a half meters above the floor, as this is the approximate height of the head.

Beyond the standardized measurements in the context of workplace safety is the objective of the measurements in the IVF laboratory, which aims at identifying exposure of vulnerable human cells to VOCs during in vitro culture.

17.2.5 Measuring with thermal desorption tubes (e.g., Tenax TA®)

The method is based on the use of thermal desorption tubes, for example, Tenax TA thermal desorption tubes, in combination with a pump followed by thermal desorption (TD) of the compounds and separation by means of gas chromatography (GC) analysis and identification through a flame ionization detector (FID) and/or a mass spectrometry detector.[4]

The Tenax® method is suitable for measurements of nonpolar and weakly polar VOCs in the mass concentration range of less than 1 mg per cubic meter up to several milligrams per cubic meter. On the basis of the principal mechanism of action, VOCs and some very volatile organic compounds (VVOCs) and semivolatile organic compounds (SVOCs) can also be analyzed by this method.

The various VOCs are classified into specific categories according to their boiling point:

- SVOC having a boiling point in the range of 240–260°C to 380–400°C.
- VOC having a boiling point in the range of 50–100°C to 240–260°C.
- VVOC having a boiling point in the range of less than 0°C to 50–100°C.

The World Health Organization established this classification.[5] However, there are many other definitions in use, depending on country, institution, association, and organization, which have historically established differing definitions.

17.2.5.1 Total volatile organic compounds (TVOCs)

The amount of VOCs in indoor air, often called total volatile organic compounds (TVOCs) can be sampled for various purposes and by using different techniques, which also yield different measurement results. For the purpose of the IVF air analysis described herein, the TVOC will be defined as TVOCs collected by Tenax TA and this will thus include all TVOCs from n-hexane to n-hexadecane. The compounds are detected by means of an ionization detector (TVOC-FID) or a mass spectrometer (TVOC-MS). The details of the measurement results are presented as "toluene-equivalents" using the total area of the chromatogram based on the "analytical window" of the toluene.[4]

It is common practice to generate a single concentration value in order to characterize the total mass of VOC in the air. This value is referred to as the "TVOC value." It should be emphasized that this TVOC value will depend on the applied sampling and analytical method. Therefore, the presented TVOC values should always give a reference to the sampling and analytical method used.

17.2.5.2 Short description of the method

A well-defined sample volume of gas is drawn from the ambient air with a pump (Figure 17.1). The gas is therewith lead over one (or more) sorbent tubes filled with the Sorbent Tenax TA (Figure 17.2). The VOCs are retained in the sorbent tube. The analysis of the tubes subsequently takes place in a specialized laboratory. The collected VOCs are thermally desorbed from the sorbent, and rinsed with a cold trap or a filled sorbent trap by using an inert carrier gas stream to a gas chromatograph. The gas chromatograph consists of a capillary column and a detector.

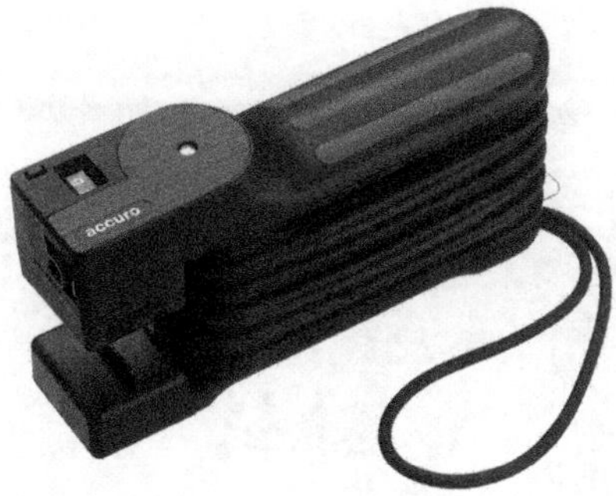

Figure 17.1 **(See color insert.)** Hand pump for Tenax TA thermo desorption tube. (Drägerwerk AG & Co. KGaA, Lübeck, Germany.)

Figure 17.2 Tenax TA thermo desorption tube. (Drägerwerk AG & Co. KGaA, Lübeck, Germany.)

All needed instruments are commercially available, and can usually also be rented from distinct laboratories conducting the later analysis. As a result of the laboratory analysis, a written report of the measurement values should be requested. However, one cannot expect the laboratory to provide an assessment of the potential impact of the results. Only the sponsor of the analysis is able to and, in principle, allowed to interpret the analysis findings and to determine the needs for action. We want to highlight that no threshold values have as yet been defined above which an adverse effect of individual VOCs or groups of VOCs is to be expected in the context of human cell culture.

Direct-reading meter. Direct-reading meters in general could estimate air contaminants by one of several detection principles. The contaminants may react to specific chemicals (e.g., CO_2 to infrared light), chemical groups (e.g., certain volatile organics to photo-ionization), or general pollutant categories (e.g., all respirable particles of scattered light).

17.2.6 VOC probe—Photo ionization detector (PID)

To get an overview of existing sources of emissions in the laboratory, it is advisable to perform a screening measurement using a handheld VOC-probe.

Commercially available VOC measurement instruments are used for such a purpose, which can determine the TVOC concentrations by the photo-ionization detection (PID) method (Figure 17.3). This method has the advantage that the results are obtained immediately and that no laboratory is required for the analysis. A disadvantage is that only the TVOC concentration is determined, that is, the total concentration of all the VOCs in a defined measuring range. The device itself is not able to qualify the different VOCs and to quantify them separately.

In order to systematically carry out such a measurement in the laboratory with the VOC probe, the hand piece should be held nearby the surfaces to be investigated, thereby slowly screening the equipment, furnishings, and other potential VOC emitters. Increases in the total concentrations can be immediately recognized and considered further for later

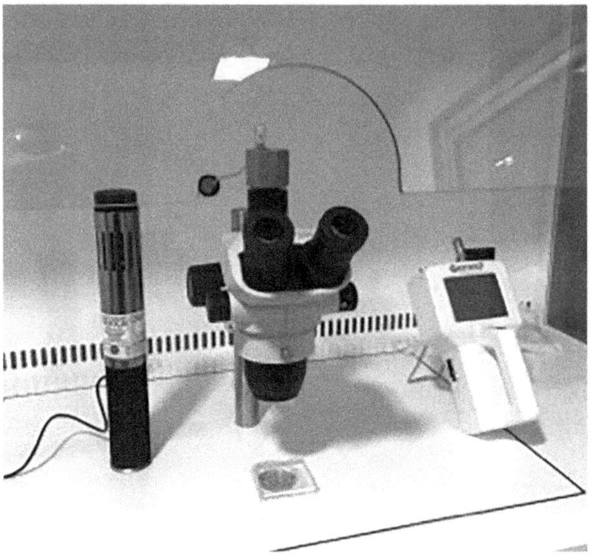

Figure 17.3 VOC probe with handheld reading meter in an IVF workbench. (Sparmed ApS, Farum, Denmark.)

measurements. Moreover, the reproducibility of a given result in relation to a potential source of emission can be checked immediately. After a complete screening of the laboratory has taken place, a summary of the test results should be written down and potentially critical equipment, surfaces, etc., should be identified. This can then serve as the basis on which measures aiming at the reduction of TVOCs are taken and surveyed for their effectiveness.

In addition to screening measurements, which should be understood as ad-hoc spot measurements, long-term measurements and analyses are also possible with such a VOC-meter. For example, one might want to monitor how the daily work routine affects the VOC-load in a given room. Often operating rooms and IVF laboratories are localized adjacent to one another. Once a procedure in the operation theater starts, significant fluctuations in VOC contamination in the IVF laboratory, for example, as a result of the use of disinfectants or anesthetics, could be detected by a constant measurement with a handheld probe.

By use of a handheld VOC probe, it is also possible to take measurements from within an incubator. For this purpose, it is important that the incubator is not loaded with cells because it is necessary that the air humidity is down regulated and the CO_2 supply is shut off. These factors would otherwise affect the results or even impede the measurement method itself. It should be noted, however, that most incubators in use in IVF laboratories take 94–95% of their indoor air from the ambient air of the room and only about 5% from gas cylinders. It should be ascertained that the gas contained in a supply container has a high and well-defined purity. The preparation of technical gases (in contrast to medical gases) is often not fully transparent. Accordingly, there is no guarantee that other excipients have been used and a routine testing for organic compounds or metallic contaminants has usually not been undertaken to control the quality and purity of the end product. Accordingly, many incubator manufacturers offer their products with special air filters that aim at purifying the air inside the incubator. It is a necessity that laboratory personnel routinely use medical grade gases and have knowledge and insight about the air purity and how this can be affected by the use of distinct materials inside the incubator.

17.3 Microbiological testing and monitoring

The risks of microbial contamination are well known in every laboratory. A wide variety of hygienic measures and staff training at regular intervals has been implemented to prevent microbial contaminations. Patient screening can minimize the risk of introducing infections into the laboratory when indicated by medical history or when mandatory according to guidelines and laws. However, pretreatment screening will not provide complete safety because of "silent" infections prior to detectable sero-conversion. Nevertheless, most national and also international guidelines recommend that patients undergoing ART treatment should be routinely tested for HIV, as well as hepatitis B and C. Screening for genital infections, that is, chlamydia, syphilis, gonorrhea, herpes simplex, cytomegalovirus, human papilloma virus, and vaginal infections should be considered case-by-case or within the context of specific patient populations under treatment and prevalence of distinct diseases.

17.3.1 Sampling methods

Passive microbial air monitoring with the help of settle plates or contact plates is a useful complement to active air sampling methods. Settle plates allow a semi-quantitative determination of microbial contaminations in the air. They are also suitable for personnel monitoring (e.g., gloves). Plates furthermore enable continuous monitoring during production processes. Since they are fairly small, they can also be used conveniently in confined spaces.

Alternatively, active air monitoring systems are available from many companies. They work nearly automatically and allow an overview over the microbial room contamination.

17.3.2 Testing and monitoring with contact and settle plates

Extensive and effective implementation of hygiene measurements like cleaning and maintenance schedules, together with strict adherence to aseptic techniques should make routine microbiological testing in principal unnecessary. However, testing may be required in order to identify a source of contamination in a culture system. Beyond that, routine microbiological testing may also be a necessity in the context of a quality management system (i.e., ISO 9000 series). In such quality management systems, one has to define and document all quality relevant processes and procedures, and this may well encompass the monitoring of the absence of microbial contaminations.

For testing the efficiency of such defined processes, constant data-driven monitoring of procedure performance is required. For hygienic measures like cleaning and maintenance, settle plates are regarded as an adequate and accepted method of verifying the expected effectiveness of a given procedure.

17.3.2.1 Sample equipment

Solid growth media (e.g., settle and contact plates), prepared according to a standardized formulation, may be obtained from or via a hospital microbiology department or a specialized laboratory. Materials that are purchased from a commercial manufacturer should, however, be preferred, because they will be manufactured to a suitable consistency and are available in a variety of formats (e.g., irradiated). Commercially available materials are batch prepared with an appropriate specification and quality controlled to test the growth capabilities of the media. Growth media should be demonstrated as "growth supporting" for the time and conditions under which exposure occurs. The quality of test materials should be checked thoroughly prior to using them. Spurious high counts may arise from the use of inadequately controlled microbiological test materials. Consideration should be given to purchasing irradiated materials for use in critical zones. Irradiated materials need not be pre-incubated and can be used immediately in critical zones. If nonirradiated materials are obtained from a commercial source, then pre-incubating to check media sterility prior to use should be considered.

It is preferable to use a growth medium with low selectivity, that is, capable of supporting a broad spectrum of microorganisms, including aerobes, anaerobes, fungi, yeast, and molds. When deemed necessary, a selective culture medium capable of detecting or searching for a particular type of microorganism should be used. It might even be advisable to consult with a medical microbiology expert for advice.

The recommended size of solid media is 90 mm in diameter (approximate internal area 64 cm^2) for settle plates and 55 mm (surface area 25 cm^2) for contact plates.[6]

17.3.2.2 *Sampling method*

Sampling should be undertaken at prespecified frequencies and locations. It is preferable to retrieve samples in the operational modus of the lab, for example, with equipment running and personnel performing routine operations.

A frequently used method of sampling has been to swab workplace surfaces, incubators, workbenches, etc., and to cultivate the samples thereafter. After this sampling, the routine cleaning of the laboratory should be done with the cleaning agents routinely used. After cleaning, the sampling should be repeated.

17.3.2.3 *Incubation conditions*

Following sample retrieval, the samples should be incubated as soon as possible (within 24 hours of sampling; same day is preferred) and should be held at room temperature. If the medium is dropped or touched by an operator, then this should be reported and the sample should be marked accordingly and treated as usual. Under no circumstances should samples be refrigerated before testing.

Incubation of samples, inverted, at 30–35°C for at least two days is suitable for the growth of bacteria. Incubation of samples, inverted, at 20–25°C for at least five days is suitable for the growth of mold and fungi. Other incubation conditions may be used if it can be shown that the conditions promote the growth of (all) microorganisms that may have been recovered during the sampling procedure. Incubation conditions should be monitored to ensure that the appropriate incubation temperature is maintained throughout the incubation phase.

17.3.2.4 *Settle plates*

Settle plate sampling is a direct method of assessing the number of microorganisms attached to a product or surface at a given time. It is based on the observation that, in the absence of any kind of influence, airborne microorganisms, typically attached to larger particles, will attach to open culture plates. Microorganisms are usually found in the air of occupied rooms in conjunction with shed human skin epithelial cells. The airborne microbial particle will deposit, by gravity, onto surfaces at a rate of approximately 1 cm/s.

17.3.2.5 *Results and reading of samples*

In settle plate sampling, Petri dishes containing agar medium are opened and exposed for a given period of time, thus allowing microbe-bearing particles to deposit onto them.

Petri dishes with 90 mm diameter are most commonly used. The number of microbe bearing particles deposited onto the agar surface of the plate over the period of exposure is analyzed by incubation of the plate and counting the number of microbial colonies, more commonly known as colony forming units (CFUs). The microbial deposition rate may be reported as the number deposited in a given area per unit time. Separate colony counts may be tabulated for mold and bacteria. Colony types may be identified if this is considered appropriate. For exact classification of the type of contamination, a suitable hygiene institute or test laboratory may be consulted.

17.3.3 Contamination of the culture media

The culture media itself should routinely be monitored to detect early signs of possible microbial contamination or deterioration. All manufacturers of common culture media express in their instructions for use precautions and warnings like "Do not use if cloudy" or "Do not use if product becomes discolored or shows any evidence of microbial contamination." Furthermore, culture media have to be used within a prespecified time period after opening of the culture media vial. In the above cited cases, when the media in the bottle change color or show any evidence of microbial contamination, a prompt and professional action in the form of an extensive root cause analysis is needed.

Among others, it should be investigated what media are affected, where were the media used, which are the possible implications, how can the error and its impacts be fixed, how can the recurrence be prevented, and so on. Also, it is possible to culture the media without cells in an open system to analyze the incubator for microbial contamination.

17.3.4 Active air monitoring systems

Active air monitoring systems are devices that can be purchased from one of the manufacturers, or alternatively rented from an analytical laboratory. The main advantage of such systems is that they run nearly automatically in a short time. The systems have to be loaded with special plates and after doing this, the system starts to run and draw a defined volume of gas over the plate. After this, the plates must be cultured and analyzed nearly in the same way as the passive contact and settle plates.

References

1. Cohen, J., Gilligan, A., Esposito, W., Schimmel, T., and Dale, B. Ambient air and its potential effects on conception in vitro. *Hum. Reprod.* 1997;12:1742–9.
2. Indoor Air Quality in Commercial and Institutional Buildings, 2011. Occupational Safety and Health Administration U.S. Department of Labor OSHA 3430-042011. http://www.osha.gov/Publications/3430indoor-air-quality-sm.pdf.
3. International Organization for Standardization, 2004. ISO 16000-1: Indoor air—Part 1: General aspects of sampling strategy (ISO 16000-1:2004).
4. International Organization for Standardization, 2011. ISO 16000-6: Indoor air—Part 6: Determination of volatile organic compounds in indoor and test chamber air by active sampling on Tenax TA® sorbent, thermal desorption and gas chromatography using MS or MS-FID (ISO 16000-6:2011).
5. World Health Organization, 2010. WHO Guidelines for indoor air quality: Selected pollutants. http://www.euro.who.int/__data/assets/pdf_file/0009/128169/e94535.pdf.
6. Guidelines on test methods for environmentalist monitoring for aseptic dispensing facilities. A working group of the Scottish quality assurance specialist interest group, 2nd ed., February 2004.

section four

Quality management in clean room assisted reproductive units

chapter eighteen

Regulatory requirements for air quality control in reproductive laboratories

Sandro C. Esteves and Fabiola C. Bento

Contents

Abstract

This chapter discusses the existing regulations regarding specific requirements for air quality control in reproductive laboratories. At present, such regulations exist for the 27 member states within the European Union (EU) and Brazil. While regulatory directives aim to safeguard public health in line with the precautionary principle, thus preventing transmission of infectious diseases via transplanted tissues and cells, they require different strategies to mitigate the potential risks associated with laboratory air contamination. A common feature of both the EU and Brazilian directives is the filtration of particulate matter and microbial contamination control, but only the Brazilian directive requires the filtration of toxic gases (volatile organic compounds [VOCs]). Studies reporting in vitro fertilization outcomes after implementation of air quality control as per regulatory directives are scarce, but the existing ones indicate that operating under such environmental conditions is both feasible and effective.

18.1 Introduction

A few regulatory agencies have issued directives that include specific requirements for air quality control in embryology laboratories. Fertility centers holding assisted reproductive technology (ART) units in countries where such regulations are in place should operate in conformance with these directives. The basis for mandating ambient air quality control is to safeguard public health by preventing the transmission of infectious diseases via transplanted tissues and cells, according to the premises of the precautionary principle.[1]

The precautionary principle is used when measures are needed in the face of a possible danger to human health where scientific data do not allow a complete evaluation of the risk.

The European Union Tissues and Cells Directive[2] and the Brazilian Cell and Tissue Directive[3] cover a wide spectrum of systems aiming at increasing quality in all units performing ART through mandatory implementation of a quality management system that involves the presence of adequately trained and certified staff, full documentation and formulation of standard operating procedures, quality control, and quality assurance. Both directives dictate specific requirements for air quality control within reproductive laboratories (reviewed by Esteves and Bento).[4]

18.2 European Union Tissues and Cells Directive (EUTCD)

With regard to air particle filtration, the EUTCD requires a clean air zone equivalent to the Grade A standards in the European commission guide to good manufacturing practice in the critical areas where tissues or cells are exposed to the environment during processing with a background environment at least equivalent to Grade D.[5] The background environment represents clean areas for carrying out less critical stages. Grade A air quality is defined by the concentration of the permitted maximum number of particles of a given size and is equivalent to ISO 14644 class 5. It means that a level of particle cleanliness of not more than 3500 particles of a size ≥0.5 μm or greater, and not more than 20 particles of a size ≥5.0 μm or greater per cubic meter of air, should be detected. Grade D air quality is equivalent to ISO 14644 class 8, meaning that not more than 3,520,000 of a size ≥0.5 μm or greater and not more than 29,300 of a size ≥5.0 μm or greater per cubic meter of air should be detected (Table 18.1).

In order to ensure that these standards are met, a filtered air supply should maintain a positive pressure and airflow relative to surrounding areas of lower air quality under all operational conditions and should flush the area effectively. Of note, there is a proviso for a lower quality clean zone air grade, if such a level of particle cleanliness can be justified through risk assessment.

Control of microbial contamination should also be ensured in addition to air particle filtration. The maximum permissible microorganisms determined by the number of colony forming units (CFUs) in a Grade A area are as follows: air sample (CFU/m^3: <1), 90 mm diameter settle plates (CFU/4 h: <1), 50 mm diameter contact plates (CFU/plate: <1), 5-finger glove print (CFU/glove: <1). The limits for microbial contamination in a Grade D area are air sample (CFU/m^3: 200), 90 mm diameter settle plates (CFU/4 h: 100), 50 mm diameter contact plates (CFU/plate: 50), 5-finger glove print (CFU/glove: not defined) (Table 18.1).

With regard to control of toxic gases in the laboratory air environment, the EUTCD has issued no specific requirement.

18.3 Brazilian Cell and Tissue Directive (BCTD; ANVISA, RDC23)

The Brazilian directive dictates that laboratory air quality for particulates should be at least equivalent to ISO class 5 in the critical areas where tissues or cells are exposed to the environment during processing.[6] One of the following methods is recommended to achieve such conditions: (1) biological safety cabinet class II type A; (2) unidirectional laminar flow workstation; (3) a clean room at least equivalent to ISO 5.

Table 18.1 Ambient air quality requirements for in vitro fertilization laboratories operating under regulatory directives in the European Union and Brazil

Region (directive)	European Union (EU directive 2004/23/EC; 2006/86/EC)	Brazil (ANVISA RDC33/2006; amended by RDC23/2011)
Particle filtration	Equivalent to GMP[a] Grade A air quality in the critical areas where tissues or cells are exposed to the environment during processing with a background environment at least equivalent to Grade D[b]	At least equivalent to ISO class 5 (NBR/ISO 14644-1) in the critical areas where tissues or cells are exposed to the environment during processing
Microbial contamination	Maximum colony forming units (CFUs) in Grades A and D air quality environments defined as follows: air sample (CFU/m^3: <1 and 200), 90 mm diameter settle plates (CFU/4 h: <1 and 100), 50 mm diameter contact plates (CFU/plate: <1 and 50), 5-finger glove print (CFU/glove: <1 and "not defined")	Microbiological monitoring required; specifications not defined
VOCs filtration	Not required	Ventilation systems should be equipped with filters imbedded with activated-carbon

Source: Adapted from Esteves and Bento. *Reprod Biomed Online*. 2013; 26: 9–21.

Note: GMP: European commission guide to good manufacturing practice revision to annex 1 (EU 2003/94/EC).

[a] GMP Grades A and D air quality for particulates are equivalent to International Standard ISO 14644-1 classes 5 and 8, respectively.

[b] A less stringent environment may be acceptable in the following cases: (1) where it is demonstrated that exposure in a Grade A environment has a detrimental effect on the required properties of the tissue or cell concerned; (2) where it is demonstrated that the mode and route of application of the tissue or cell to the recipient implies a significantly lower risk of transmitting bacterial or fungal infection to the recipient than with cell and tissue transplantation; (3) where it is not technically possible to carry out the required process in a Grade A environment (e.g., due to requirements for specific equipment in the processing area that is not fully compatible with grade A).

Laboratory background air, which includes indoor air in areas for carrying out less critical stages, should be pressurized and filtered for particulate matter when biological safety cabins and unidirectional laminar flows rather than clean rooms are applied. For this, air volume flow rates of 15 and 45 [m^3/h]/m^2 or greater for outside and total air, respectively, and a filtration system composed of at least G3 + F8 filters are required. G3-type filters are the primary filters used to collect coarse dust with a dust spot efficiency of 80–90%, while F8 are secondary filters that collect and retain small particle dust with an average and minimum spot efficiency for 0.4 μm particles of 90–95% and 55%, respectively.[7]

Areas in which oocytes/reproductive tissue/sperm are surgically retrieved should be pressurized as well with outside and total air volumes of 6 and 18 [m^3/h]/m^2 or greater, respectively. In addition, inflow air from outside should be filtered for particulates using at least G4 class dust filtration, which collects coarse dust with a dust spot efficiency at least 90%.

In addition to particle filtration, ventilation systems should be equipped with filters embedded with activated carbon to remove VOCs. However, specific instructions about the minimum requirements of such filtration systems have not been determined (Table 18.1). Last, microbial control should be ensured but likewise VOC filtration, no specifications were defined.

18.4 Implications for practice

ART units providing assisted reproduction treatments involving in vitro manipulation of gametes and embryos that operate in the EU and Brazil are obliged to comply with specific regulatory requirements, as defined by standards of quality and safety for the donation, obtaining, testing, processing, preservation, storage, and distribution of human tissues and cells. In Europe, the EUTCD has been in place since 2004, and it affects all in vitro fertilization (IVF) centers of member states, namely, Austria, Belgium, Bulgaria, Cyprus, Czech Republic, Denmark, Estonia, Finland, France, Germany, Greece, Hungary, Ireland, Italy, Latvia, Lithuania, Luxembourg, Malta, the Netherlands, Poland, Portugal, Romania, Slovakia, Slovenia, Spain, Sweden, and the United Kingdom.[2]

In Brazil, the National Agency for Sanitary Surveillance (ANVISA) passed a similar regulatory directive in 2006 that was subsequently amended in 2011.[3] While regulatory directives aim to safeguard public health in line with the precautionary principle,[1] thus preventing transmission of infectious diseases via transplanted tissues and cells, they require different strategies to mitigate these risks, as shown in Table 18.1, but do not specifically address how periodic testing and validation should be carried out.[8]

With the publication of the aforesaid directives, a debate has started in which several practitioners challenged the feasibility and effectiveness of such strict requirements. Some of them even argued that there could be a likely adverse impact of applying clean room air quality standards to IVF laboratories.[9–11] In brief, it had been hypothesized that laminar flow cabinets do not provide optimized conditions for the control of both temperature and pH, which are crucial in IVF procedures. In addition, the vibration from laminar flow cabinets would greatly compromise micromanipulation of the gametes, and the high volume airflow would create a cooling effect that would be difficult to countereffect with microscope warm stages. Last, large oscillations in temperature and humidity due to the airflow would jeopardize embryo development because of the need to remove them from incubators for grading purposes. Nevertheless, a contrary opinion has been presented by investigators who reported improvement in ART effectiveness after implementation of air quality controls as per the EU and Brazilian directives (reviewed by Esteves and Bento).[12] In one study involving infertile couples undergoing IVF in the United Kingdom, Knaggs et al. evaluated the outcomes of IVF carried out in a newly constructed laboratory facility in accordance with the EUTCD requirements for air quality control. Analysis of key performance indicators in a period prior to and after the move into the new embryology facility indicated that implantation and pregnancy rates increased after the move into the clean room.[13] In another study conducted in the United States, Heitmann et al. observed that live birth rates were increased by improvements in air quality after the installation of a centered system supplying filtered air (both particulate and VOC air filtration) to the IVF laboratory and related critical areas.[14] We have also evaluated the outcomes of 2315 IVF cycles over a nine-year period before and after air quality control implementation according to the Brazilian Tissue and Cell Directive. In our observational analytic cohort study, live birth rates increased (35.6% vs. 25.8%, $p = 0.02$) while miscarriage rates decreased (28.7% vs. 20.0%, $p = 0.04$) after clean room implementation.[4] Despite the debate regarding the role of air quality control in IVF, the aforementioned regulatory authorities in both the European Union and Brazil amended their directives in 2006 and 2011, respectively, and kept the requirements for air quality control in the environments in which gametes and embryos are handled.

18.5 Conclusions

ART units in both the European Union and Brazil operate under regulatory directives that require clean room standards to reproductive laboratories. A common ground of these directives is the need to supply pressurized and filtered air for particulate matter into the areas where gametes and embryos are handled, in addition to microbial contamination control. However, the directives differ with regard to VOC filtration. While these regulatory directives aim to safeguard public health in line with the precautionary principle, thus preventing transmission of infectious diseases via transplanted tissues and cells, they do not specifically address how periodic testing and validation of these areas should be carried out. Few centers operating under such regulations have presented reassuring IVF outcomes, but further information should be collected from other units practicing within the same framework. Guidelines on the target limits and best practice statements on how to implement air quality control to IVF are still lacking.

References

1. Commission of the European Union Communities, 2000. Communication from the Commission on the precautionary principle. http://eur-lex.europa.eu/smartapi/cgi/sga_doc?smartapi!celexplus!prod!DocNumber&lg=en&type_doc=COMfinal&an_doc=2000&nu_doc=1 (accessed May 14, 2015).
2. Commission of the European Parliament, 2004. Directive 2004/23/EC of the European Parliament and of the Council of 31 March 2004 on setting standards of quality and safety for the donation, procurement, testing, processing, preservation, storage and distribution of human tissues and cells. http://eur-lex.europa.eu/LexUriServ/LexUriServ.do?uri=CELEX:32004L0023:EN:NOT (accessed May 15, 2015).
3. ANVISA. Brazilian National Agency for Sanitary Surveillance, 2006. Resolução no. 33 da Diretoria colegiada da Agência Nacional de Vigilância Sanitária (amended by RDC23 of May 27, 2011 on setting standards of quality and safety for the donation, procurement, testing, processing, preservation, storage and distribution of human tissues and cells). http://bvsms.saude.gov.br/bvs/saudelegis/anvisa/2011/res0023_27_05_2011.html (accessed May 15, 2015).
4. Esteves SC, Bento FC. Implementation of air quality control in reproductive laboratories in full compliance with the Brazilian Cells and Germinative Tissue Directive. *Reprod Biomed Online.* 2013; 26: 9–21.
5. European Commission, 2003. EC guide to good manufacturing practice revision to annex 1. http://ec.europa.eu/health/files/eudralex/vol-4/pdfs-en/revan1vol4_3_en.pdf (accessed June 6, 2015).
6. International Organization for Standardization, 1999. ISO NBR 14644-1:2005 on cleanrooms and associated controlled environments. Associação Brasileira de Normas Técnicas (ABNT), Brasilia, DF, Brasil.
7. Esteves SC, Agarwal A. Explaining how reproductive laboratories work. In: Bento F, Esteves S, Agarwal A, eds. *Quality Management in ART Clinics: A Practical Guide.* 1st ed., Springer Science+Business Media, New York, pp. 79–127, 2013.
8. Esteves SC, Bento FC. Implementation of cleanroom technology in reproductive laboratories: The question is not why but how. *Reprod Biomed Online.* Oct 20, 2015. pii: S1472-6483(15)00486-1. doi: 10.1016/j.rbmo.2015.09.014. [Epub ahead of print].
9. Mortimer D. A critical assessment of the impact of the European Union Tissues and Cells Directive (2004) on laboratory practices in assisted conception. *Reprod Biomed Online* 2005; 11: 162–76.
10. Hartshorne GM. Challenges of the EU 'tissues and cells' directive. *Reprod Biomed Online* 2005; 11: 404–7.

11. Bhargava PM. Commentary on the critical assessment of the impact of the recent European Union Tissues and Cells Directive. *Reprod Biomed Online* 2005; 11: 161.
12. Esteves SC, Bento FC. Air quality control in the ART laboratory is a major determinant of IVF success. *Asian J Androl.* Nov 10, 2015. doi: 10.4103/1008-682X.166433. [Epub ahead of print].
13. Knaggs P, Birch D, Drury S, Morgan M, Kumari S, Sriskandakumar R et al. Full compliance with the EU directive air quality standards does not compromise IVF outcome. *Hum Reprod* 2007; 22 (Suppl.1): i164–5.
14. Heitmann RJ, Hill MJ, James AN, Schimmel T, Segars JH et al. Live births achieved via IVF are increased by improvements in air quality and laboratory environment. *Reprod Biomed Online* 2015; 31: 364–71.

chapter nineteen

Risk management in clean room assisted reproductive units

Adrianne K. Pope

Contents

Abstract

Quality management systems can play a significant role in ensuring effective, efficient, and safe delivery of care in assisted reproductive technology (ART) with a focus on customer service. The ISO 31000:2009 standard is recognized as the necessary tool to determine, analyze, and treat risks. It can be successfully applied to reproductive technology and it is becoming common to include a risk management system in ART units. As air quality is a major risk to the success of ART, identifying potential environmental risks is essential to aid in developing strategies to address volatile organic compounds (VOCs) and particulate matter that may impact embryo development and safety. Risk management systems may be utilized across all aspects of ART service delivery. In this chapter, the emphasis will be on risk management systems and their use in managing air quality in ART units.

19.1 Introduction

The need for international standards has long been recognized, and in February 1947 the International Organization for Standardization (ISO) was established. It was named ISO after the Greek ISOS meaning equal. It is an independent, nongovernmental membership organization and the world's largest developer of voluntary international standards. Based in Geneva, the ISO has now developed over 19,500 international standards. These standards make things work by giving world-class specifications for products, services, and systems to ensure efficacy, efficiency, and safety. This aids in facilitating international trade.

One of the most commonly utilized standards is ISO 9001:2008. This standard has been revised and a new version was released in 2015. This is a generic business standard that may be utilized by any business, be it manufacturing or service provision. ISO 9001 is the quality management standard designed to provide confidence in an organization's ability to provide products or services that fulfill customer needs and expectations. It forms the basis of quality management systems (QMSs) and has been utilized by the assisted reproductive technology (ART) industry. The standard forms the backbone of good practice in ART. Michael Alper described the importance of ISO 9001 in ART as providing a sense of transparency within an organization, a clearer understanding of how service is provided to patients and the framework to allow continual improvement.[1] Much has now been written about the value of QMS in ART and slowly the concept is being embraced by ART units globally.

In 2004, the European Union developed a Tissues and Cells Directive 2004/23/EC. This directive sets standards of quality and safety for the donation, procurement, testing, processing, preservation, storage, and distribution of human tissues and cells intended for human application. Only licensed centers in the EU are allowed to handle human tissues and cells intended for human application. This introduced an international alignment with bodies such as the U.S. Food and Drug Administration (FDA) and the Australian Therapeutic Goods Administration (TGA). However, the EU Tissues and Cells Directive, and subsequent Technical Directives 2006/17/EU and 2006/86/EU, included ART units and described some very specific compliance requirements for ART units, including air quality.[2] The standards were concerned with minimizing risk and improving quality.[3–5] This was achieved through the implementation of QMSs. The European Society of Human Reproduction and Embryology (ESHRE) Revised guidelines for good practice in IVF laboratories, the Australian Fertility Society Reproductive Technology Accreditation Committee (RTAC) Code of Practice March 2014, and the American Society for Reproductive Medicine (ASRM) Revised guidelines for human embryology and andrology laboratories also outline the current best practice requirements for ART units.[6–8] The Australian RTAC Code of Practice is based on QMSs and risk management with particular focus on high risk activities in ART.

Historically, risk management was aligned with occupational health and safety, insurance, and litigation. In 1993, risk management took on a business focus in the United Kingdom after the release of the Cadbury and Turnbull reports on internal control and risk management. The introduction of the U.S. Government Performance and Results Act 1993 continued the trend. Risk management became a focus in both the public and private sectors.

The widespread use of air travel and the exponential increase in air traffic has placed an emphasis on air safety over the years and the aviation industry has been instrumental in establishing safety standards. In 1999, the Joint Standards Australia and Standards New Zealand developed AS/NZS 4360—Risk management—a standard on identifying, assessing, and mitigating risk. Following a revision in 2004 the ISO developed the first international risk management standard ISO 31000:2009 based on AS/NZS 4360. The current version, ISO 31000:2009, defines risk as the effect of uncertainty on objectives.[9] Risk management is aligned with the organization's culture, strategic objectives, values, resources, structure, processes, and policies. Risk management is effective based on the principles described in Table 19.1.

This standard provides ART units with an excellent tool to identify, analyze, evaluate, and treat risks in a clinical setting. Dominique de Ziegler and colleagues described the benefits of risk and safety management in ART.[10] The emphasis is on reducing medical errors and increasing the quality of care. David Meldrum and colleagues, and Richard Scott and

Table 19.1 Risk management principles

ISO 31000:2009 Risk management	
a. Creates and protects value	g. Tailored to organization
b. Integral part of all organizational processes	h. Human and cultural factors are taken into account
c. Part of decision making	i. Transparent and inclusive
d. Explicitly addresses uncertainty	j. Dynamic, iterative, and responsive to change
e. Systematic, structured, and timely	k. Facilitates continual improvement of the organization
f. Based on the best available information	

colleagues suggested ART should follow the aviation industry and consider the establishment of Safety Boards for ART, similar to those in the aviation industry.[11,12] ART is recognized for its highly complex procedures with extreme risks. The Human Fertilisation and Embryology Authority (HFEA) in the United Kingdom recently released a report detailing the risks identified in IVF units in the United Kingdom between 2010 and 2012.[13] Among the incidents identified were those relating to equipment failure and operator error. These are of particular importance when considering air quality and the instrumentation necessary to minimize risk. Such reports are valuable when identifying the risks associated with individual IVF laboratories.

19.2 ISO 31000:2009

ISO 31000:2009 is recognized as the necessary tool to determine, analyze, and treat risks.[9] It can be successfully applied to ART units and it is becoming common to include a risk management system into ART units. It will be compulsory in any standard reflecting a QMS. The standard provides the principles and generic guidelines on risk management and the process is outlined in Figure 19.1. Risk management systems now include compliance and governance along with risk. This highlights an organization's need to be familiar with any relevant legislation, regulations, or guidelines impacting on the business. It also encourages internal governance review. This allows a confidence that company policies and procedures comply with external legislation and regulation and that staff also comply. Risk management systems may be utilized across all aspects of ART service delivery. In this chapter, the emphasis will be on risk management systems and their use in managing air quality in ART units.

The standard defines the steps in developing an integrated governance, risk management, and compliance system. These steps are depicted in Figure 19.2.

19.2.1 Communicate and consult

When initiating a risk management system implementation project, it is essential to identify the appropriate project team members and to help define the context of the risk management system. Communication with key stakeholders, both internal and external, is helpful in identifying the areas of expertise required. A consultative approach helps to define the context of the system, ensure risks are identified effectively, and that the appropriate experts are working together to analyze the risks. Communication allows discussion with all stakeholders, thus providing a more balanced approach to risk analysis and mitigation. It may be valuable to develop links with external stakeholders such as regulators, patients/customers, or suppliers to ensure compliance and feasibility of any risk mitigation strategies.

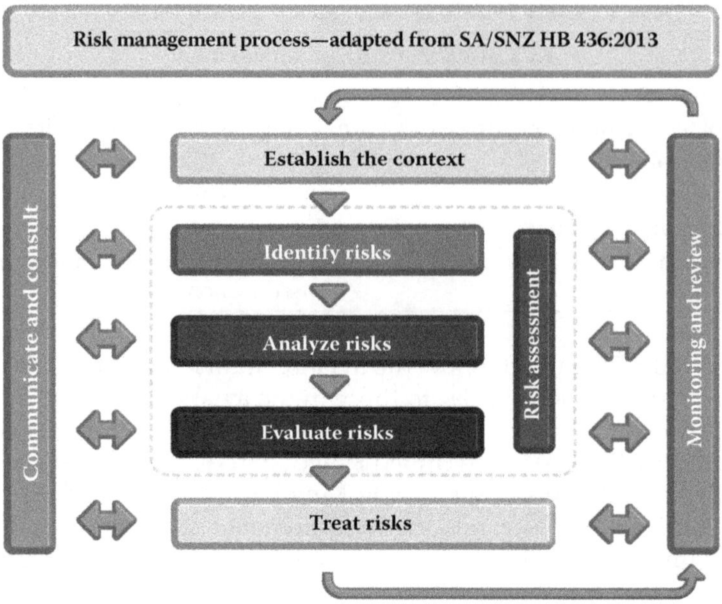

Figure 19.1 **(See color insert.)** Risk management process.

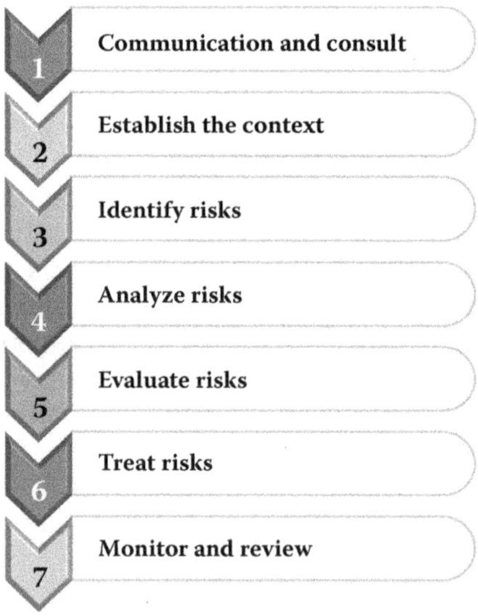

Figure 19.2 Risk management steps.

It is essential to identify risk "owners," those people with the expertise and authority to take responsibility. These people may not necessarily be directly involved in specific risk mitigation but by taking full responsibility will ensure that all necessary activities are undertaken.

Open communication encourages staff to take an active involvement in risk management and proactively assist in risk prevention. Managers should facilitate the engagement of stakeholders and ensure managerial support. One of the eight principles of quality management is leadership, and it is critical that all staff members appreciate the significance and high level support of risk management systems. In some countries, the ultimate responsibility for the mitigation of risk and compliance now falls on company directors under corporate law. Thus, many company boards are requesting specific information on risk management systems and reporting. Consideration should be given as to how risks will be monitored as the risk management systems are developed.

19.2.2 Context

Establishing the context of the risk management system is determined by a number of factors. These may include but not be limited to:

- Legislative or regulatory compliance requirements
- External context—strengths, weaknesses, opportunities, and threats
- ART units strategic objectives
- Components of ART unit to which the system will apply
- Internal capabilities and resources
- Financial constraints or opportunities
- Environmental factors
- Political, ethical, social, or cultural parameters
- Internal governance
- ART units risk tolerance appetite

Under the context of air quality in ART units, consideration should be given to compliance issues. ART units compliant with licensing specifying the requirements for laboratory air quality must ensure such legislation and regulation is part of the risk management system. Failure to comply with all requirements is a risk that may result in the loss of a licence. Air quality may be governed by ISO standards such as ISO 14644 used for the specification of air cleanliness in clean rooms.[14] The EU Commission Directive 2006/86/EC Section D (Facilities/Premises 2 and 3) stipulates[5]:

- When these activities include processing of tissues and cells while exposed to the environment, this must take place in an environment with specified air quality and cleanliness in order to minimize the risk of contamination, including cross-contamination between donations. The effectiveness of these measures must be validated and monitored.
- Unless otherwise specified in point 4,[5] where tissues and cells are exposed to the environment during processing, without a subsequent microbial inactivation process, an air quality with particle counts and microbial colony counts equivalent to those of Grade A as defined in the European Guide to Good Manufacturing Practice (GMP), Annex 1, and Directive 2003/94/EC is required with a background environment appropriate for the processing of tissue/cell concerned but at least to GMP Grade D in terms of particles and microbial counts.

If legislation or regulation is not a compliance issue, consideration should still be given to international standards (ISO 14644) and good practice recommendations from international authorities.[6–8]

It is essential when identifying and assessing risk to have clearly defined objectives. When considering air quality, the following are examples of possible air quality objectives (Table 19.2).

Table 19.2 ART laboratory air quality objectives

GOAL (compliance with)	Particulate matter (maximum permitted number of particles per m³ equal to or greater than the tabulated size)	Volatile organic compounds	Limits of microbial contamination
ISO 14644 Part 1: **ISO Class 5** EU Grade A = ISO Class 5 EU Grade D = ISO Class 8	0.1 μm: 100,000 0.2 μm: 23,700 0.3 μm: 10,200 0.5 μm: 3520 1.0 μm: 832 5.0 μm: 29	Not stipulated	Not stipulated
EU Good Manufacturing Practice Directive 2003/94/EC—Grade A[15] **High risk activities**	***At rest:*** 0.5 μm: 3520 5.0 μm: 29 ***In operation:*** 0.5 μm: 3520 5.0 μm: 29	Not required	• **Air sample** (CFU/m³): <1 • **Settle plates** (diam. 90 mm; CFU/4 h): <1 • **Contact plates** (diam. 55 mm; CFU/plate): <1 • **Glove print 5 fingers** (CFU/glove): <1
EU Good Manufacturing Practice Directive 2003/94/EC—Grade D[15] **Clean Areas—Controlled aseptic processing**	***At rest:*** 0.5 μm: 3,520,000 5.0 μm: 29,000 ***In operation:*** 0.5 μm: Not defined 5.0 μm: Not defined	Not required	• **Air sample** (CFU/m³): 200 • **Settle plates** (diam. 90 mm; CFU/4 h): 100 • **Contact plates** (diam. 55 mm; CFU/plate): 50 • **Glove print 5 fingers** (CFU/glove): Not defined

(*Continued*)

Table 19.2 (Continued) ART laboratory air quality objectives

GOAL (compliance with)	**Particulate matter (maximum permitted number of particles per m^3 equal to or greater than the tabulated size)**	**Volatile organic compounds**	**Limits of microbial contamination**
ESHRE Guidelines for good practice in IVF laboratories[6]	Not specified but should be considered; *Section 3.1: Laboratory design*	Not specified but should be considered; *Section 3.1: Laboratory design*	Not specified but should be considered; *Section 3.3: Infectious agents*
ASRM Revised guidelines for human embryology & andrology laboratories[8]	Not specified but should be considered; *Section III: Laboratory Space & Design*	Not specified but should be considered; *Section III: Laboratory Space & Design*	Not specified but should be considered; *Section V: Laboratory Safety & Infection Control*
Fertility Society of Australia RTAC Code of Practice 2014[7]	Critical Criteria: *10. Data Monitoring; 4. Adverse Events* Good Practice Criteria *1. QMS*	Critical Criteria *10. Data Monitoring; 4. Adverse Events* Good Practice Criteria *1. QMS*	Critical Criteria *13. Management of Infection Risk*
United Kingdom Human Fertilisation & Embryology Authority[16]	Class II flow cabinets delivering Grade C (ISO Class 7/8) quality air; with background Grade D (ISO Class 8) air quality	Class II flow cabinets delivering Grade C (ISO Class 7/8) quality air; with background Grade D (ISO Class 8) air quality	Class II flow cabinets delivering Grade C (ISO Class 7/8) quality air; with background Grade D (ISO Class 8) air quality

Table 19.3 Tolerance levels

Tolerance levels	Measures	Considerations
1. Avoid the risk	Decide not to proceed with an activity that is likely to generate risk	Alternatively, consider another option to reach the same outcome that doesn't involve risk
2. Reduce the risk	Reduce the likelihood of occurrence by:	• Changes in procedures • Quality control processes • Auditing • Compliance with legislation and regulation • Staff training • Regular maintenance
	Reduce the impact if the risk occurs:	• Emergency procedures • Data backup • Minimizing exposure to source of risk • Using public relations to address public dissatisfaction
3. Transfer the risk	It may be possible to shift the risk to another party through:	• Insurance • Outsourcing • Joint ventures or partnerships
	Risks may be transferred by:	• Cross-training staff so that more than one person is skilled in the task • Identifying alternate suppliers • Keeping old equipment, practice doing things manually in case of computer network or equipment failure
4. Adequate insurance	Insurance should cover the requirements of the business, including:	• Loss of property/facility—natural disasters • Loss of income—business continuity insurance • Professional indemnity • Injury—public liability • Key person insurance • Worker's compensation • Travel interruption—travel insurance
5. Accept the risk	Accept that the risk cannot be avoided, reduced or transferred	Risks may be rare and therefore impractical or expensive to treat
		Develop an incident response plan and disaster recovery plan to deal with the consequences if the risk occurs

Consideration should be given to the ART unit's tolerance for risk. This will aid in determining risk mitigation strategies. A risk management profile register may include a tolerance rating. There are a number of ways to manage risk, as provided in Table 19.3.

Establishing the context for a risk management system for air quality in an ART unit may include:

- Regulatory and physical environment
- Atmospheric conditions—pollution, proximity to emissions
- Future urban planning
- Construction work in close proximity

- Storage and delivery of supplies
- Staff safety
- Contamination
- Age and structure of building
- New or start-up facility

19.2.3 Risk identification

Organizations must determine the relevant risks to the ART unit. Ask the question: "What could happen?" or "What can go wrong?" This can be undertaken in a number of ways, which may include brainstorming with a group of stakeholders; reviewing internal incidents or from other organizations; identifying reports outlining common risks in the industry, or discussing "what if" scenarios. Identification of risks relies on corporate history, lateral thinking, and experience in the field. It should involve a broad spectrum of people with a variety of skill sets. Jacqueline Jeynes[17] suggests all risks should be considered strategically at the most senior level, including:

- Health and safety risks
- Environmental risks
- Security risks
- Financial risks
- Competitive risks
- Political risks

There are tools available to assist in determining risks (Figure 19.3).[17,18] They provide prompts. Risk identification may be based on culture, industry practice, and compliance. Methods may include:

- Risk charting—Developing a register by listing resources at risk
- Objective based—Related to organizational strategy, goals, or project plans
- Scenario based—Developing different scenarios to assess potential risks
- Common risk checking—Based on historical data or industry knowledge

A register of all the risks (based on previous exposure, a history in the industry, or experience) is developed and each risk identified and recorded. A register may include (Table 19.4):

1. Risk unique identifier
2. Risk category (operational, strategic, etc.)
3. Risk description
4. Consequence
5. Causes
6. Risk owner (person responsible)

Initial risk assessment information should include (Table 19.5):

- Initial impact (severity)
- Initial likelihood
- Initial overall risk rating

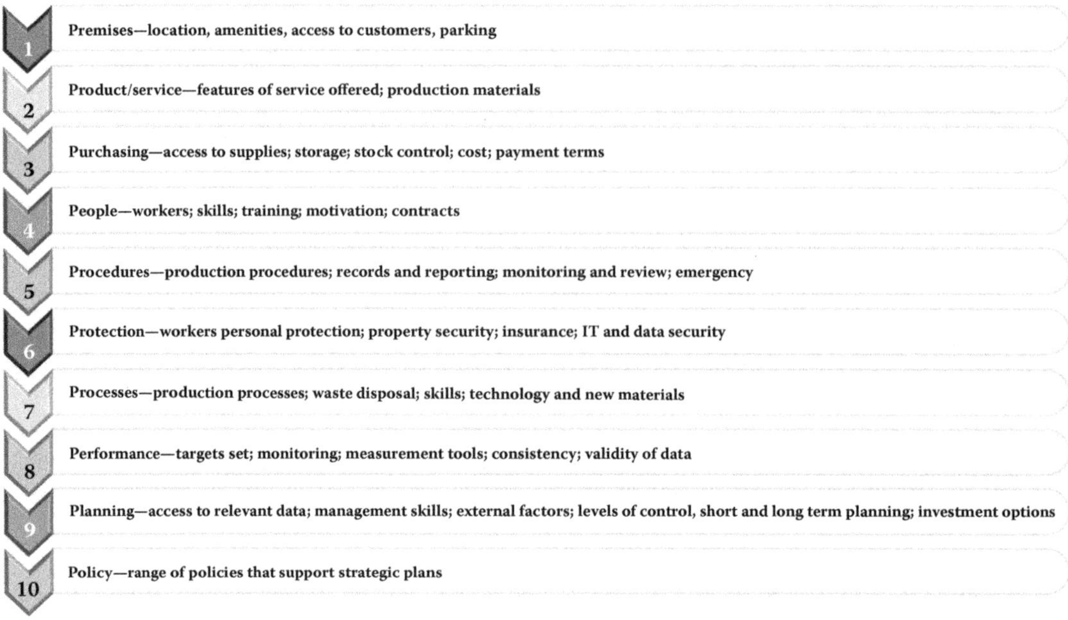

Figure 19.3 Ten business risk areas—the 10 Ps.

- Triggers
- Risk treatment strategy

After identifying and mitigating the risk, some risk will remain at a certain level. This is what is termed "residual risk." Residual risks are assessed the same way you perform the initial risk assessment, but taking into account the influence of controls so both the likelihood of an incident and its impact are decreased. Residual risk assessment information should include (Table 19.6):

- Residual impact—severity
- Residual likelihood
- Residual overall risk rating
- Risk treatment strategy responsibility
- Monitoring and reporting
- Risk treatment strategy status
- Risk treatment strategy (date raised)
- Risk treatment strategy (due date)
- Risk treatment strategy review period
- Risk tolerance

This may simply be in the form of an excel spreadsheet or sophisticated risk management software designed for recording and managing risks. However, the register is only as good as the information provided.

Risks associated with air quality will be unique to each laboratory. Factors influencing air quality risk may include the ones listed below:

- Age of laboratory—off-gassing of equipment and construction materials
- Construction of laboratory—materials used in construction
- Air filtration systems in place—HEPA, potassium permanganate; activated carbon or coconut shell activated carbon; UV decontamination; filter replacement; validation and testing
- Air flow ducts—input and output; location to possible contaminants
- Fragrances and cosmetics—may contain sodium, magnesium, silicon calcium, potassium or iron and may emit VOCs[19]
- Disposable products utilized in laboratory—Styrene[20] off-gassing
- Air filtration systems in equipment
- Humidity, pressure, and room temperature
- Protective clothing and foot wear—lint and shedding
- Toluene, formaldehyde from insulation; refrigerant gases[19]
- Incubators: VOC levels and microbial contaminants; sinks (oil; humidity pans) to absorb VOCs—VOCs oil soluble
- Measurement instruments for VOC levels: measure parts per billion; analysis technique[19]
- Laboratory furniture: chemicals used in manufacture
- Gas bottle distance of cylinders from incubators[21]
- Location of laboratory
- Styrene, acetone, benzene, toluene, octane, n-decane, freon, aldehydes; nonane, methylcyclohexane and butane levels in laboratory and incubators
- Levels of aromatic hydrocarbons—toluene; benzene and xylene
- In solvent; paints; dyes printing solutions
- Levels of alkanes—propane, hexane in glues; acetylene gas torches
- Technology and equipment to address air quality; preventative and for measurement
- Sterilization methods: ethylene oxide, etc.[22]
- Cross-contamination risks: use of biosafety cabinets

- What chemicals, VOCs, particulates and microbial contaminants impact IVF outcomes?
- Environmental pollution levels: coal burning; biomass burn off; mining; roads; freeways; heating; air conditioning
- Proximity to construction work—paints and glues; dust
- Storage of consumables: cardboard; plastic ware (ethylbenzene and benzaldehyde[19]); plasticizers (phthalates)[20,23]
- Cleaning products: alcohols; ammonia based; chemical composition
- Levels of halocarbons (isoflurane)
- Proximity to anaesthetic gases
- Air pressure of laboratory
- Number of people in laboratory
- Benzene levels in CO_2 cylinders[24]; inline gas filters; cleaning of cylinders
- Isopropyl alcohol fumes[25]; proximity to theatre; blood collection areas
- Gas lines: plumbing copper or stainless steel; lead in solders and radiation shielding
- Laboratory plumbing: sinks; microbial contamination risks
- Paper and pens: chemicals used in manufacture
- Formaldehydes created from the chemical reactivity between ozone and other VOCs during the use of PCs, laser printers and photocopiers[26]
- Use and effectiveness of surgical masks
- Levels of aldehydes: nonanal; decanal in fragrances and flavorings
- Levels of alcohols: ethanol; propanol and phenol
- In cleaning agents; wipes; pens
- Levels of styrenes: ethylbenzine; benzaldehyde in plastic ware
- Time necessary to off-gas plastic ware, incubators etc.
- Use of horizontal or vertical laminar flow; clean bench equipment
- Water sources: contamination; chlorination; fluoride

Table 19.4 Example of risk register

Risk ID	Risk category	Operational/ strategic	Risk description	Consequence	Causes	Risk owner—accountable manager
R001:	Environmental	Operational	No method to detect or remove VOC levels in IVF laboratory or determine any detrimental effect	High levels of VOCs may impact fertilization and embryo development; decreasing pregnancy rates	No procedure or equipment to assess or prevent VOC levels; limitations of testing methods	Scientific director

Table 19.5 Example of risk register—Initial

Initial impact—severity	Initial likelihood	Initial overall risk rating/ evaluation	Triggers	Risk treatment strategy (RTS)
Catastrophic (rating value = 5)	Almost certain (rating value = 5)	Critical (risk score = 25)	No equipment, procedure for monitoring or prevention Inability to determine effects on patient outcomes	• Investigate equipment and solutions for minimizing VOC levels • Purchase equipment within financial/ budget constraints • Implement protocols

Particulate matter includes dirt, dust, smoke, soot, and liquid droplets.[27] Natural particles include bushfires, dust storms, pollens, and sea sprays. Those related to human activity include motor vehicle emissions, industrial processes (e.g., electricity generation, incinerators, stone crushing), unpaved roads, biomass burn off—crop stubble, forest residues, and wood heaters. Particulate matter varies in size from coarse (10 to 25 μm in diameter) to fine particles (smaller than 2.5 μm) and ultrafine particles (smaller than 0.1 μm). By comparison, the diameter of hair is 70 μm. The toxicity of particles depends on their size and chemical composition. Particulate pollution, described as exposure to pollutants such as airborne particulate matter and ozone, has been associated with increased mortality.[28] Particulates or particulate matter are classified by aerodynamic diameter (PM). A 10 μm ($1\ \mu m = 10^{-6}$ m) particle is PM_{10}; a 2.5 μm is $PM_{2.5}$. In practical terms, PM_{10} are thoracic particles smaller than 10 μm which may penetrate the lower respiratory system; $PM_{2.5}$ are respirable particles smaller than 2.5 μm that can penetrate into the gas exchange region of the lung, and ultrafine particles are smaller than 100 nm (0.1 μm) $PM_{0.1}$.[28] Sandro Esteves and colleagues suggest particles between 0.1 and 10 μm are of interest in IVF laboratories.[29] It is accepted that particles of 0.3 μm or larger should be targeted for particulate contamination control in ART as bacteria and other contaminants can attach to particles. Air filtration allows for the initial removal of larger particles followed by high efficiency particulate air (HEPA) or ultra low penetration air (ULPA) filtering to trap the smaller particles. HEPA filtration aids in the removal of microbial contamination such as bacteria, viruses, and spores. Table 19.7 details some particle size comparisons.

Volatile organic compounds (VOCs) are the result of organic chemical compounds that enable evaporation under normal indoor atmospheric conditions.[29,30] The *volatile* refers to ease of evaporation and *organic compounds* as in containing carbon atoms. Table 19.8 details the U.S. Agency for Toxic Substances & Disease Registry (ATSDR) list of some common VOCs and the government's health risk information.[30] Little evidence-based information about the effect of VOCs on early embryo development in the IVF laboratory is known at present, but a preventative approach may aid in risk mitigation. However, VOCs have been linked to reduced outcomes in ART,[29,31] including aromatic hydrocarbons (benzene, xylene, and toluene), alcohols (ethanol, propanol, and phenol), alkanes (propane and hexane), and aldehydes (nonanal and decanal).[19] Pollution control law in Japan defines a VOC as one that becomes gas in atmosphere.[32] VOCs can occur as both gases and particles.[33]

Table 19.6 Example of risk register—Residual risk

Residual impact—severity	Residual likelihood	Residual overall risk rating/evaluation	RTS responsibility	Monitoring and reporting	RTS status	RTS—date raised	RTS due	RTS review period	Risk tolerance
Insignificant (rating value = 1)	Possible (rating value = 3)	Low (risk score = 3)	Scientific director	3 Monthly audits	Pending	3.5.15	1.6.15	6 monthly	Reduction

Table 19.7 Particle size comparison

Particle size	Item
10 nm (0.01 μm)	Lower size of tobacco smoke
42 nm (0.042 μm)	Diameter of Hep. B virus
55–65 nm (0.055–0.065 μm)	Diameter of Hep. C virus
80 nm (0.08 μm)	Diameter of Ebola virus
80–120 nm (0.08–0.12 μm)	Influenza A virus
100 nm (0.1 μm)	Greatest particle size to fit through a surgical mask
100 nm (0.1 μm)	90% of particles in wood smoke smaller
120 nm (0.12 μm)	Diameter of HIV
120 nm (0.12 μm)	Greatest particle size to fit through a ULPA filter
300 nm (0.3 μm)	Greatest particle size to fit through a HEPA filter
120 nm (0.12 μm)	Diameter of HIV
200 nm (0.2 μm)	Size of *Mycoplasma* bacterium
600–800 nm (0.6–0.8 μm)	Size of *Staph. aureus* bacteria

These organic components are used in manufacturing and react with indoor ozone to produce harmful by products. The major sources of VOCs include vehicle exhaust, gasoline evaporation, solvent use, natural gas emissions, and industrial processes. They are 100–1000 times smaller than the effective pore size of HEPA filters. Activated carbon filters are used to trap VOCs.[29] Alcohols and ketones are oxidized using potassium permanganate as not easily removed by carbon.[29] Richard Legro and colleagues noted the effects of declining air quality on reproductive outcomes after IVF are variable but increased nitrogen dioxide (NO_2) is consistently associated with lower live birth rates.[34] Fine particulate matter ($PM_{2.5}$) in the IVF laboratory during embryo culture was associated with decreased conception rates.

Air pollutants such as carbon monoxide, lead, nitrogen dioxide, ozone, particles, and sulfur dioxide can lead to increases in the incidence of cancer, birth defects, genetic damage, central nervous system defects, immunodeficiency, and disorders of the respiratory and nervous systems.[35]

Biomass burning releases carbon monoxide. Benzene and formaldehyde are also present in the smoke.[36] Philippe Grandjean and colleagues identified industrial chemicals, such as lead, methylmercury, polychlorinated biphenyls, arsenic, toluene, manganese, fluoride, chloropyrifos, dichlorodiphenyltrichloroethane, tetrachloroethylene, and polybrominated diphenyl ethers as neurotoxicants.[23]

Concern is also rising over the safety of phthalates used in consumer products such as medical devices (plastic tubing and intravenous storage bags), food wrap, building materials, packaging, automotive parts, children's toys, and articles made from polyvinyl chloride (PVC). The addition of phthalates to PVC makes the brittle plastic more durable and flexible. Phthalates are also found in fragrances, cosmetics, nail polish, and hairspray, and to make products more effectively penetrative. Phthalates have been identified as reproductive and developmental toxicants. The U.S. EPA classifies di-(2-ethylexyl) phthalate (DEHP) and benzyl butyl phthalate (BBP) as probable and possible human carcinogens, respectively.[37] BBP is found in vinyl flooring, sealants, adhesives, artificial leather, and food wrapping. DEHP is common in plastic shoes (flip-flops), raincoats, furniture, automobile upholstery, and floor tiles.

Table 19.8 U.S. Agency for Toxic Substances & Disease Registry (ATSDR) common volatile organic compounds list

Name/possible health risk	Source	Name/possible health risk	Source
1,1,1-Trichloroethane In animals, it has been shown that 1,1,1-trichloroethane can pass from the mother's blood into a fetus. When pregnant mice were exposed to high levels of 1,1,1-trichloroethane in air, their babies developed more slowly than normal and had some behavioral problems. However, whether similar effects occur in humans has not been demonstrated.	Solvent; household products such as spot cleaners, glues, and aerosol sprays	Chlorobenzene Animal studies indicate that the liver, kidney, and central nervous system are affected by exposure to chlorobenzene. Effects on the central nervous system from breathing chlorobenzene include unconsciousness, tremors, restlessness, and death. Longer exposure has caused liver and kidney damage. The limited data available indicate that chlorobenzene does not cause birth defects or infertility.	Used in the past to make other chemicals, such as phenol and DDT. Now chlorobenzene is used as a solvent for some pesticide formulations, to degrease automobile parts, and as a chemical intermediate to make several other chemicals.
1,1,2,2-Tetrachloroethane Some effects have been observed in animals born to females exposed to 1,1,2,2-tetrachloroethane during pregnancy. This occurred at exposure levels that were also toxic to the mothers. A very small number of studies in animals do not suggest that 1,1,2,2-tetrachloroethane is a developmental toxin.	Industrial solvent to clean and degrease metals; an ingredient in paints and pesticides	Chloroethane Not known whether chloroethane exposure can affect development in people. In animal studies, the babies of mice exposed to chloroethane during pregnancy had delayed development. It is not known whether children differ from adults in their susceptibility to chloroethane.	Used in leaded gasoline, but strict government regulations have reduced that use dramatically. It is used in the production of cellulose, dyes, medicinal drugs, and other commercial products, and as a solvent and refrigerant. It is also used to numb the skin before medical procedures such as ear piercing and skin biopsies and as a treatment in sports injuries.

(*Continued*)

Table 19.8 (Continued) U.S. Agency for Toxic Substances & Disease Registry (ATSDR) common volatile organic compounds list

Name/possible health risk	Source	Name/possible health risk	Source
1,1,2-Trichloroethane Not known whether 1,1,2-trichloroethane can affect reproduction in people. Animal studies have not shown the chemical to affect normal reproduction and development.	Solvent; a chemical intermediate in industry	Chloroform It is not known whether chloroform causes reproductive effects or birth defects in people. Animal studies have shown that miscarriages occurred in rats and mice that breathed air containing 30 to 300 ppm chloroform during pregnancy and also in rats that ate chloroform during pregnancy. Offspring of rats and mice that breathed chloroform during pregnancy had birth defects. Abnormal sperm were found in mice that breathed air containing 400 ppm chloroform for a few days.	In the past, chloroform was used as an inhaled anesthetic during surgery, but it isn't used that way today. Today, chloroform is used to make other chemicals and can also be formed in small amounts when chlorine is added to water.
1,1-Dichloroethane Not known whether 1,1-Dichloroethane can produce birth defects in humans. Minor skeletal problems were observed in the fetuses of rats breathing 1,1-dichloro-ethane; decreases in body weight were also observed in the mothers.	Used mostly as an intermediate in the manufacture of 1,1,1-trichloroethane, and to a lesser extent, vinyl chloride and high vacuum rubber. In the past, it was used as a surgical anesthetic.	Chloromethane Not known if chloromethane exposure will harm developing fetuses or young children. Animal studies show that female rats exposed to chloromethane during pregnancy had young that were smaller than normal, with underdeveloped bones, and possibly abnormal hearts (this effect remains uncertain).	Some chloromethane is produced by industry. Most of the chloromethane that is released into the environment is from natural sources, such as chemical reactions that occur in the oceans. It is also given off when materials like grass, wood, charcoal, and plastics are burned. It is present in lakes and streams and has been found in drinking water.

(Continued)

Table 19.8 (Continued) U.S. Agency for Toxic Substances & Disease Registry (ATSDR) common volatile organic compounds list

Name/possible health risk	Source	Name/possible health risk	Source
		Some animal studies showed that animals that breathed low levels of chloromethane experienced slower growth and had brain damage. In other animal studies, males that were exposed to chloromethane were less fertile, or even sterile, or produced damaged sperm. Females that became pregnant by these males lost their developing young.	Other sources of exposure are cigarette smoke, polystyrene insulation, aerosol propellants, and chlorinated swimming pools.
1,1-Dichloroethene Animals that breathed high levels of 1,1-dichloroethene had damaged livers, kidneys, and lungs. The offspring of some of the animals had a higher number of birth defects. Not known if birth defects occur when people are exposed to 1,1-dichloroethene. Animals that ingested high levels of 1,1-dichloroethene had damaged livers, kidneys, and lungs. There were no birth defects in animals that ingested the chemical.	Used to make certain plastics, such as flexible films like food wrap, and in packaging materials. It is also used to make flame retardant coatings for fiber and carpet backings, and in piping, coating for steel pipes, and in adhesive applications.	Dichlorobenzenes There is no reliable evidence suggesting that dichlorobenzenes cause birth defects, although animal data raise concern for effects of 1,4-dichlorobenzene on postnatal development of the nervous system.	Used to make herbicides, insecticides, medicine, and dyes. 1,4-Dichlorobenzene, the most important of the three chemicals, is a colorless to white solid with a strong, pungent odor.

(Continued)

Table 19.8 (Continued) U.S. Agency for Toxic Substances & Disease Registry (ATSDR) common volatile organic compounds list

Name/possible health risk	Source	Name/possible health risk	Source
1,2,3 Trichloropropane Not known if 1,2,3-trichloropropane damages people's ability to reproduce or if it causes birth defects. When rats breathed low levels for several weeks or swallowed a large amount for a few days there were no effects on their ability to reproduce and there was no increase in birth defects.	Used to make other chemicals. Some of it is also used as an industrial solvent, paint and varnish remover, and cleaning and degreasing agent.	Dichloropropenes Not known whether dichloropropenes can cause birth defects in humans. Pregnant rats that inhaled 1,3-dichloropropene gave birth to fewer pups or pups with lower body weight. This occurred at exposures high enough to be toxic to the mothers.	Used mainly in farming as a pesticide.
1,2-Dibromo-3-Chloropropane Studies on workers have shown that men may produce fewer sperm, produce sperm that results in more girl than boy babies, and eventually become unable to father children. It can also cause headaches, nausea, light headedness, and weakness in workers. Animals breathing high levels of the chemical were not able to reproduce and had damaged stomachs, livers, kidneys, brains, spleens, blood, and lungs. Breathing low to moderate levels also caused damage to the reproductive system.	Used to make another chemical that is used to make materials that resist burning. Large amounts of 1,2-dibromo-3-chloropropane were used in the past on certain farms to kill pests that harmed crops. No longer used in some countries.	Ethylbenzene Not known if ethylbenzene will cause birth defects in humans. Minor birth defects and low birth weight have occurred in newborn animals whose mothers were exposed to ethylbenzene in air during pregnancy.	It is naturally found in coal tar and petroleum and is also found in manufactured products such as inks, pesticides, and paints. Ethylbenzene is used primarily to make another chemical, styrene. Other uses include as a solvent, in fuels, and to make other chemicals.

(Continued)

Table 19.8 (Continued) U.S. Agency for Toxic Substances & Disease Registry (ATSDR) common volatile organic compounds list

Name/possible health risk	Source	Name/possible health risk	Source
The ability of people to reproduce was not affected by drinking water contaminated with low levels of 1,2-dibromo-3-chloropropane and there was no increase in the number of birth defects. Rats exposed to high levels did, however, have an increase in birth defects. It can also cause skin and eye damage from direct contact.			
1,2-Dibromoethane Although very little is known about the effects from breathing 1,2-dibromoethane over a long period of time, some male workers had reproductive effects including damage to their sperm. No other long-term effects are known in people. In rats, death occurred from breathing high levels for a short time. Lower levels caused liver and kidney damage. When rats breathed air or ate food containing 1,2-dibromo-ethane for short or long periods of time, they were less fertile or had abnormal sperm.	Used as a pesticide in soil, and on citrus, vegetable, and grain crops. Most of these uses have been stopped by the Environmental Protection Agency (EPA) since 1984. Another major use was as an additive in leaded gasoline; however, since leaded gasoline is now banned, it is no longer used for this purpose. Uses today include treatment of logs for termites and beetles, control of moths in beehives, and as a preparation for dyes and waxes.	Formaldehyde Studies in animals suggest that formaldehyde will not cause birth defects in humans.	It is produced by both human and natural sources. Small amounts of formaldehyde are naturally produced by plants, animals, and humans. It is used in the production of fertilizer, paper, plywood, and urea-formaldehyde resins. It is also used as a preservative in some foods and in many products used around the house, such as antiseptics, medicines, and cosmetics.

(*Continued*)

Table 19.8 (Continued) U.S. Agency for Toxic Substances & Disease Registry (ATSDR) common volatile organic compounds list

Name/possible health risk	Source	Name/possible health risk	Source
Changes in the brain and behavior were also seen in young rats whose male parents had breathed 1,2-dibromoethane, and birth defects were observed in the young of animals that were exposed while pregnant. 1,2-Dibromo-ethane is not known to cause birth defects in people.			
1,2-Dichloroethane In laboratory animals, breathing or ingesting large amounts of 1,2-dichloroethane have also caused nervous system disorders and liver, kidney, and lung effects. Animal studies also suggest that 1,2-dichloroethane may damage the immune system. Kidney disease has also been seen in animals ingesting low doses of 1,2-dichloroethane for a long time. Studies in animals indicate that 1,2-dichloroethane does not affect reproduction.	Most common use of 1,2-dichloroethane is in the production of vinyl chloride which is used to make a variety of plastic and vinyl products including polyvinyl chloride (PVC) pipes, furniture and automobile upholstery, wall coverings, housewares, and automobile parts. It is also used to as a solvent and is added to leaded gasoline to remove lead.	Gasoline, Automotive There is not enough information available to determine if gasoline causes birth defects or affects reproduction.	Typically, gasoline contains more than 150 chemicals, including small amounts of benzene, toluene, xylene, and sometimes lead. How the gasoline is made determines which chemicals are present in the gasoline mixture and how much of each is present. The actual composition varies with the source of the crude petroleum, the manufacturer, and the time of year.

(Continued)

Table 19.8 (Continued) U.S. Agency for Toxic Substances & Disease Registry (ATSDR) common volatile organic compounds list

Name/possible health risk	Source	Name/possible health risk	Source
1,2-Dichloroethene The long-term (365 days or longer) human health effects after exposure to low concentrations of 1,2-dichloroethene aren't known. One animal study suggested that an exposed fetus may not grow as quickly as one that hasn't been exposed. Exposure to 1,2-dichloroethene hasn't been shown to affect fertility in people or animals.	Used to produce solvents and in chemical mixtures.	Hexachlorobutadiene Studies in mice have shown irritation of the nose when large amounts were breathed over a short time. The only other effect noted in animals from breathing hexachlorobutadiene was a reduction in the body weights of foetuses when their mothers breathed high levels of the chemical. There are no studies which looked at animals breathing low levels of hexachlorobutadiene over a long time. Rats and mice that drank low levels of hexachlorobutadiene over both short and long periods had kidney and liver damage. No effects on reproduction or on the developing foetuses were seen when rats and mice drank hexachloro-butadiene. Studies in rabbits found kidney and liver damage from contact with the chemical on the skin for a short time.	Used to make rubber compounds. It is also used as a solvent, and to make lubricants, in gyroscopes, as a heat transfer liquid, and as a hydraulic fluid.

(*Continued*)

Table 19.8 (Continued) U.S. Agency for Toxic Substances & Disease Registry (ATSDR) common volatile organic compounds list

Name/possible health risk	Source	Name/possible health risk	Source
1,2-Dichloropropane Animal studies indicate that breathing low levels of 1,2-dichloropropane over short- or long-term periods causes damage to the liver, kidney, and respiratory system. Breathing high levels causes death. Similar effects have been reported when animals were given 1,2-dichloropropane by mouth. Some studies indicate that ingesting 1,2-dichloropropane may cause reproductive effects. One study reported a delay in bone formation of the skull in foetal rats following exposure of the mother rats to 1,2-dichloropropane.	Used in the past as a soil fumigant, chemical intermediate, and industrial solvent and was found in paint strippers, varnishes, and furniture finish removers. Most of these uses were discontinued. Today, almost all of the 1,2-dichloropropane is used as a chemical intermediate to make perchloroethylene and several other related chlorinated chemicals.	Hexachloroethane Hexachloroethane is not a very toxic substance. If exposed to a large amount for a long time, your liver could be affected. There is also a slight chance that your kidneys could be damaged. Animal studies have not shown hexachloroethane to cause birth defects or to affect reproduction.	Its vapours smell like camphor. In the United States, about half of the hexachloroethane is used by the military for smoke-producing devices. It is also used to remove air bubbles in melted aluminium. Hexachloroethane may be present as an ingredient in some fungicides, insecticides, lubricants, and plastics. Can be formed by incinerators when materials containing chlorinated hydrocarbons are burned. Some hexachloroethane can also be formed when chlorine reacts with carbon compounds in drinking water.
1,3-Butadiene Not known if exposure to 1,3-butadiene will result in birth defects or other developmental effects in people. Animal studies showed that breathing 1,3-butadiene during pregnancy can decrease foetal weights and increase the number of skeletal defects.	Used to make synthetic rubber. Synthetic rubber is widely used for tires on cars and trucks. 1,3-Butadiene is also used to make plastics including acrylics. Small amounts are found in gasoline.	Hydrazines Breathing hydrazines for short periods may cause coughing and irritation of the throat and lungs, convulsions, tremors, or seizures. Breathing hydrazines for long periods may cause liver and kidney damage, as well as serious effects on reproductive organs. Eating or drinking small amounts of hydrazines may cause nausea, vomiting, uncontrolled shaking, inflammation of the nerves, drowsiness, or coma.	Most hydrazines are manufactured for use as rocket propellants and fuels, boiler water treatments, chemical reactants, medicines, and in cancer research.

(Continued)

Table 19.8 (Continued) U.S. Agency for Toxic Substances & Disease Registry (ATSDR) common volatile organic compounds list

Name/possible health risk	Source	Name/possible health risk	Source
2-Butanone Serious health effects in animals have been seen only at very high levels. When breathed, these effects included birth defects, loss of consciousness, and death. When swallowed, rats had nervous system effects including drooping eyelids and uncoordinated muscle movements. There was no damage to the ability to reproduce.	Nearly half of its use is in paints and other coatings because it will quickly evaporate into the air and it dissolves many substances. It is also used in glues and as a cleaning agent. 2-Butanone occurs as a natural product. It is made by some trees and found in some fruits and vegetables in small amounts. It is also released to the air from car and truck exhausts.	Methyl Mercaptan Not known whether long-term exposure to low levels of methyl mercaptan can result in harmful health effects.	Methyl mercaptan is released from decaying organic matter in marshes and is present in the natural gas of certain regions, in coal tar, and in some crude oils. It is manufactured for use in the plastics industry, in pesticides, and as a jet fuel additive. It is also released as a decay product of wood in pulp mills. It is a natural substance found in the blood, brain, and other tissues of people and animals. It is released from animal feces. It occurs naturally in certain foods, such as some nuts and cheese.
2-Hexanone In one study, pregnant rats that breathed 2-hexanone did not gain as much weight during their pregnancy, had fewer babies, and had babies that were smaller and less active than the rats that were not exposed. Not known if breathing 2-hexanone affects human reproduction or causes birth defects.	It was used in the past in paint and paint thinners, to make other chemical substances, and to dissolve oils and waxes. It is no longer made or used in the United States because it has harmful health effects. It is formed as a waste product resulting from industrial activities such as making wood pulp and producing gas from coal, and in oil shale operations.	n-Hexane In laboratory studies, animals exposed to high levels of n-hexane in air had signs of nerve damage. Some animals also had lung damage. In other studies, rats exposed to very high levels of n-hexane had damage to sperm-forming cells.	The major use for solvents containing n-hexane is to extract vegetable oils from crops such as soybeans. These solvents are also used as cleaning agents in the printing, textile, furniture, and shoemaking industries. Certain kinds of special glues used in the roofing and shoe and leather industries also contain n-hexane. Several consumer products contain n-hexane, such as gasoline, quick-drying glues used in various hobbies, and rubber cement.

(Continued)

Table 19.8 (Continued) U.S. Agency for Toxic Substances & Disease Registry (ATSDR) common volatile organic compounds list

Name/possible health risk	Source	Name/possible health risk	Source
Not known whether touching or ingesting 2-hexanone would affect your health. Animal studies have shown that ingesting high levels of 2-hexanone harms the nervous system. Also, animals that ingested 2-hexanone experienced decreased body weight and effects on reproduction.			
Acetone Health effects from long-term exposures are known mostly from animal studies. Kidney, liver, and nerve damage, increased birth defects, and lowered ability to reproduce (males only) occurred in animals exposed long-term.	Acetone is used to make plastic, fibers, drugs, and other chemicals. It is also used to dissolve other substances. It occurs naturally in plants, trees, volcanic gases, forest fires, and as a product of the breakdown of body fat. It is present in vehicle exhaust, tobacco smoke, and landfill sites. Industrial processes contribute more acetone to the environment than natural processes.	Nitrobenzene Animal studies have reported effects on the blood and liver from exposure to nitrobenzene. A single dose of nitrobenzene fed to male rats resulted in damage to the testicles and decreased levels of sperm.	Most of the nitrobenzene produced in the United States is used to manufacture a chemical called aniline. Nitrobenzene is also used to produce lubricating oils such as those used in motors and machinery. A small amount of nitrobenzene is used in the manufacture of dyes, drugs, pesticides, and synthetic rubber.
Acrolein In animal studies, ingestion of very large amounts of acrolein during pregnancy caused reduced birth weights and skeletal deformities in newborns. However, the levels causing these effects were often fatal to the mother.	Small amounts of acrolein can be formed and can enter the air when trees, tobacco, other plants, gasoline, and oil are burned. Acrolein is used as a pesticide to control algae, weeds, bacteria, and molluscs. It is also used to make other chemicals.	Stoddard Solvent It is not known whether Stoddard solvent can cause birth defects or affect reproduction.	Stoddard solvent is a petroleum mixture that is also known as dry cleaning safety solvent, petroleum solvent, and varnoline. It is a chemical mixture that is similar to white spirits. Stoddard solvent is used as a paint thinner; in some types of photocopier toners, printing inks, and adhesives; as a dry cleaning solvent; and as a general cleaner and degreaser.

(Continued)

Table 19.8 (Continued) U.S. Agency for Toxic Substances & Disease Registry (ATSDR) common volatile organic compounds list

Name/possible health risk	Source	Name/possible health risk	Source
Benzene Some women who breathed high levels of benzene for many months had irregular menstrual periods and a decrease in the size of their ovaries, but we do not know for certain that benzene caused the effects. It is not known whether benzene will affect fertility in men. Benzene can pass from the mother's blood to a foetus. Animal studies have shown low birth weights, delayed bone formation, and bone marrow damage when pregnant animals breathed benzene.	Some industries use benzene to make other chemicals that are used to make plastics, resins, and nylon and other synthetic fibers. Benzene is also used to make some types of rubbers, lubricants, dyes, detergents, drugs, and pesticides. Natural sources of benzene include emissions from volcanoes and forest fires. Benzene is also a natural part of crude oil, gasoline, and cigarette smoke.	Styrene Studies in workers have examined whether styrene can cause birth defects or low birth weight; however, the results are inconclusive. No birth defects were observed in animal studies.	Styrene is widely used to make plastics and rubber. Products containing styrene include insulation, fiberglass, plastic pipes, automobile parts, shoes, drinking cups and other food containers, and carpet backing. Most of these products contain styrene linked together in a long chain (polystyrene) as well as unlinked styrene.
Bromodichloromethane Animal studies indicate that the liver, kidney, and central nervous system are affected by exposure to bromodichloromethane. The effects of high doses on the central nervous system include sleepiness and incoordination. Longer exposure to lower doses causes damage to the liver and kidneys. There is some evidence from animal studies that bromodichloromethane may cause birth defects at doses high enough to make the mother sick.	Most bromodichloromethane is formed as a by-product when chlorine is added to drinking water to kill bacteria.	Tetrachloroethylene (PERC) Results from some studies suggest that women who work in dry cleaning industries where exposures to tetrachloroethylene can be quite high may have more menstrual problems and spontaneous abortions than women who are not exposed. However, it is not known if tetrachloroethylene was responsible for these problems because other possible causes were not considered.	Widely used for dry cleaning of fabrics and for metal-degreasing. It is also used to make other chemicals and is used in some consumer products.

(Continued)

Table 19.8 (Continued) U.S. Agency for Toxic Substances & Disease Registry (ATSDR) common volatile organic compounds list

Name/possible health risk	Source	Name/possible health risk	Source
It is not known if lower doses would cause birth defects.		Results of animal studies, conducted with amounts much higher than those that most people are exposed to, show that tetrachloroethylene can cause liver and kidney damage. Exposure to very high levels of tetrachloroethylene can be toxic to the unborn pups of pregnant rats and mice. Changes in behavior were observed in the offspring of rats that breathed high levels of the chemical while they were pregnant.	
Bromoform and Dibromochloromethane Animals exposed to high amounts of bromoform or dibromochloromethane developed liver and kidney injuries. Exposure to low levels of bromoform or dibromochloromethane do not appear to seriously affect the brain, liver, or kidneys. Not known if bromoform or dibromochloromethane affect fertility in humans, but studies in animals suggest that the risk of doing so is low.	These chemicals were used in the past as solvents and flame retardants, or to make other chemicals, but now they are used mainly as laboratory reagents. By products when chlorine is added to drinking water to kill bacteria.	Toluene Breathing very high levels of toluene during pregnancy can result in children with birth defects and retard mental abilities, and growth. Not known if toluene harms the unborn child if the mother is exposed to low levels of toluene during pregnancy.	Toluene occurs naturally in crude oil and in the tolu tree. It is also produced in the process of making gasoline and other fuels from crude oil and making coke from coal. Toluene is used in making paints, paint thinners, fingernail polish, lacquers, adhesives, and rubber and in some printing and leather tanning processes.

(Continued)

Table 19.8 (Continued) U.S. Agency for Toxic Substances & Disease Registry (ATSDR) common volatile organic compounds list

Name/possible health risk	Source	Name/possible health risk	Source
Bromomethane Not known if it affects our ability to reproduce. Studies in animals suggest that bromomethane does not cause birth defects and does not interfere with reproduction, except at high exposure levels.	Used to kill a variety of pests including rats, insects, and fungi. It is also used to make other chemicals or as a solvent to get oil out of nuts, seeds, and wool.	Trichloroethylene (TCE) Drinking small amounts of trichloroethylene for long periods may cause liver and kidney damage, impaired immune system function, and impaired fetal development in pregnant women, although the extent of some of these effects is not yet clear.	Used mainly as a solvent to remove grease from metal parts, but it is also an ingredient in adhesives, paint removers, typewriter correction fluids, and spot removers.
Carbon Disulfide Studies in animals indicate that carbon disulfide can affect the normal functions of the brain, liver, and heart. After pregnant rats breathed carbon disulfide in the air, some of the newborn rats died or had birth defects.	In nature, small amounts of carbon disulfide are found in gases released to the earth's surface as, for example, in volcanic eruptions or over marshes. Commercial carbon disulfide is made by combining carbon and sulfur at very high temperatures.	Vinyl Chloride Animal studies have shown that long-term exposure to vinyl chloride can damage the sperm and testes.	Used to make polyvinyl chloride (PVC). PVC is used to make a variety of plastic products, including pipes, wire and cable coatings, and packaging materials.
Carbon Tetrachloride A few survey-type studies suggest that maternal drinking water exposure to carbon tetrachloride might possibly be related to certain birth defects. Studies in animals showed that carbon tetrachloride can cause early foetal deaths, but did not cause birth defects. A study with human breast milk in a test tube suggested that it would be possible for carbon tetrachloride to pass from the maternal circulation to breast milk, but there is no direct demonstration of this occurring.	Used in the production of refrigeration fluid and propellants for aerosol cans, as a pesticide, as a cleaning fluid and degreasing agent, in fire extinguishers, and in spot removers. Because of its harmful effects, these uses are now banned and it is only used in some industrial applications.	Xylenes Studies of unborn animals indicate that high concentrations of xylene may cause increased numbers of deaths, and delayed growth and development.	It occurs naturally in petroleum and coal tar. Chemical industries produce xylene from petroleum. Xylene is used as a solvent and in the printing, rubber, and leather industries. It is also used as a cleaning agent, a thinner for paint, and in paints and varnishes. It is found in small amounts in airplane fuel and gasoline.

Source: Adapted from http://www.atsdr.cdc.gov/substances/toxchemicallisting.asp?sysid=7.

Table 19.9 provides a list of some of the chemicals and substances suspected of causing health-related problems in humans. There is limited data on the effects during fertilization and early embryo development, so most information relates to pregnancy, children, and adult exposure. A risk register presents an opportunity to consider and record potential risks and implement a preventative approach without having all the necessary data to support the action. Such risks would be regularly reviewed to assess additional evidence.

Following the risk identification process, it is necessary to determine the material risks, that is, risks that could impact significantly on the business. Risk identification is an evolving process with new risks being added in response to incidents, compliance changes, opportunities, and experiences from other businesses. Staff and relevant external stakeholders need to be knowledgeable about the business activities being reviewed. Risks are allocated to individuals—risk owners.

19.2.4 *Risk analysis*

Risk analysis is concerned with determining the potential consequences of risk events. It is a process to comprehend the nature of the risk and determine the level of the risk. ISO 31000:2009 provides tools to assist in analyzing risk based on the likelihood of an event occurring and the severity. As likelihood and severity are subjective measures, it is essential to develop robust, coherent measures to allow objective analysis.

A risk assessment form may be utilized to aid in the analysis of risks (Figure 19.4). The use of questions can help prompt the person assessing the risk. Some useful questions are listed below. Forms may be designed to aid the user and thus ensure conformity in evaluation.

- What could cause harm?
- What could go wrong?
- Evaluate the likelihood and consequence.
- What controls are currently in place?
- What additional controls are required?
- How and when will this risk be measured and monitored?

The commonly used risk matrix process includes classifications and the ability to arbitrarily allocate values. The *likelihood* of an event occurring is multiplied by the *severity* of the event to provide an overall *risk rating* (Table 19.10).

1. Analyze risks using the risk assessment tools
   a. *Likelihood*
      i. Almost certain (5)
      ii. Likely (4)
      iii. Possible (3)
      iv. Unlikely (2)
      v. Rare (1)
   b. *Severity*
      i. Catastrophic (5)
      ii. Major (4)
      iii. Moderate (3)
      iv. Minor (2)
      v. Insignificant (1)

Table 19.9 Potential air quality risks in ART laboratories—chemically active contaminants (CACs)

No.	Compound	Occurrence	Particle/ CACs	Volatile organic compounds	Microbial contamination	Possible adverse effects	Reference number
1	Dust	PM_{10} and $PM_{2.5}$—Particular concern; traffic related pollution	✓		✓	Exposure during pregnancy associated with autism	33
2	Bacteria/viruses	HEPA and ULPA filters trap bacteria	✓		✓		
3	Pollen/spores	HEPA and ULPA filters trap particles	✓		✓		
4	Smoke	Biomass burning; indoor cooking; crop burn off	✓		✓		
5	Particles—dirt; liquid droplets; soot	Air pollutant—matter from combustion composed of organic carbon species; elemental or black carbon and trace metals (e.g. lead, arsenic) Range in diameter 0.2 to 1 μm Ultrafine particles linked to fresh combustion and traffic related pollution	✓			Neurotoxicants	33; 36
6	Diesel emissions	Fine particulate matter ($PM_{2.5}$) containing polycyclic aromatic hydrocarbons (PAH)	✓	✓		Carcinogens; Intrauterine growth retardation (IUGR)	33; 38
7	Ozone O_3—many VOCs contribute to the formation and thinning of ozone	Air pollution—gas produced in presence of sunlight and VOCs from combustion of fossil fuels	✓			Neurotoxicants	36

(Continued)

Table 19.9 (Continued) Potential air quality risks in ART laboratories—chemically active contaminants (CACs)

No.	Compound	Occurrence	Particle/ CACs	Volatile organic compounds	Microbial contamination	Possible adverse effects	Reference number
8	Nitrogen dioxide (NO_2)	Air pollutants	✓			Neurotoxicants; NO_2—Incidence of cancer; birth defects; genetic damage; central nervous system defects; immunodeficiency; respiratory and nervous system disorders; adverse birth outcomes	34; 36
9	Carbon monoxide (CO)	Air pollutants; traffic; smoke—biomass burning	✓			Neurotoxicants	36
10	Sulfur dioxide (SO_2)	Air pollutants; high sulfur content coal used in indoor cooking	✓			Neurotoxicants	38
11	Lead	Air pollutants—gas produced in presence of sunlight and VOCs from combustion of fossil fuels; dust; paint	✓	✓		Lead is a neurotoxin, a poison that acts on the nervous system; elevated blood lead is linked to permanent cognitive impairment measured in decreased IQ and has also been linked to a greater likelihood to commit crime later in life	33; 36; 39

(*Continued*)

Table 19.9 (Continued) Potential air quality risks in ART laboratories—chemically active contaminants (CACs)

No.	Compound	Occurrence	Particle/ CACs	Volatile organic compounds	Microbial contamination	Possible adverse effects	Reference number
12	Formaldehyde Increases in temperature and humidity result in increases in formaldehyde	Smoke; inside incubators. Insulation—air handling systems; refrigerant gases; building materials; furniture; household cleaners; paints and wallpapers; textiles; medicinal and personal care products; pesticides; products with sealed surfaces emit less; emissions generally decrease as product ages; formaldehyde can be created from the chemical reaction between ozone and other VOCs during the use of computers, laser printers and photocopiers		✓		High levels associated with cancer in humans	26; 35; 40
13	Arsenic Arsine gas AsH_3 Gallium Arsenade	Dust, water run-off; volcanoes; wood preservatives; glass; pesticides; microchip industry—arsine gas; laser light—gallium arsenade	✓			Neurotoxicants; Skin, lung, liver, lymphatic cancer; infertility, miscarriage	36; 41; 42

(*Continued*)

Table 19.9 (Continued) Potential air quality risks in ART laboratories—chemically active contaminants (CACs)

No.	Compound	Occurrence	Particle/ CACs	Volatile organic compounds	Microbial contamination	Possible adverse effects	Reference number
14	Mercury converted to methyl mercury	Fish—Methyl mercury; Coal fired power	✓			Neurotoxicants; May harm developing nervous system; may affect fetus—brain damage; mental retardation; blindness; seizures; inability to speak; Cancer—Methyl mercury; Adverse effects on immune; reproductive, nervous and endocrine systems	33; 36; 43; 44
15	Polychlorinated biphenyls (manmade organic chemicals)	Transformers and capacitors; electrical equipment; fluorescent light ballasts; adhesives and tapes; oil based paint; plastics; carbonless copy paper; pigments and dyes	✓			Neurotoxicants; Developmental delay; reduced intellectual capacity in exposed children	36; 45

(*Continued*)

Table 19.9 (Continued) Potential air quality risks in ART laboratories—chemically active contaminants (CACs)

No.	Compound	Occurrence	Particle/ CACs	Volatile organic compounds	Microbial contamination	Possible adverse effects	Reference number
16	Propylene	Propylene glycols used for paints, household detergents and automotive brake fluids. Polypropylene fibers for indoor/outdoor carpeting. Polyurethane systems for rigid foam insulation and flexible foam seat cushions; ABS resins for telephones and molded automotive trim parts. In addition to its use as a chemical intermediate, propylene is produced and consumed in refinery operations for the production of gasoline components.	✓	✓			30
17	Manganese—Manganese chloride Manganese sulphate Potassium permanganate	Used in steel production; manganese dioxide used in production of dry cell batteries, matches, fireworks; manganese sulfate 18 is used in fertilizer; glazes; varnishes and ceramics; potassium permanganate in filters	✓			Studies of manganese workers have not found increases in birth defects or low birth weight in their offspring. No birth defects were observed in animals exposed to manganese.	36; 46

(Continued)

Table 19.9 (Continued) Potential air quality risks in ART laboratories—chemically active contaminants (CACs)

No.	Compound	Occurrence	Particle/ CACs	Volatile organic compounds	Microbial contamination	Possible adverse effects	Reference number
						Exposure to high levels of manganese in air can cause lung irritation and reproductive effects. Nervous system and reproductive effects have been observed in animals after high oral doses of manganese.	
18	Chlorpyrifos—Organophosphate	Pesticides insecticide, acaricide and miticide used to control foliage and soil-borne insect pests on a variety of food and feed crops	✓			There is no information at present to show that chlorpyrifos either effects the ability of humans to reproduce or causes human birth defects.	36; 47; 48
19	Dichlorodiphenyl-trichloroethane (DDT)	Insecticide used in agriculture—used to control mosquitoes that spread malaria in some parts of the world; Exposure from food—eating; breathing or touching contaminated products	✓			Animal studies show effects on the liver and reproduction; DDT is considered a possible human carcinogen.	36; 49

(Continued)

Table 19.9 (Continued) Potential air quality risks in ART laboratories—chemically active contaminants (CACs)

No.	Compound	Occurrence	Particle/ CACs	Volatile organic compounds	Microbial contamination	Possible adverse effects	Reference number
20	Fluoride	Drinking water	✓			Prolonged high intake of fluoride, at any age, can result in skeletal fluorosis, a condition that may increase bone brittleness, and in a potential increase in risk of bone fracture. In high-dose cases, severe bone abnormalities can develop, crippling the affected individual.	36; 50
21	Polybrominated diphenyl ethers—209 possible PBDE compounds/ congeners (BDE —number)	PBDEs are a class of brominated flame retardants that are added to plastics, polyurethane foam, textiles (clothing; carpet, furniture fabric, upholstery, mattresses), and electronic equipment (computers) to reduce the likelihood of ignition and to slow the burn rate if the products do catch fire; dust; food/water ingestion	✓			PBDEs—concerns regarding liver, thyroid, developmental and reproductive toxicity and developmental neurotoxicity EPA—BDE 209—suggestive evidence of carcinogenic potential	36; 51–53

(Continued)

Table 19.9 (Continued) Potential air quality risks in ART laboratories—chemically active contaminants (CACs)

No.	Compound	Occurrence	Particle/ CACs	Volatile organic compounds	Microbial contamination	Possible adverse effects	Reference number
22	Tetrachloroethylene C_2Cl_4–PERK; PERC; ethylene tetrachloride	Used in dry cleaning industry; dry cleaned clothes; aerosol paints; typewriter correction fluid; waterproofing compounds; paint and varnish removers; furniture polish and cleaners; hard surface cleaners; rug, carpet and upholstery cleaners; lubricating greases and oils; agricultural and automotive chemicals; pulp and paper manufacture; manufacture of inks; exposure—breathing contaminated air; eating; drinking; when released into soil will evaporate or leach into ground water	✓			High concentrations of tetrachloroethylene in air may cause central nervous system effects; narcotic at high levels; Worksafe Australia reports as suspected carcinogen	36; 54
23	Di-(2-ethylexyl) phthalate (DEHP)	Articles made from poly-vinyl chloride (PVC)—medical devices (IV tubing and bags); flip flops—plastic shoes; furniture; rain coats; automobile upholstery; floor tiles	✓			Reproductive and developmental toxicants; probable human carcinogen	23; 37; 55

(Continued)

Table 19.9 (Continued) Potential air quality risks in ART laboratories—chemically active contaminants (CACs)

No.	Compound	Occurrence	Particle/ CACs	Volatile organic compounds	Microbial contamination	Possible adverse effects	Reference number
24	Benzyl butyl phthalate (BBP)	Articles made from polyvinyl chloride (PVC)—vinyl floors; sealants; adhesives; artificial leather; food wraps	✓			Reproductive and developmental toxicants; probable human carcinogen	23; 37
25	Alcohols: ethanol-acetaldehyde (immediate metabolite)	Inside incubators; laboratory cleaning products		✓		Teratogenesis; malformation of the face and brain, growth retardation	25; 56
26	Alcohols: Phenol	Phenol is used primarily in the production of phenolic resins and in the manufacture of nylon and other synthetic fibres. Used in slimicides (chemicals that kill bacteria and fungi in slimes), as a disinfectant and antiseptic, and in medicinal preparations such as mouthwash and sore throat lozenges.		✓		Phenol has caused minor birth defects and low birth weight in animals generally at exposure levels that also were toxic to the pregnant mothers. Phenol can have beneficial effects when used medically as an antiseptic or anesthetic.	57
27	Alcohols: Propanol (Also known as: ethyl carbinol; 1-propanol; propyl alcohol)	Solvents; alcohol swaps; rubbing alcohol; printing; inks; medications; sanitizing wipes; nebulizers and inhalants; cosmetics; nail varnish remover		✓			

(*Continued*)

Table 19.9 (Continued) Potential air quality risks in ART laboratories—chemically active contaminants (CACs)

No.	Compound	Occurrence	Particle/ CACs	Volatile organic compounds	Microbial contamination	Possible adverse effects	Reference number
28	Aldehydes: Nonanal	Used in food flavorings; fragrances; essential oils; citrus and rose oils		✓			
29	Aldehydes: Decanal	Used in food flavorings and fragrances		✓			
30	Polycyclic aromatic hydrocarbons (PAH)	Vehicle exhaust		✓			33
31	Alkanes: n-Hexane	Solvents containing n-hexane used to extract vegetable oils from crops such as soybeans. Used as cleaning agents in the printing, textile, furniture, and shoemaking industries. Certain kinds of special glues used in the roofing and shoe and leather industries also contain n-hexane. Several consumer products contain n-hexane, such as gasoline, quick-drying glues used in various hobbies, and rubber cement.		✓		In laboratory studies, animals exposed to high levels of n-hexane in air had signs of nerve damage. Some animals also had lung damage. In other studies, rats exposed to very high levels of n-hexane had damage to sperm-forming cells.	58

(Continued)

Table 19.9 (Continued) Potential air quality risks in ART laboratories—chemically active contaminants (CACs)

No.	Compound	Occurrence	Particle/ CACs	Volatile organic compounds	Microbial contamination	Possible adverse effects	Reference number
32	Alkanes: Propane	A by-product of natural gas processing and petroleum refining, it is commonly used as a fuel for engines, oxy-gas torches, barbecues, portable stoves, and residential central heating. Propane is one of a group of liquefied petroleum gases (LP gases).		✓			
33	Aromatic hydrocarbon: Benzene	Inside incubators; gas cylinders; crude oil; gasoline; cigarette smoke; volcanoes; forest fires; smoke; plastics; resins; nylon and synthetic fibers; lubricants; rubbers; dyes; detergents; drugs a pesticides; laser printers; automobile exhaust; CO_2 cylinders		✓		Harmful effects on bone marrow; may cause menstrual irregularities; decreased ovarian size; low birth weights and delayed bone formation in animals; carcinogenic	24; 33; 35; 59;

(Continued)

Table 19.9 (Continued) Potential air quality risks in ART laboratories—chemically active contaminants (CACs)

No.	Compound	Occurrence	Particle/ CACs	Volatile organic compounds	Microbial contamination	Possible adverse effects	Reference number
34	Aromatic hydrocarbon: Toluene—Methylbenzene; toluol; phenylmethane	Insulation—air handling systems; refrigerant gases; solvents; acrylic paints; gasoline; varnishes; lacquers; paint thinners; adhesives; glues; shoe polish; airplane glues		✓		Breathing very high levels of toluene during pregnancy can result in children with birth defects and retarded mental abilities, and growth. Not known if toluene harms the unborn child if the mother is exposed to low levels of toluene during pregnancy. EPA Group D—nonclassifiable as to carcinogenicity in humans.	30; 33; 36; 60; 61
35	Aromatic hydrocarbon: Xylene	It occurs naturally in petroleum and coal tar. Chemical industries produce xylene from petroleum. Xylene is used as a solvent and in the printing, rubber, and leather industries. It is also used as a cleaning agent, a thinner for paint, and in paints and varnishes. It is found in small amounts in airplane fuel and gasoline.		✓		Studies of unborn animals indicate that high concentrations of xylene may cause increased numbers of deaths, and delayed growth and development.	30; 33

(Continued)

Table 19.9 (Continued) Potential air quality risks in ART laboratories—chemically active contaminants (CACs)

No.	Compound	Occurrence	Particle/ CACs	Volatile organic compounds	Microbial contamination	Possible adverse effects	Reference number
36	Styrenes: Ethylbenzene C_8H_{10} Benzaldehyde	Emitted from laboratory plastic ware—Petri dishes; carpet backing; insulation; resins; tobacco; fuels; solvent; constituent of asphalt and naphtha; naturally in fruits, vegetables, nuts, meats and beverages		✓		Animal studies report central nervous system toxicity; pulmonary, liver, kidney and eye (irritation) effects from acute inhalation; EPA classified as Group D—not classifiable as to human carcinogenicity	20; 33; 62; 63
37	Acetone (also known as dimethyl ketone, 2-propanone, beta-ketopropane)	Inside incubators; used to make plastic, fibers, drugs, and other chemicals; solvent. Occurs naturally in plants, trees, volcanic gases, forest fires, and as a product of the breakdown of body fat. Present in vehicle exhaust, tobacco smoke, and landfill sites.		✓		Health effects from long-term exposures are known mostly from animal studies. Kidney, liver, and nerve damage, increased birth defects, and lowered ability to reproduce (males only) occurred in animals exposed long-term.	64
38	Acetylene	Welding	✓				
39	Ammonia	Naturally occurring; produced by human activity; bacteria; used in smelling salts; household cleaners; window cleaners; dissolves in water; found in soil, air, food	✓			Not known if exposure to ammonia causes birth defects.	33; 65

(Continued)

Table 19.9 (Continued) Potential air quality risks in ART laboratories—chemically active contaminants (CACs)

No.	Compound	Occurrence	Particle/ CACs	Volatile organic compounds	Microbial contamination	Possible adverse effects	Reference number
40	Butane	Butane is a hydrocarbon and a highly flammable, colorless, odorless, easily liquefied gas. It is typically used as fuel for cigarette lighters and portable stoves, a propellant in aerosols, a heating fuel, a refrigerant, and in the manufacture of a wide range of products. Butane is also found in liquefied petroleum gas (LPG). Since 1987, hydrocarbons have replaced chlorofluorocarbons (CFCs) as the propellant used in most aerosols. Butane is one of the commonly used propellants in household and industrial aerosols and therefore can be found in numerous aerosol products. However, the packaging of many aerosols products will commonly identify the propellant as "hydrocarbon," not specifically identifying butane.		✓			

(*Continued*)

Table 19.9 (Continued) Potential air quality risks in ART laboratories—chemically active contaminants (CACs)

No.	Compound	Occurrence	Particle/ CACs	Volatile organic compounds	Microbial contamination	Possible adverse effects	Reference number
41	Pentane	Fuel; solvents; properties similar to butanes and hexanes		✓			
42	Ethylene oxide	Sterilizing agent; ethylene oxide is a man-made chemical that is used primarily to make ethylene glycol (a chemical used to make antifreeze and polyester). A small amount (less than 1%) is used to control insects in some stored agricultural products and a very small amount is used in hospitals to sterilize medical equipment and supplies.		✓		There is some evidence that exposure to ethylene oxide can cause a pregnant woman to have a miscarriage. Animal studies indicate that in addition to irritation of the respiratory passages, nervous system effects, and reproductive effects, the kidneys, adrenal gland, and skeletal muscles may be affected from long-term exposure to ethylene oxide.	22

(*Continued*)

Table 19.9 (Continued) Potential air quality risks in ART laboratories—chemically active contaminants (CACs)

No.	Compound	Occurrence	Particle/CACs	Volatile organic compounds	Microbial contamination	Possible adverse effects	Reference number
43	Freon is a brand name for chlorofluoro-carbon—CFC113	Used as a coolant in air conditioning; as a blowing agent in aerosols; high temperature lubricants and fluorocarbon resins; Most commonly used CFS include CFC-11, CFC-12, CFC-113, CFC-114, and CFC-115; chlorofluorocarbons (CFCs) are being phased out worldwide	✓				
44	Halocarbon—Isoflurane 1-chloro-2,2,2-trifluoroethyl difluoromethyl ether	Anesthetic	✓				
45	Methylcyclohexane	Used in solvents; correction fluids	✓				
46	Writing instruments, felt tip marking pens	May contain acetone; butanol; methanol; ethanol; isopropanol, 1-propanol; methyl isobutyl ketone; and several other ketones; esters and acetates; phthalates	✓	✓			66; 67

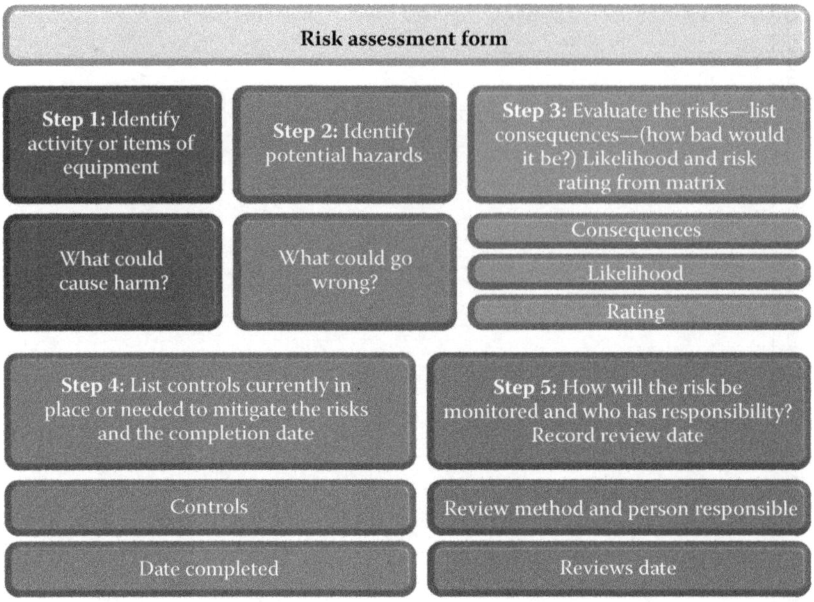

Figure 19.4 **(See color insert.)** Example of risk assessment form.

Table 19.10 Risk evaluation example

Likelihood of an event occurring (rating value)	Severity of event (rating value)	Overall risk rating (risk score)
Possible (3)	Moderate (4)	High (12)

c. *Overall Risk Rating Matrix—Determined by multiplying* ***Likelihood × Severity***
   i. Critical (20–25)
   ii. High (10–16)
   iii. Medium (5–9)
   iv. Low (1–4)

As likelihood and severity will vary between organizations, it is important to tailor the tools to the organization. A catastrophic event to one organization may be moderate to another. Table 19.11 provides an example of a "likelihood table" and Table 19.12 an example of a "severity table." These are developed to meet the specifications of a business or ART unit or the context under which they were utilized.

19.2.5 *Risk evaluation*

Risk evaluation utilizes the initial analysis information to compare, prioritize, and rank risks. The initial risk analysis takes into consideration the processes in place to currently manage the actual, potential, or perceived risk. It aids in identifying risks with "high" to "catastrophic" risk ratings and allows the organization to focus attention on treatment strategies for these specific risks. This phase is identified as "Initial Risk" and is

Table 19.11 Likelihood rating guidelines

Rating value	Rating	Description
5	Almost certain	There is little doubt that the event will occur (once every three months) History of regular occurrence at ART clinic and/or similar businesses
4	Likely	There is a strong possibility that the event will occur (once every 3 to 6 months) History of occurrence at ART clinic and/or similar businesses
3	Possible	There is a possibility that the event will occur (every 6 to 12 months) History of casual occurrence at ART clinic and/or similar businesses
2	Unlikely	There is a slight possibility that the event will occur (once every year to five years) History of casual occurrence at similar businesses
1	Rare	It is highly unlikely that the event will occur (>5 years)

compared to "Residual Risk" after the treatment of identified risks. A risk rating matrix as depicted in Figure 19.5 can be utilized to compare and quantify risks within the ART unit. Consideration should be given to processes that clearly define corrective action following a risk assessment. Many organizations report high and catastrophic risks to senior management review committees or corporate boards (Table 19.13). These are reviewed after the implementation of "risk treatment strategies" to determine residual risk. High risk activities may be assessed for tolerance and continually reviewed in relation to the organization's objectives.

19.2.6 Risk treatment

The treatment of risks involves identifying options and considering the potential benefits and costs of addressing the risk (Figure 19.6).

A cost–benefit analysis of the options in treating the risk is essential. If the cost of addressing the risk far outweighs the benefit, another treatment option may be necessary. Risk treatment strategies once prioritized need to be implemented and plans established. The plans include the timelines, available resources, and a repeated risk assessment to determine any residual risk. Table 19.14 provides an overview of possible treatment options for managing air quality in an IVF laboratory. This provides information on the effectiveness of the mitigation plans and allows a decision on the level of any residual risk that is acceptable or will be tolerated. Not all risk can be eliminated but if the residual risk is high, it can be monitored more closely.

19.2.7 Monitoring and review

Risk is constantly evolving and although the establishment of a risk management system provides a sound basis to control unexpected events, risks will continue to develop and change. Thus, systems to monitor and review risks are necessary. In addition to considering new risks, the treatment strategies in place to manage the identified risks are continually reviewed to ensure efficacy, efficiency, and safety. Regular review includes the risk management process, the risks and opportunities the organization faces, the effectiveness and adequacy of existing control, and the implementation of risk treatment strategies.[18]

Table 19.12 Severity rating guidelines

Rating value	Rating	Description
5	Catastrophic	• Long term (>3 months) cessation of core activities • Financial losses > USD 20,000,000 • Loss of patients (>50% of total number or secured work) • Major disruption to business activities following loss or failure of equipment >3 months • Microbial contaminants > acceptable levels for three months or more • ISO Class 5 particulate levels > acceptable levels for three months or more • Key person major injury or illness resulting in >3 months' time off work
4	Major	• Short term (2–3 months) cessation of core activities • Financial losses between USD 10,000,000 and 20,000,000 • Loss of patients (30–50% of total number or secured work) • Major disruption to business activities following loss or failure of equipment for 2–3 months • Microbial contaminants > acceptable levels for 2–3 months • ISO Class 5 particulate levels > acceptable levels for 2–3 months • Key Person Major injury or illness resulting in 2–3 months' time off work
3	Moderate	• Short term (1–2 months) cessation of core activities • Financial losses between USD 5,000,000 and 10,000,000 • Loss of patients (20–30% of total number or secured work) • Major disruption to business activities following loss or failure of equipment for 1–2 months • Microbial contaminants > acceptable levels for 1–2 months • ISO Class 5 particulate levels > acceptable levels for 1–2 months • Key Person Moderate injury or illness resulting in 1–2 months' time off work
2	Minor	• Short term (one month) cessation of core activities • Financial losses between USD 1,000,000 and 5,000,000 • Loss of patients (10–20% of total number or secured work) • Major disruption to business activities following loss or failure of equipment for one month • Microbial contaminants > acceptable levels for one month • ISO Class 5 particulate levels > acceptable levels for one month • Key person Injury or illness resulting in one months' time off work
1	Insignificant	• Short term (<1 month) cessation of core activities • Financial losses < USD 1,000,000 • Loss of patients (<10% of total number or secured work) • Major disruption to business activities following loss or failure of equipment for <1 month • Microbial contaminants > acceptable levels for <1 month • ISO Class 5 particulate levels > acceptable levels for < 1 month • Key person minor injury or illness resulting in <1 months' time off work

Likelihood					
Almost certain (5)	Medium (5)	High (10)	High (15)	Critical (20)	Critical (25)
Likely (4)	Low (4)	Medium (8)	High (12)	High (16)	Critical (20)
Possible (3)	Low (3)	Medium (6)	Medium (9)	High (12)	High (15)
Unlikely (2)	Low (2)	Low (4)	Medium (6)	Medium (8)	High (10)
Rare (1)	Low (1)	Low (2)	Low (3)	Low (4)	Medium (5)
	Insignificant (1)	*Minor (2)*	*Moderate (3)*	*Major (4)*	*Catastrophic (5)*
	Severity				

Figure 19.5 **(See color insert.)** Risk rating matrix.

Table 19.13 Example risk assessment action process

Risk score	Risk rating	What should I do?
20–25	Critical	Immediate action required
10–16	High	Action plan required, senior management attention needed
5–9	Medium	Specific monitoring or procedure required, management responsibility specified
1–4	Low	Manage through routine procedures

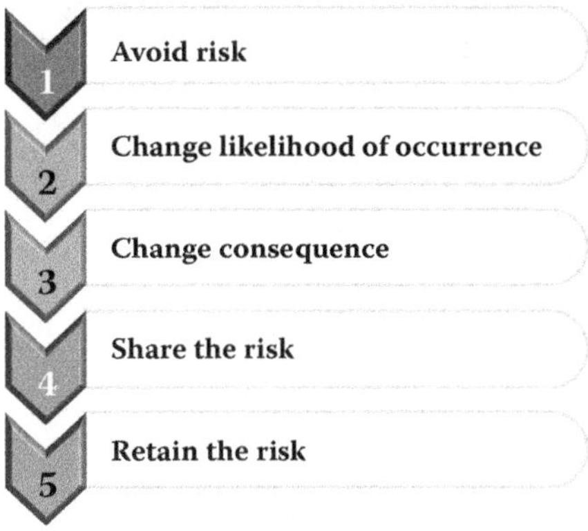
1
Avoid risk
2
Change likelihood of occurrence
3
Change consequence
4
Share the risk
5
Retain the risk

Figure 19.6 Risk treatment options.

Table 19.14 Possible treatment options

	High efficiency particulate air (HEPA) or ultra low penetration air (ULPA) filtration (trap particles as small as 0.3 μm)	Activated carbon	Filters Impregnated with potassium permanganate	UV light for decontamination	Oil overlays on culture media (act as sinks to capture VOCs—oil soluble)	Biological safety cabinets[a]: Class I Class II	Laminar flow clean bench systems[a]: horizontal; vertical	Positive pressure differential
Infectious agents: bacteria; fungi; spores; pollens	✓ HEPA filters 99.97% particle collective efficiency			✓		✓	✓ Product protection	
Alcohols and ketones		✓	✓					
Benzene		✓			✓			
Formaldehyde		✓			✓			
Particles 0.3 μm or larger	✓					✓	✓ Product protection	✓

[a] Biological Safety Cabinets:[68] Class I—Utilizes HEPA filtration and negative pressure to protect the operator; useful for containing moderate to high risk microbiological agents; aerosols, etc. Confers personnel protection; Class II—Utilizes HEPA filtration and unidirectional air flow for a very clean environment; downward laminar airflow minimizes cross contamination. Confers personnel, product and environmental protection; laminar flow—Utilizes HEPA filtration with either horizontal or vertical airflow. Confers product protection only.

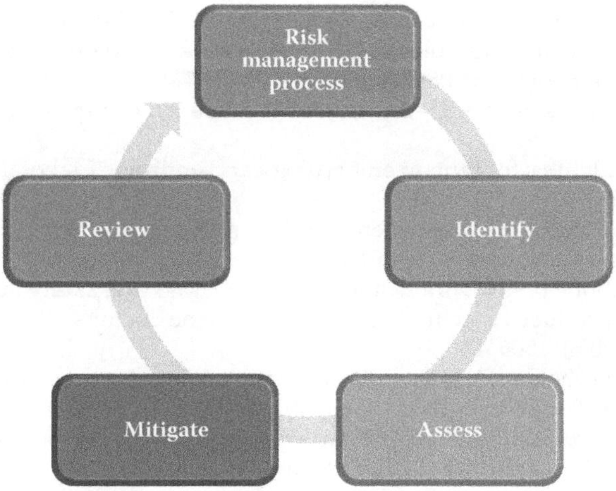

Figure 19.7 Risk management cycle.

Monitoring activities are embedded in the treatment plans to encourage ongoing review (Figure 19.7). These may include quality control and quality assurance activities, audits, incident/near miss/adverse event reporting, customer satisfaction surveys, review of suppliers/services, and complaints.

In regard to air quality in IVF laboratories, monitoring measures are clearly defined and documented to ensure risks are mitigated or minimized and that the data and processes necessary to minimize risk are part of the normal routine. This may include scheduled air quality testing, replacement of filters, maintenance of equipment, and daily temperature and humidity reporting. Staff need to be aware of the significance of the risk and the processes in place to mitigate.

In conclusion, risk management systems provide valuable tools in identifying risks and implementing systems to prevent or minimize the consequences. Although the system will not eliminate all risks, it will ensure a level of confidence and consistency in the delivery of care.

References

1. Alper MM. Experience with ISO quality control in assisted reproductive technology. *Fertil Steril* 2013; 100(6): 1503–8.
2. ESHRE position paper on the EU Tissues and Cells Directive EC/2004/23. November 2007. https://www.eshre.eu/Guidelines-and-Legal/ESHRE-Position-Papers.aspx.
3. European Union Directive 2004/23/EC of the European Parliament and of the Council of March 31, 2004 on setting standards of quality and safety for the donation, procurement, testing, processing, preservation, storage and distribution of human tissues and cells. http://eur-lex.europa.eu/LexUriServ/LexUriServ.do?uri=CELEX:32004L0023:EN:NOT.
4. Commission Directive 2006/17/EC of 8 February 2006 implementing Directive 2004/23/EC of the European Parliament and of the Council as regards certain technical requirements for the donation, procurement and testing of human tissues and cells. http://eur-lex.europa.eu/legal-content/EN/TXT/?uri=celex:32006L0017.
5. Commission Directive 2006/86/EC of 24 October 2006 implementing Directive 2004/23/EC of the European Parliament and of the Council as regards traceability requirements, notification of serious adverse reactions and events and certain technical requirements for the coding, processing, preservation, storage and distribution of human tissues and cells. http://eur-lex.europa.eu/legal-content/EN/TXT/?uri=CELEX:32006L0086.

6. Magli C, Van den Abbeel E, Lundin K, Royere D, Van der Elst J et al. For Committee of the Special Interest Group on Embryology ESHRE Pages—Revised guidelines for good practice in IVF laboratories. *Hum Reprod* 2008; 23(6): 1253–62.
7. Fertility Society of Australia—RTAC Code of Practice 2014. http://www.fertilitysociety.com.au/rtac/.
8. ASRM revised guidelines for human embryology and andrology laboratories. *Fertil Steril* 2008; 90(Suppl 3): S45–59.
9. SA/SNZ HB 436:2013. Risk Management Guidelines: Companion to AS/NZS ISO 31000:2009 Risk management—Principles and guidelines.
10. de Ziegler D, Gambone J, Meldrum D, and Chapron C. Risk and safety management in infertility and assisted reproductive technology (ART): From the doctor's office to the ART procedure. *Fertil Steril* 2013; 100(6): 1509–17.
11. Meldrum D and de Ziegler D. Risk and safety management in infertility and assisted reproductive technology. *Fertil Steril* 2013; 100(6): 1497–8.
12. Scott R and De Ziegler N. Could safety boards provide a valuable tool to enhance the safety of reproductive medicine? *Fertil Steril* 2013; 100(6): 1518–23.
13. HFEA 2014. Adverse incidents in fertility clinics: Lessons to learn 2010–2012. http://www.hfea.gov.uk/docs/INCIDENTS_REPORT.pdf.
14. ISO 14644. Cleanrooms and associated controlled environments. http://www.iso.org/iso/iso_catalogue/catalogue_tc/catalogue_tc_browse.htm?commid=54874.
15. European Commission Volume 4 EU Guidelines to Good Manufacturing Practice Medicinal Products for Human and Veterinary Use—Annex 1 Manufacture of Sterile Medicinal Products (corrected version) November 25, 2008. http://ec.europa.eu/health/files/eudralex/vol-4/2008_11_25_gmp-an1_en.pdf.
16. United Kingdom Human Fertilisation & Embryology Authority. http://www.hfea.gov.uk.
17. Jeynes J, PhD., MBA. Consultant, Opal Services, Principles of Risk Management—The 10 P's. 12 Knight St, St. John's, Worcester WR2 5DB, England [personal communication].
18. Standards Australia HB158 (2010). Delivering assurance based on ISO 31000:2009 Risk management: Principles and guidelines. http://infostore.saiglobal.com/store/details.aspx?ProductID=1396045.
19. Esteves SC and Bento FC. Implementation of air quality control in reproductive laboratories in full compliance with the Brazilian Cells and Germinative Tissue Directive. *Reprod BioMed Online* 2013; 26: 9–21.
20. Gilligan A, Schimmel T, Esposito Jr B, and Cohen J. Release of volatile organic compounds such as styrene by sterile petri dishes and flasks used for in vitro fertilization. 53rd Annual Meeting of the American Association for Reproductive Medicine October 1997 (Abstract 21; S52–S53).
21. Khoudja R, Xu Y, Li T, and Zhou C. Better IVF outcomes following improvements in laboratory air quality. *J Assist Reprod Genet* 2013; 30: 60–76.
22. United States of America Government Agency for Toxic Substances & Disease Registry: Ethylene Oxide. ToxFAQs March 3, 2011. http://www.atsdr.cdc.gov/substances/toxsubstance.asp?toxid=133.
23. Grandjean P and Landrigan PJ. 2014. Neurobehavioural effects of developmental toxicity. *Lancet Neurol* 2014; 13(3): 330–8.
24. Schimmel T, Gilligan A, Garrisi GJ, Esposito B, Cecchi M, Dale B et al. Removal of Volatile Organic Compounds from incubators used for gamete and embryo culture. *Fertil Steril* 1997; 1001: S165.
25. Chen S, Periasamy A, Yang B, Herman B, Jacobson K, and Sulik K. Differential sensitivity of mouse neural crest cells to ethanol-induced toxicity. *Alcohol* 2000; 20: 75–81.
26. United Sates of America Consumer Product Safety Commission: An update on formaldehyde, 2013. Revision 012013. https://www.cpsc.gov/PageFiles/121919/AN%20UPDATE%20ON%20FORMALDEHYDE%20final%200113.pdf.
27. Australian Government Department of Environment Particles: Air quality fact sheet 2005. https://www.environment.gov.au/resource/particles.
28. Brunekreef B and Holgate ST. Air pollution and health. *Lancet* 2002; 360: 1233–42.

29. Esteves SC and Agarwal A. Explaining how reproductive laboratories work. In: Bento F, Esteves S, and Agarwal A, eds. *Quality Management in ART Clinics: A Practical Guide.* 1st ed., Springer Science+Business Media, New York, pp. 79–127, 2013.
30. United States of America Government Agency for Toxic Substances & Disease Registry (ATSDR) Volatile Organic Compounds. http://www.atsdr.cdc.gov/substances/toxchemical listing.asp?sysid=7.
31. Cohen J, Gilligan A, Esposito W, Schimmel T, and Dale B. Ambient air and its potential effects on conception in vitro. *Hum Reprod* 1997; 12(8): 1742– 9.
32. Okada Y, Nakagoshi A, Tsurukawa M, Matsumura C, Eiho J, and Nakano T. Environmental risk assessment and concentration trend of atmospheric volatile organic compounds in Hyogo Prefecture, Japan. *Environ Sci Pollut Res* 2012; 19: 201–13.
33. Climate and Health Alliance Submission to Senate Standing Committees Community Affairs: Inquiry into the impacts on health of air quality in Australia, March 2013. http://www.caha.org.au.
34. Legro RS, Sauer MV, Mottla GL, Richter KS, Li X, Dodson WC et al. Effect of air quality on assisted human reproduction. *Hum Reprod* 2010; 25(5): 1317–24.
35. Australian Government Department of Environment Air Toxics. Air quality fact sheet, 2005. https://envirojustice.org.au/sites/default/files/files/Submissions%20and%20reports/Enviro justice_air_pollution_report_final.pdf.
36. Australian Government Department of Environment: Smoke from biomass burning. Air quality fact sheet, 2005. https://www.environment.gov.au/resource/smoke-biomass-burning.
37. Phthalates and their alternatives: Health and Environmental Concerns, Technical Briefing. Lowell Center for Sustainable Production, University of Massachusetts, January 2011. http://www.sustainableproduction.org/downloads/PhthalateAlternatives-January2011.pdf.
38. Ritz B and Wilhelm M. Ambient air pollution and adverse birth outcomes: Methodological Issues in an Emerging Field. *Basic Clin Pharmacol Toxicol* 2008; 102(2): 182–90.
39. United States of America Government Agency for Toxic Substances & Disease Registry: Lead. ToxFAQs March 3 2011. http://www.atsdr.cdc.gov/substances/toxsubstance.asp?toxid=22.
40. Possanzini M, Di Palo V, and Cecinato A. Sources and photodecomposition of formaldehyde and acetaldehyde in Rome ambient air. *Atmospheric Environment* 2002; 36: 3195–201.
41. Lenntech Information Sheet: Arsenic—As. http://www.lenntech.com/periodic/elements /as.htm.
42. United States of America Government Agency for Toxic Substances & Disease Registry (ATSDR): Arsenic. ToxFAQs August 2007. http://www.atsdr.cdc.gov/toxfaqs/tfacts2.pdf.
43. United States of America Environmental Protection Agency: Mercury Basic Information 11/03/14. http://www.epa.gov/mercury/about.htm.
44. United States of America Government Agency for Toxic Substances & Disease Registry: Mercury. ToxFAQs August 2014. http://www.atsdr.cdc.gov/toxfaqs/tfacts46.pdf.
45. United States of America Environmental Protection Agency. Polychlorinated biphenyls (PCBs) basic information, 09/04/2013. http://www.epa.gov/wastes/hazard/tsd/pcbs/about.htm.
46. United States of America Environmental Protection Agency. Manganese compounds hazard summary. Created in April 1992; Revised in February 16, 2010. http://www.epa.gov/ttnatw01 /hlthef/manganes.html.
47. United States of America Environmental Protection Agency. Chlorpyrifos facts, February 2002. http://www.epa.gov/oppsrrd1/REDs/factsheets/chlorpyrifos_fs.htm.
48. United States of America Government Agency for Toxic Substances & Disease Registry. Chlorpyrifos. ToxFAQs October 2011. http://www.atsdr.cdc.gov/tfacts84.pdf.
49. US Centers for Disease Control. Environmental Health Dichlorodiphenyltrichloroethane (DDT), November 2009. http://www.cdc.gov/biomonitoring/pdf/DDT_FactSheet.pdf.
50. United States of America Environmental Protection Agency. New fluoride risk assessment and relative source contribution documents, January 2011. http://water.epa.gov/action/advisories /drinking/fluoride_index.cfm.
51. United States of America Environmental Protection Agency. Polybrominated diphenyl ethers (PBDEs): Action plan summary. 30/10/2014. http://www.epa.gov/oppt/existingchemicals /pubs/actionplans/pbde.html.

52. National Center for Environmental Assessment Office of Research and Development. An exposure assessment of polybrominated diphenyl ethers. US Environmental Protection Agency, Washington DC, May 2010. file:///Users/sandroesteves/Downloads/PBDE_FINAL_MAY2010.PDF.
53. Australian Government. Polybrominated diphenyl ether flame retardants (PBDEs). http://www.environment.gov.au/system/files/resources/8e81d7e1-a379-4590-b296-19e14a72d909/files/factsheet.pdf.
54. Australian Government Department of the Environment. National pollutant inventory tetrachloroethylene: Fact sheet. http://www.npi.gov.au/resource/tetrachloroethylene.
55. United States of America Government Agency for Toxic Substances & Disease Registry. Di(2-ethylhexyl) phthalate (DEHP). ToxFAQs March 3, 2011. http://www.atsdr.cdc.gov/substances/toxsubstance.asp?toxid=65.
56. Wynter JM, Walsh DA, Webster WS, McEwen SE, and Lipson AH. Teratogenesis after acute alcohol exposure in cultured rat embryos. *Teratog Carcinog Mutagen* 1983; 3(5): 421–8.
57. United States of America Government Agency for Toxic Substances & Disease Registry. Phenol. ToxFAQs March 3, 2011. http://www.atsdr.cdc.gov/toxfaqs/tf.asp?id=147&tid=27.
58. United States of America Government Agency for Toxic Substances & Disease Registry. n-Hexane. ToxFAQs March 3, 2011. http://www.atsdr.cdc.gov/toxfaqs/tf.asp?id=392&tid=68.
59. Centers for Disease Control and Prevention. Facts about benzene, Feb. 14, 2013. http://www.bt.cdc.gov/agent/benzene/basics/facts.asp.
60. McKeown NJ. Medscape. Toluene toxicity. Feb. 8, 2013. http://emedicine.medscape.com/article/818939-overview.
61. United States of America Government Agency for Toxic Substances & Disease Registry. Toluene. ToxFAQs March 2014. http://www.atsdr.cdc.gov/toxfaqs/tf.asp?id=160&tid=29.
62. United States of America Environmental Protection Agency Technology Transfer Network. Air toxics web site ethylbenzene hazard summary. Created in April 1992; Revised in January 2000. http://www.epa.gov/ttnatw01/hlthef/ethylben.html.
63. United States of America Government Agency for Toxic Substances & Disease Registry (ATSDR). Ethylbenzene. March 3 2011. http://www.atsdr.cdc.gov/substances/toxsubstance.asp?toxid=66.
64. United States of America Government Agency for Toxic Substances & Disease Registry. Acetone. ToxFAQs July 8, 2013. http://www.atsdr.cdc.gov/toxfaqs/tf.asp?id=4&tid=1.
65. United States of America Government Agency for Toxic Substances & Disease Registry. Ammonia. ToxFAQs February 12 2013. http://www.atsdr.cdc.gov/toxfaqs/tfacts126.pdf.
66. Anderson R and Anderson J. Acute toxicity of marking pen emissions. 9th International Conference on Indoor Air Quality and Climate Proceedings: Indoor Air, 2002. http://www.irbnet.de/daten/iconda/CIB6679.pdf.
67. Mehta JG. Media and quality control in IVF laboratory. In: Jain K and Talwar P, eds. IVF Techniques for Beginners. Jaypee Brothers Medical Publishers (P) Ltd, New Delhi, pp. 36–64, 2013.
68. Elder K and Dale B. The clinical in-vitro fertilization laboratory. In: Elder K and Dale B, eds. *In-Vitro Fertilization*. 3rd. ed., Cambridge University Press, Cambridge, pp. 109–38, 2011.

chapter twenty

Troubleshooting aspects in clean room assisted reproductive units

Ronny Janssens and Johan Guns

Contents

Abstract

Most modern human IVF clinics now have their embryology laboratory located in a clean room. This strategy ensures a low level of environmental pollutants and high air purity, as well as low microbiological contamination, so that the IVF "production process" complies with regulations and licensing requirements. Early in the design phase, attention should be given to proper dimensioning and design, and a risk analysis should be done to identify potential problems and possible interruptions of normal functioning. At commissioning, special attention should be given to operational procedures and an SLA should be agreed on for monitoring, preventive maintenance, and repair. The clean room should be monitored according to ISO 14644 and if environmental monitoring indicates problems, extra cleaning and disinfection might be necessary.

20.1 Introduction

Over the last decades, practice in in vitro fertilization (IVF) has seen drastic changes. Current standards and regulatory requirements for embryology laboratories such as the European Union Tissues and Cells Directive (EUTCD) are getting more and more strict.[1] In Commission Directive 2006/86/EC it states that the air quality should be a GMP defined Grade A on a background air quality of Grade D.[2] Due to these changes in regulations, the facilities where embryology laboratories are housed are evolving toward good manufacturing practice (GMP) like facilities. Most modern human IVF clinics now have their embryology laboratory located in a clean room in order to ensure a low level of environmental pollutants and high air purity and low limits for microbiological contamination, so that the IVF "production process" complies with regulations and licensing requirements.

The purpose of a clean room is to maintain particulate-free air through the use of either high efficiency particulate air (HEPA) or ultra low penetration air (ULPA) filters employing laminar or turbulent air flow principles, and this requires a rather complicated heating, ventilation, and air conditioning (HVAC) installation with regular maintenance and risks of breakdown or deficiency. In an ideal world, troubleshooting should not be necessary because we should be able to avoid problems (prevention). Troubleshooting the clean room is something that any laboratory manager wishes to avoid at all times. As for any clinical treatment, we should be able to guarantee continuous and optimal functioning of all essential equipment, including the clean room. Any interruption of the normal function of the clean room may lead to impaired quality, increased infection risk, and reduced efficiency of the treatment and should be avoided at any time. The IVF process takes several days and oocytes and embryos have an extremely high emotional value for patients. It is hard to explain to patients undergoing assisted reproductive technology (ART) treatment that their cycle is being interrupted or compromised by a failure in the clean room.

Unfortunately, an HVAC installation is technically quite complex and comprises multiple pumps, filters, valves, humidifiers, etc. Hence, when problems arise with this complex machinery, embryology laboratories are completely dependent on fast support from a technical service or a maintenance company. Also, sometimes a clean room needs to be shut down for preventive maintenance. In contrast to an ART laboratory, which is organized in such a way that 24-hour service is guaranteed, any technical service or maintenance company is less organized to achieve a rapid intervention or is organized to do necessary interventions out of regular working hours.

Therefore, the best policy to avoid shutdown and problems is by taking enough preventive measures. Already in the early design phase of a clean room, attention should be given to proper dimensioning and design, and identifying potential problems and interruptions. This prevention is usually done by performing a risk analysis. Remember Murphy's Law: "If anything can go wrong, it will go wrong!" Many things can and will go wrong, including (1) lack of preventive maintenance and regular servicing, (2) inadequate filter changing frequency, (3) incorrect temperature or humidity, (4) incorrect differential air pressure, (5) accidental defects, (6) release of volatile organic compounds (VOCs), and (7) power failure.

But how can we beat Murphy's Law? The answer is by assuring that the technical staff is properly trained and educated, that there are documented and detailed written standard operating procedures (SOPs) and logbooks for clean room operation and maintenance. All these measures should be defined and written down in a service level agreement (SLA) with a technical service or maintenance company defining maximum intervention times in case of breakdown and this SLA should be revised periodically.

20.2 *Preventive measures early in the design phase*

The design of a clean room is not the topic of this chapter, but it is crucial that a new clean room and the HVAC installation are designed and dimensioned such that the desired environmental parameters and air quality (particulate contamination, VOC) can be achieved at all times. The HVAC unit should be designed to ensure that it meets user requirement specifications, acceptable tolerances for parameters, and capacity. Variables to be taken into account to calculate HVAC dimensions and capacity are (1) volume of clean room, (2) number of staff working simultaneously, (3) desired air quality (ISO classification or GMP class), (4) temperature and relative humidity (RH) in the clean room, (5) outside air temperature and RH (hot and humid outside air in summer and cold and dry during winter), (6) environmental pollution, (7) size and dimensions of laboratory equipment, (8) heat generation of laboratory equipment, (9) air movement and airflow direction, and (10) endogenous VOC generation (out-gassing of plastics, equipment). All these elements should be considered carefully, written down in user requirements specifications, and this document should be an integral part of the SLA.

For safety, mechanical or electronic door interlocking systems should have a manual override system to open the doors so in case of defect or failure (or fire), staff still can leave the clean room.

According to international professional guidelines and standards[3,4] and ISO 15189[5] there should be a backup of critical equipment. The HVAC installation of a clean room is certainly classified as critical and measures should be taken to ensure continuity. Taking this into account, when we rebuilt the Centre for Reproductive Medicine at UZ Brussel in 2011, we decided to duplicate the installation and we constructed two identical clean rooms for embryology work, with two completely independent HVAC units, ensuring continuity of service. If budget allows, it is also a good idea to anticipate future expansion by building the clean room larger than strictly necessary to accommodate future capacity increases or the application of new technology.

20.3 *Preventive measures during commissioning and qualification*

Not only prior to the design but also before commissioning an HVAC installation, it is appropriate to perform a second risk analysis to assess the functioning of this critical equipment to determine critical and noncritical parameters, components, subsystems, and controls and identify possible areas of concern.

Items to take into consideration in this phase are (1) frequency of control of filters, (2) maintenance frequency, (3) presence of fire detection in clean room and ducts, (4) presence of fire extinguishers, (5) electrical installation, and (6) presence of emergency power supply and (7) operational processes.

Table 20.1 ISO 14644 clean room tests

Test parameter	Objective	Maximum time interval	Test procedure
Particle count	Verify cleanliness	6 months or 12 months depending on Class	Particle counter
Air pressure differential	Verify absence of cross-contamination	12 months	Measure pressure difference
Airflow volume	Verify air change rates	12 months	Measure supply and return air, air change rate
Airflow velocity	Verify unidirectional airflow	12 months	Velocity measurements

At this stage, special attention should go to operational processes. An example of such an important operational process to be considered is the starting and shutdown sequence of motors after a planned or accidental down period of the HVAC unit. To avoid negative pressure and influx of particles and external air into the clean room, the air inlet (pulsation) motors should always be started before the extraction motors start and at shutdown, and under no circumstances should the extraction motor be allowed to work when the pulsation motor is down.

Before commissioning, installation records and documented evidence of measure capacities of the system, operation and maintenance manuals, schematic drawings, protocols, and test reports should be handed over and approved by the end user.

Before a newly built clean room can be used, it needs to be qualified and validated "as built" (an empty room, without equipment or personnel), "at rest" (with equipment but no operators present), and "in operation" (the normal process with equipment and personnel). Parameters included in this qualification (or validation) are (1) temperature, (2) humidity (RH), (3) air supply, (4) return and exhaust air quantities, (5) room air change rates and room pressures (pressure differentials), (6) room clean-up rate, (7) particle counts, (8) microbial counts of air and surfaces, (9) HEPA filter integrity tests, and (10) tests of warning and alarm systems.

The methods for qualification and testing are defined in the ISO 14644 norm (International Organization for Standardization, 2001).[6] This set of standards advises a schedule of tests to demonstrate continuing compliance, as shown in Table 20.1. In addition to the tests listed in Table 20.1, filter leakage, containment leakage, recovery time, and airflow visualization testing can be carried out.

20.3.1 Operational processes and training

Proper training of technical and laboratory staff is crucial. Even the best-designed clean room will be inefficient when the proper operation processes are not known or not respected. Laboratory staff should understand the principles and functioning in a clean room, the function of an airlock, dress code and changing procedures, personnel hygiene, and disinfection. Special attention should be given to the daily cleaning procedures. Dedicated cleaning personnel should be appointed and trained in proper cleaning and disinfection. Ordering and inventory management should be able to ensure sufficient supply of clean room dresses and personal protective equipment (overshoes, gloves). At regular intervals, staff should be tested on their knowledge of the operational processes and retraining should be provided. All the aforesaid are part of a risk assessment analysis, as shown in Table 20.2.

Table 20.2 Example of a risk assessment checklist on operational processes

Is there a system of operational procedures defining different tasks, responsibilities (ISO 14644-5 §4)?	Yes/No
Is staff trained in working in a clean room?	Yes/No
Is a written SOP easily available/accessible?	Yes/No
Is staff tested on their knowledge of these SOPs?	Yes/No
Is regular retraining organized?	Yes/No
Are there clear instructions in the airlock/entry doors?	Yes/No
Are there clear instructions to change protective clothes (ISO 14644-4 §D.2.4.3)?	Yes/No
Are there clear instructions for hand hygiene (ISO 14644-4 §D.2.4.3)?	Yes/No
Is there a mirror to check protective cloths (ISO 14644-4 §D.2.4.3)?	Yes/No
Are there sufficient cover shoes?	Yes/No
Clean room dress: sufficient number and sizes?	Yes/No
Clean room monitoring ISO 14644-1 (§4.2.1)	Max 6 months ISO <5 Max 12 months ISO >5
Frequency of leakage tests HEPA (ISO 14644-2 annex A)	Max 24 months
Visualization airflow (ISO 14644-2 annex A)	Max 24 months
Recuperation (ISO 14644-2 annex A)	Max 24 months
Leakage test air isolation in-out (ISO 14644-2 annex A)	Max 24 months
Instructions for cleaning (SOP) available?	Yes/No
List of dedicated cleaning staff?	Yes/No
Is cleaning staff trained?	Yes/No

20.3.2 Clean room monitoring

Performance control and function monitoring of an HVAC unit should be carried out by a facility or building monitoring system. Additional factors that should be monitored are planned shutdown, replacement of filters, and preventive maintenance. Topics to include in an SLA are (1) the normal operating ranges, (2) alert and action limits and responsibilities for the facility monitoring system, (3) contacts in case of alarm, (4) actions when exceeding established limits, (5) responsibilities for maintenance and failure, (6) maximal intervention times, (7) procedures, (8) program and records for planned preventive maintenance, (9) filter changing frequency, and (10) registration of interventions. Each ART establishment must establish "warning limits" and "action limits" for each clean room area. These limits can be determined and adjusted based on trends observed during validation and monitoring. In general, the mean is ±1 or 2 standard deviations (SDs).

20.3.3 Volatile organic compounds (VOCs)

VOCs are natural or synthetic chemicals that can vaporize under normal atmospheric conditions. The compounds that the human nose can smell are generally VOCs. In 1997, Cohen was the first to report a negative correlation between VOC levels and human embryo development.[7] Ideally, the lab is equipped with an over-pressured heating, ventilation, and air conditioning (HVAC) system with pretreatment of air with active carbon and oxidation using potassium permanganate and/or photo oxidation as well as physical filtration to remove eventual VOCs from outside air and the same filters in the air recirculation circuit to remove endogenous generated VOCs. Filter efficiency needs to be monitored on a regular basis because saturated filters gradually release their accumulated VOCs into the filtered air. Saturated active carbon filters will no longer retain VOCs, but will gradually release bound VOCs back into laboratory air so filters need to be replaced before their maximum absorption capacity is reached. The filter change frequency depends on outside air quality and levels of endogenous VOC generation by medical gasses, staff (perfumes), equipment, cleaning agents, and out-gassing of plastics. The saturation grade of the VOC filters can be determined by regular analysis of used filters and the filter change frequency can be adjusted accordingly.

It is now possible to install very sensitive VOC meters (able to detect in the ppm or ppb range), connected to equipment or a building monitoring system so the VOC content in the laboratory air can be monitored continuously.

20.4 Troubleshooting issues

20.4.1 Ambiguous responsibility

Clean rooms are used by many operators, and they will be busy with different aspects of the ART treatment. To ensure a quick response to faults, it is crucial that it is clearly defined who is responsible for all aspects of facility or building monitoring systems, reaction to alarms, and the normal functioning and technical interventions necessary so that no precious time is lost in case of malfunctioning due to late or no reaction to alarms. These responsibilities are an integral part of the operators' job descriptions and an SLA with a technical company.

20.4.2 HVAC unit

Air quality management in the IVF laboratory aims to prevent (cross) contamination of reproductive tissues and cells, as well as exposure of laboratory personnel to communicable disease agents. A good air-handling unit ensures the adequate filter of air to control contaminants and maintains specific airflows from more clean to less clean areas and minimizes condensation on critical surfaces. Critical parameters of the air-handling unit can pose risks and should be monitored and recorded by a building monitoring system.

Problems that can occur are (1) blocked or faulty flow rate controllers, (2) poorly adjusted control dampers, (3) bad water and steam quality in the humidifier, (4) poor drainage of humidifier, (5) no elimination of condensed water and poor drainage of the cooling battery, and (6) broken or badly installed filters and problems with duct material and internal insulator. Needless to say, all incidents and/or interventions should be registered in detailed logbooks.

20.4.2.1 Temperature and relative humidity

If the environment of a clean room is cold and dry, microbiological contaminants will not grow. Decreasing the ambient temperature in the environment of IVF facilities is not an option due to the side effects on the fertilization rates, slow cleavage rates, embryo fragmentation, and the human comfort of the operators.[7] However, moister control solutions are technically possible. If the ambient relative humidity of the clean room environment exceeds 50%, the risk of bacteria growth increases. On the other hand, humidity that is below 35% promotes static electricity, personal discomfort, and irritation of mucous membranes and eyes. Ambient RH between 40 and 50% minimizes the impact of bacteria and respiratory infections and provides a comfortable working environment.

The air-handling unit should have the capability of providing humidification and dehumidification. Design should be such that these humidifiers do not become sources of contamination. Temperature and relative humidity should be continuously monitored and recorded and minimum and maximum limits need to be defined. If the temperature and/or relative humidity in the clean room are not up to specifications, then it might be that relevant environmental sensors are not calibrated, and therefore it is important to ensure that calibration records are up to date.

20.4.2.2 Pressurization

IVF laboratories work under positive pressure to the outside to prevent infiltration of unfiltered, contaminated air from outside. Most clean rooms are designed with airlocks with differential pressure and interlocking doors to maintain over-pressure. Positive differential pressurization between the critical areas and adjacent areas of different classifications maintains an airflow that avoids infiltrations of contaminants of less cleaner areas. When dealing with hazardous tissues or cells, a negative differential pressure is maintained between the critical areas and the airlock and hatches. The latter are in overpressure against the less clean areas. In general, a differential pressure between 5 and 15 Pa is recommended.[8]

Pressure drops and pressure fluctuations are common problems caused by poorly fine-tuned HVAC installations. Quite often the origin of the problem is over-pressurization and/or uncontrolled leakage areas. The higher the pressurization, the higher the uncontrolled leakage of air by door undercuts, walls, ceilings, and duct joints, resulting in a higher demand of fresh filtered air and higher exploitation costs.

A pressure drop should not necessarily lead to the destruction of the reproductive tissues processed during this failure; however, one might not ignore that the risk of contamination increases. In these circumstances, additional sterility controls of the tissue products are recommended (microbiological controls of spent culture media).

20.4.3 (Cross-)contamination

(Cross-)contamination refers to contamination of a starting material, intermediate product, or finished product with another starting material or product during production or processing (= cross-contamination) or from the environment or operators. In embryology laboratories, (cross-)contamination can lead to infections in culture dishes and may lead to loss of gametes or embryos.

Several studies in tissue banks and industrial clean rooms showed that more than half of the recovered bacteria on the surfaces in controlled environments belong to the normal skin flora of humans.[9–12] The human body can shed up to approximately 10,000 colony forming units (CFUs)/minute.[13] This not only affects the microbial load of the air surrounding the operator, but provides a source for contamination by touch. Cobo and Concha showed that incorrectly applied aseptic techniques entail a greater risk than the surrounding environment.[9] This risk (of using a wrong aseptic technique) decreases when the techniques are performed in a clean room.[14] The operator can either directly or indirectly represent a source of microbial contamination. Therefore, controls should be done "in operation" to monitor this main contamination factor, that is, the operator. To date, only a limited number of published reports indicate that the source of the infection can be attributed to the environment in which the processing of the tissues and cells took place.

Known factors leading to contamination can be design errors of the HVAC and dust extraction systems, poorly operated or maintained HVAC systems, inadequate procedures for, and movement of personnel, materials, and equipment, and inefficient cleaning procedures of insufficiently cleaned equipment.

(Cross-)contamination can be minimized by:

- Applying strict personnel procedures (dress code, using personnel protection, gowning)
- Adequate premises (design)
- Use of closed production systems
- Adequate, validated cleaning procedures
- Appropriate levels of product protection
- Correct air pressure cascade

By regular environmental monitoring and microbiological testing as per ISO 14698, changing trends of microbial count and microflora within a clean room provide information about the functioning of the HVAC unit, the construction of the clean room, staff respect of operational procedures and personnel cleanliness, gowning practices, the equipment, and cleaning operations.[15] If environmental monitoring indicates problems, corrective action should be taken. Extra cleaning and disinfection of the clean room might be necessary. If problems are persistent, then the installation of impervious barriers such as spot ventilation and capture hoods can be considered in some cases.

Most standards regarding environmental monitoring, including ISO14644 and ISO 14698, derive from pharmaceutical or electronic industry guidelines and are not familiar with ART. Well-known pitfalls in setting up a microbiological monitoring program are insufficient number of samples, sampling frequency, sampling technique, sampling time, selection of microbiological culture media, and incubation conditions.

20.4.3.1 *Number of samples*

For classification purposes, the number of samples is described in the ISO14644-1 and should be evenly distributed throughout the area.[6,15] The number of samples within a microbiological monitoring program may differ from these guidelines and should be considered on the basis of a risk analysis in function of ART specific processes. Once the sample locations are selected we suggest applying them permanently during the whole monitoring program which allows you to compare monitoring results over time.

20.4.3.2 *Sample frequency*

Most standards do not go into detail. The EU GMP asks for frequent monitoring while the U.S. cGMP states that near and long-term oversights depend on the classification of the clean room.[2,16]

It is generally accepted that the processing of tissue or cells in ART implies a significantly lower risk of transmitting bacterial or fungal infections to the recipient than embryo transfer. Publications and case reports dealing with infected ART culture dishes are scarce. The added value of routine aseptic process monitoring (in operation) seems therefore questionable. However, this low incidence may be partly due to underreporting. Kastrop routinely performed microbiological examination in all turbid culture dishes for an eight-year period from 1997 onward.[17] He registered infected cultures in 0.68% IVF and ICSI cycles combined, and exclusively occurring in IVF cycles with an incidence of 0.86%. Interestingly, in the aforementioned study, one-third of them, the same microorganism, based on antibiotic resistance, was isolated from semen. In two-thirds of ART culture infections, the source was elsewhere. Regular environmental monitoring of the process core and background is therefore recommended.

20.4.3.3 Sampling technique

The EU GMP and U.S. cGMP consider monitoring of airborne viable particles, using an air sampler, as the standard method for microbiological monitoring of classified environments.[2,18] However, Friberg and colleagues did not find any correlation between the occurrence of wound infections and microbiological contamination of the immediate environment in operating theaters with laminar airflow using an air sampler, although this relationship was determined using sedimentation plates.[19,20] In operating rooms with turbulent air flow, a correlation between wound infection and microbiological contamination is observed with an air sampler.[19] Whyte came to a similar conclusion in pharmaceutical production environments. He found that the use of the sedimentation plates was the best method for quantifying possible microbiological contamination in filling systems under laminar flow.[21] The use of a microbiological "air sampler" has in addition a direct impact on the environment of measurement by their physical presence, and it is very difficult to ensure the sterility of an air sampler.[22] Since the use of an air sampler entails a potential risk of infection, the method is not recommended for monitoring and validation of environments that are in direct contact with tissues or cells.

20.4.3.4 Sampling time with sedimentation plates

The use of sedimentation plates is a cost-effective and easy-to-establish monitoring method. The results are reported as a number of colony formed units per four-hours exposure time. In practice, four hours of exposure is not always realistic due to dehydration of the culture medium characterized by broken and parched soils after several days of incubation. Dehydration depends on the composition and volume of culture medium, but also on the airflow rate and pattern. The weight loss to the original weight of 30-mL Tryptic soy agar plates increases with exposure time to 9.3–11.7% after four-hours exposure,[11] which has been shown to be correlated with an 8% loss of viability of test organisms.[23] We advise an exposure time of a maximum of two hours. For longer processes, you could replace the sedimentation plates with new plates.

20.4.3.5 Microbiological culture media

The first international standard for biocontamination control in clean rooms and associated environments ISO14698-1:2003 advises the use of a nonselective culture medium containing additives to overcome the residual effect of biocides and cleaning agents, thus allowing growth of the expected microorganisms.[15] The eventual need for a selective culture medium for yeast and molds, such as Sabouraud Dextrose agar, has been a matter of debate for years.[24] But the USP has now proposed the soybean-casein digest (SCD) agar or TSA as an all-purpose solid medium for the recovery and quantification of most environmental microorganisms in clean rooms, both bacteria and fungi.[18,24] The use of only one type of culture medium will simplify the monitoring program and minimize the costs.

20.4.3.6 Incubation conditions

Recovery and incubation conditions have to be compatible with the sampling method in order to permit growth and identification of viable microorganisms, and validated as such. Ideal culture conditions differ between microorganisms, two to five days at 30–35°C for bacteria versus five to seven days at 20–25°C for fungi and molds.[15,16,24] Therefore, some centers collect duplicate samples, which doubles sampling time and reagent costs. Alternatively, one general culture medium such as TSA can be incubated under biphasic conditions.[11,12,15,25]

20.4.4 Presence of VOCs

When smells are noticed inside the laboratory and there is VOC filtration installed in the HVAC unit, it is likely that the filters are saturated and should be replaced.

Accidental release of VOCs can be the result of unauthorized use of chemicals such as alcohol or alcohol containing products. The laboratory staff should supervise cleaning staff and approve the use of detergents and cleaning/decontaminating agents and should check that cleaning staff is not using nonapproved products.

20.4.5 HVAC down after power failure

All elements of the HVAC unit should be connected to an uninterruptable power supply (UPS) so that continuous operation is not at risk after a power failure of normal testing of electricity circuits.

References

1. Commission of the European Parliament, 2004. Directive 2004/23/EC of the European Parliament and of the Council of March 31, 2004 on setting standards of quality and safety for the donation, procurement, testing, processing, preservation, storage and distribution of human tissues and cells. Commission Directive 2006/86/EC, Annex I.D. http://eur-lex.europa.eu/LexUriServ/LexUriServ.do?uri=CELEX:32004L0023:EN:NOT (accessed January 15, 2015).
2. European Union Good Manufacturing Practice, 2008 (EU GMP). Medicinal Products for Human and Veterinary Use. Annex 1 Manufacture of Sterile Medicinal Products (corrected version). 91/356/EEC, EudraLex–Volume 4 Good Manufacturing Practice (GMP) Guidelines.
3. ASRM and SART. Revised guidelines for human embryology and andrology laboratories. *Fertil Steril* 2008; 90: S45–59.
4. Magli MC, van den Abbeel E, Lundin K, Royere D, van der Elst J, and Gianaroli L. For Committee of the Special Interest Group on Embryology. *Hum Reprod* 2008; 23: 1253–62.
5. International Organization for Standardization, 2012. ISO 15189:2012. Medical Laboratories—Requirements for Quality and Competence, Geneva, Switzerland, 2012.
6. International Organization for Standardization, 1999. ISO14644-1:1999. Cleanrooms and associated controlled environments—Part 1: Classification of air cleanliness.
7. Cohen J, Gilligan A, Esposito W, Schimmel T, and Dale B. Ambient air and its potential effects on conception in vitro. *Hum Reprod* 1997; 12: 1742–9.
8. International Organization for Standardization, 2001. ISO14644-4: 2001. Cleanrooms and associated controlled environments—Part 4: Design, construction and start up.
9. Cobo F and Concha A. Environmental microbial contamination in a stem cell bank. *Letters in Applied Microbiology* 2007; 44: 379–86.
10. Favero MS, Puleo JR, Marshall JH, and Oxborrow GS. Comparative levels and types of microbial contamination detected in industrial clean rooms. *Applied Microbiology* 1966; 14: 539.
11. Guns J, Janssens R, and Vercammen M. Air quality management. In: Nagy ZP, Varghese AC, and Ashok A, eds. *Practical Manual of in Vitro Fertilization: Advanced Methods and Novel Devices*, Springer, New York, 2012.
12. Herlong JL, Reubish K, Higdon HL, and Boone WR. Quantitative and qualitative analysis of microorganisms in an assisted reproductive technology facility. *Fertil Steril* 2008; 89: 847–53.
13. Thomas M, Sanborn MD, and Couldry RIV. Admixture contamination rates: Traditional practice site versus a class 1000 cleanroom. *Am J Health-System Pharmacists* 2005; 62: 2386–92.

14. Stucki C, Sautter AM, Favet J, and Bonnabry P. Microbial contamination of syringes during preparation: The direct influence of environmental cleanliness and risk manipulations on end-product quality. *Am J Health-System Pharmacy* 2009; 66: 2032–6.
15. International Organization for Standardization, 2003. ISO14698-1: 2003. Cleanrooms and associated controlled environments—Biocontamination control—Part 1: General principles and methods.
16. Food and Drug Administration, 2004. Guidance for Industry. Sterile Drug Products. Produced by Aseptic Processing—Current Good Manufacturing Practice.
17. Kastrop PMM, de Graaf-Miltenburg LAM, Gutknecht DR, and Weima SM. Microbial contamination of embryo cultures in an ART laboratory: Sources and management. *Hum Reprod* 2007; 22: 2243–8.
18. USP 29-NF 24, 2010. Microbiological evaluation of clean rooms and other controlled environments. United States Pharmacopeia, Baltimore, MD.
19. Friberg B, Friberg S, and Burman LG. Correlation between surface and air counts of particles carrying aerobic bacteria in operating rooms with turbulent ventilation an experimental study. *J Hosp Infection* 1999; 42: 61–8.
20. Friberg B, Friberg S, and Burman LG. Inconsistent correlation between aerobic bacterial surface and air counts in operating rooms with ultra clean laminar air flows: Proposal of a new bacteriological standard for surface contamination. *J Hosp Infection* 1999; 42: 287–93.
21. Whyte W. In support of settle plates. *PDA J Pharm Sci Technol* 1996; 50: 201–4.
22. Pasquarella C, Pitzurra O, and Savino A. The index of microbial air contamination. *J Hosp Infection* 2000; 46: 241–56.
23. Deschenes PD. Viable environmental microbiological monitoring. In: Agalloco J and Carleton FJ, eds. *Validation of Pharmaceutical Processes.* Informa Healthcare, New York, pp. 357–369, 2008.
24. Clontz L. Microbial Limit and Bioburden Tests. Validation Approaches and Global Requirements. CRC Press, Taylor & Francis Group, Boca Raton, FL, 2009.
25. Moldenhauer J. Practical issues in designing and implementing an environmental control program. In: Moldenhauer J, ed. *Environmental Monitoring. A Comprehensive Handbook.* Volume 1, PDA Books, Bethesda, MD, pp. 7–26, 2005.

chapter twenty-one

Role of quality manager in clean room assisted reproductive units and policies for efficient running

Fabiola C. Bento and Sandro C. Esteves

Contents

Abstract

This chapter discusses the role of quality managers in assisted reproductive technology (ART) centers and their importance in the implementation and maintenance of a quality management system (QMS) that includes the efficient running of clean room facilities. Clear policies, teamwork, and leadership guarantee efficient running and help reduce variations and nonconformities, thus resulting in improvement of overall outcomes.

21.1 Introduction

Although many attempts have been made to define "quality," no one has been able to come up with any simple definition. Quality is a personal concept that varies according to people's feelings, faith, culture, background, and expectations, not to mention type of product or service being offered.[1]

When considering assisted reproductive technology (ART) centers and the kind of services they provide, the variation is huge. Some procedures that are offered in one country, such as donor insemination and gamete donation, are completely forbidden in another, and the relationship between doctors and patients may simply go from friendly and egalitarian to distant and authoritarian. Consequently, the demands and expectations patients have can be completely different, and the definition of quality impossible to be universal.

Therefore, each organization must analyze the services they offer and how they are offered, must understand their customer's expectations and critically evaluate their own common understanding of what it means to provide a "quality" service or product, to be able to define quality. This concept must be created internally in order to be owned by the organization and shared by the team.

According to Philip B. Crosby, famous quality guru, quality has to be defined as conformance to requirements, not as goodness. That is because the concept of "goodness" is what varies so much among people and causes such confusion. Recent international directives specifically require ART centers to implement and maintain a quality management system, including air quality control in reproductive laboratories, and even in countries where there are no such requirements, most ART centers are interested in implementing such a system due to its proven beneficial effects and improved results.

21.2 Quality management system requirements

The European Union Tissues and Cells Directive (EUTCD; Commission of the European Parliament, 2004) and the Brazilian Cell and Tissues Directive (ANVISA, 2006), for instance, require the implementation of a quality management system (QMS) aiming at increasing quality in all ART centers.[2,3] A QMS is therefore mandatory, and involves specific requirements such as certified staff, training programs, fully documented and implemented standard operating procedures (SOPs), quality control, and quality assurance, among others.

A QMS must be based on the interconnection of all processes necessary to deliver a product or service. Every process must be broken into procedures or tasks that must be standardized and formally described in order to allow reproducibility and guarantee that it is always performed in the same way, without variation. Standardization facilitates training and the establishment of goals and policies, besides leading to reduced variations and stable results, and allows outcomes to be compared and improvements to be conducted based on real and comparable data.

Understanding this interaction is necessary to determine what affects each process and what should be controlled. Critical processes or procedures can then be identified and improvement plans be implemented to guarantee quality, avoid "near miss" events, and prevent risks. Defense mechanisms to minimize the chances of errors must be in place to protect patients from harm.[4]

21.3 Controlling variation

In ART, there are many variations that cannot be controlled, such as the patient's age, cause of infertility, patient's response to the medication, etc. Cases may be similar, but never totally equal. Therefore, it is of utmost importance to reduce or eliminate all other variations, to be able to achieve quality. Dr. W. Edwards Deming, considered the number one quality guru, used to say that improved quality means reduced variation (Figure 21.1).

In ART, variation can be reduced by:

1. Prescribing the same type of medication to all patients (doses and regimens have to vary, of course, based on patients' profiles, etc., but the type of drug should be the same in order to enable comparison of results). If different drugs are prescribed, then comparisons should be made only among patients using the same type of drug.
2. Using the same types of dishes and disposable materials. If different disposables are used, results have to be analyzed separately.
3. Using the same type of culture media and applying similar incubation conditions. Again, if different media or different culture systems and incubators are used, results have to be analyzed separately.

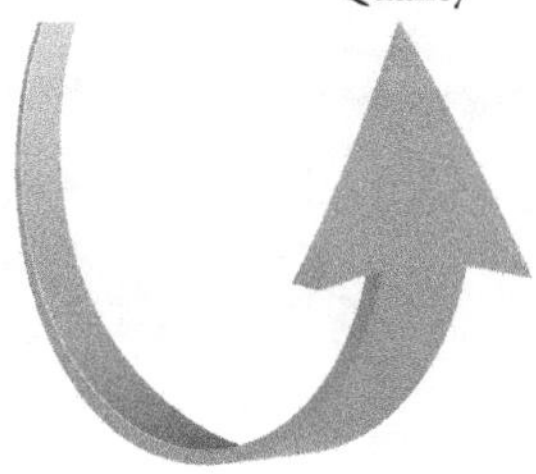

Figure 21.1 Variation X quality.

4. Following established procedures (SOPs) that guarantee standardization.
5. Training staff based on SOPs to guarantee standardization and reproducibility.
6. Run regular audits to guarantee SOPs are being followed without variation.

21.4 Quality manager role

The first role of a quality manager is to implement the quality policy and manage the QMS efficiently. That means the quality manager's main job is to guarantee that policies and objectives are fully understood by the team and to make sure that everybody is going in the same direction. An organization must operate as a genuine team, and the quality manager must encourage the team to take full ownership of the QMS, in order to be able to manage the business in the direction defined, monitor progress, and achieve required objectives.

Leadership is therefore the main skill a quality manager must have, but this leadership must be a very positive one. The focus must be on helping people perform and not on judging them. Without leadership, the quality system is very unlikely to be effective. The quality manager must lead, encourage, support, and advise the whole team, aiming at implementing, maintaining, and improving the QMS continually.

It is very important to promote two-way communication that drives away fear. Open lines of communication must be established to encourage the whole team to talk about aspects of their work that need improvements, to report mistakes or near miss events, and to seek ways of improving the QMS as a genuine team. Every suggestion must be seriously considered, discussed, and implemented whenever appropriate. The QMS belongs ultimately to the team, not to the manager or the organization, and quality must be an integral part of the organization's culture at all levels.

Another role of the quality manager is to make sure the QMS is regularly audited. The auditing process may be performed by the manager and/or by a trained quality team. Again, it is ideal to involve the whole team in the process, and developing quality personnel, who have critical views, good interpersonal skills, and quality awareness, is important to develop communication channels.

The objective of the auditing process is to verify compliancy and not to find nonconformance, as many believe.[5] Findings should be first shared and discussed with the team, in order to discuss deviations, if any were found, and evaluate changes and improvements. The final report should be presented to the board or management for their formal review and approval.

Once processes are established and procedures described, critical steps can be identified and must be the focus of prevention. The "Swiss cheese theory of error" described by James Reason presents a perfect model for preventing errors in such cases, through a series of layers

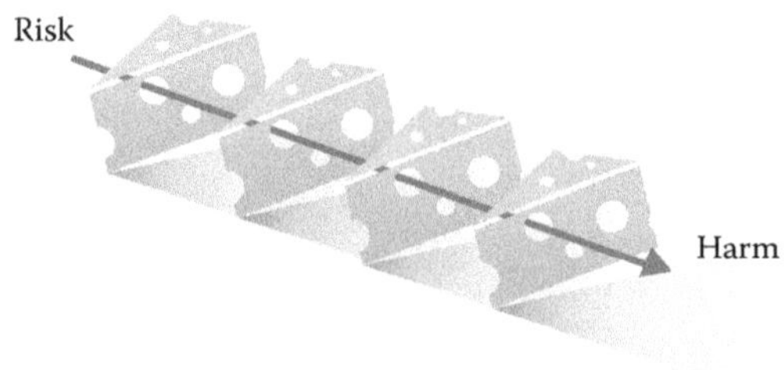

Figure 21.2 Swiss cheese model. The illustration depicts how defenses may be penetrated by an accident trajectory. The defects in multiple layers of defenses may line up to allow a risk factor to cause harm. (Adapted from Reason J. *BMJ* 2000; 320: 768.)

and barriers of defense against errors.[6,7] The quality manager has an important role in establishing these layers with the team, and making sure they follow the procedures created to avoid mistakes. The more layers of protection, the less likely errors will happen (Figure 21.2).

The quality manager should ultimately work as the center of quality expertise in the organization and should be able to understand how everybody and everything works, without necessarily knowing how to perform each procedure, to be able to discuss all aspects of the work performed by the team, suggest changes and improvements, help in the distribution of tasks and responsibilities, as well as establish good work teams and efficient work flows. The quality manager must be the catalyzer of all efforts toward total quality (Table 21.1).

21.5 Quality manager role in ART centers with clean room laboratories

The roles previously described apply to the quality manager in clean room laboratories as well. It is still the quality manager's role to implement quality policies, to manage the quality management system efficiently, to develop positive leadership, to promote communication, to audit the QMS, to focus on prevention, and to be the quality expert. However, when working in a fertility center with clean room laboratories, the quality manager has additional responsibilities. The first one is to understand what a clean room is.

Whenever possible, the quality manager should be involved in the implementation of the clean room laboratory from the beginning, before it is actually built. It is important to understand the requirements and specifications, regulatory and from the clinic itself, and also to participate in the design development and actual building work. This knowledge will enable the quality manager to verify if the installation is in accordance with the design, and later work on the regular validation of the system, and maintain the clean room operative and at the planned cleanliness level. The Association of Clinical Embryologists (ACE), based in the United Kingdom, describes three validation steps: (1) design qualification; (2) installation qualification; and (3) operational qualification; each with its importance and objectives in the clean room validation process.[8]

Table 21.2 summarizes some of the aspects included in each step of the validation. While the design qualification focuses on demonstrating that the design adheres to standards, regulatory and user's requirements, the installation qualification focuses on providing evidence that the clean rooms have been installed in accordance with the design. Finally, the operational qualification aims at providing evidence that the classified rooms function according to the design intent, and evaluates the system performance and recovery capabilities for periods of operation.[8]

Table 21.1 Quality manager role and responsibilities

QM role	Responsibilities	Additional responsibilities in clean room laboratories
Implement quality policies	• Guarantee policies and objectives are fully understood by the team. • Make sure everybody is going in the same direction and shares a unity of purpose. • Guarantee the organization operates as a genuine team that takes full ownership of the QMS.	• Train the team who will be working inside the clean room laboratory, so that they understand the demands of the clean room system, such as the correct use of special clothing and restricted access of authorized personnel. • Establish policies with details about how to work in the clean room laboratory, in order to guarantee the desired cleanliness level.
Manage the QMS efficiently	• Manage the business in the direction defined. • Monitor progress. • Achieve required objectives. • Develop quality personnel, with critical view, good teamwork, and communication skills.	• Check and replace clean room filters periodically to maintain the air quality and the laboratory classification. • Guarantee the filter replacement and clean room certification expenses are included in the annual budget.
Develop positive leadership	• Focus on helping people perform and not on judging them. • Lead, encourage, support, and advise the whole team, aiming at implementing, maintaining, and improving the QMS continually. • Guarantee quality is an integral part of the organization's culture at all levels.	
Promote communication	• Promote a two-way communication that drives away fear and promotes open discussions. • Encourage the team to talk about aspects of their work that need improvements, to report mistakes or near miss events, and to seek ways of improving the quality management system. • Consider and discuss every suggestion, and implement new ideas whenever appropriate.	• Encourage the clean room team to report any deviation and any problem that may compromise the laboratory air quality immediately.

(Continued)

Table 21.1 (Continued) Quality manager role and responsibilities

QM role	Responsibilities	Additional responsibilities in clean room laboratories
Audit the QMS	• Run audits regularly, developing a quality team that works with the manager. • Focus on verifying compliance and not on finding nonconformance.	• During the auditing process, make sure the team understands, respects, and works adequately inside the clean room laboratory, following the established policies to work in the controlled environment.
	• Share findings with the team and discuss deviations, if any were found, and evaluate changes and improvements. • Present a final report to the board or management for their formal review and approval.	• Include filter replacement checks during audits.
Focus on prevention	• Define critical steps in each process/procedure established. • Develop layers of defense barriers to prevent errors. • Make sure the team follows rules and procedures.	• Check the air quality system periodically, to ensure efficiency. • Replace filters with initial signs of saturation.
Be the quality expert	• Understand how everybody and everything works. • Be able to discuss all aspects of the work performed by the team, suggesting changes and improvements. • Help in the distribution of tasks and responsibilities. • Establish good work teams and efficient workflows. • Be the catalyzer of all efforts towards total quality.	• Understand how the clean room works, what is needed to work inside such a laboratory, and what is needed to guarantee its classification.

If the quality manager is hired later, after the clean room laboratory is built, he or she will need to have access and study all documents related to the clean room specifications and design, in order to understand the requirements to work on such an environment and also understand how to validate the clean room facility at regular intervals.

Besides understanding how the clean room works, the quality manager also needs to know what is needed to work inside such a laboratory. This is important to train the team who will be working inside the laboratory appropriately. They must be aware of the demands of the clean room system, such as the correct use of special clothing. It is of utmost importance to have a team that understands, respects, and works adequately inside the lab, not to compromise the air quality and cleanliness the system provides.

The quality manager needs to ensure that specific SOPs explaining how to work in a clean room environment have been developed. This is important to ensure appropriate training, and to enable auditing and data analysis by compliance with regulatory authorities and/or project. The personnel who work inside the clean room environment are the main

Table 21.2 Validation of clean room facilities—Aspects for design, installation, and operational qualification

Validation item	Objectives
Supporting documentation	User's requirements clearly defined; materials and personnel flow diagrams provided; client approved room data sheets; health and safety risk assessment; validation master plans.
Contractor supplied documents	Functional and/or technical specifications available; suitable air system schematic to allow assessment of the airflow and pressure philosophy; ductwork layout drawing; ceiling drawing including HEPA's and lighting.
HVAC (heating, ventilation, and air conditioning)	Appropriate type of system (recirculatory or total loss); extraction of air to remove contaminants and/or avoid cross-contamination (if necessary); suitable air input and extract located at high and low level to assist the system sweeping the areas with filtered air; air movement from clean to dirty side.
Supply and extract air handling unit plant, ductwork system, supply air terminal (HEPA)	Air handling suitably sized and specified to handle air volume's flow rates; suitable access panels for inspection, providing access to filters and components.
Facility layout	Design in accordance with material and personnel flows; layout allows space for movement of personnel, materials, equipment, etc.; room sizes meet user's requirements; no risk of cross-contamination from crossover of incoming materials and/or waste materials; compatibility between materials of construction and cleaning agents.
Floors, walls, ceilings, doors	Suitable materials for clean room facilities; suitable materials in vision panels; suitable door opening and closure (interlocking system); direction of door opening in accordance with pressure differentials.
Emergency exits	Suitable materials; proper location; emergency lighting; lighting housings compatible to clean room.
Environment parameters	Air cleanliness; air change rates; pressure differentials; temperature; humidity; noise; lighting levels.
Control systems	Air change rates and pressure differentials; calibration of measurement instruments; uninterruptible power supply considered.
Alarms and preventive maintenance	Alarms for out of limits air change rates, pressure differentials, temperature, humidity, etc.; preventive maintenance of the clean room system and HVAC.

Source: The Association of Clinical Embryologists (ACE). https://www.embryologists.org.uk/.

source of contamination, and should, therefore, do whatever is needed to maintain the clean room conditions and air quality. The ultimate goal is to have a system that operates effectively to provide air quality inside laboratories and other critical areas where manipulation of gametes and embryos take place, to reduce contamination and improve overall results.

Another important aspect, and important role of the quality manager, is that a clean room works with special filters and these must be checked and replaced periodically to maintain the level of air control needed and certified. Besides guaranteeing these regular "checks," the quality manager must guarantee the clinic has the necessary funds to pay for this service and also for the filters that may need to be replaced periodically. These expenses must be included in the annual budget.

21.6 Conclusions

Even though not all ART centers have a manager exclusively dedicated to quality management, the role of the quality manager must not be underestimated. The quality manager has many important roles, which are summarized below:

1. Define what "quality" is for the ART center together with the team.
2. Define the quality policies, benchmarks, and goals.
3. Monitor benchmarks and work with the team to achieve goals.
4. Control nonconformities in order to bring them to a minimum.
5. Design and implement improvement plans.
6. Focus on prevention, minimizing variation and risks.
7. Be fully committed to continuous quality improvement, leading and motivating the team, and making sure everybody is involved and shares the same goals.
8. Keep himself and the team well trained.
9. Understand how everything works, even without knowing how to perform all procedures, to be able to tackle problems, make suggestions, and help solve deviations.
10. Understand how the clean room laboratory works, to guarantee validation and proper operation in previously established cleanliness level.

References

1. Bento F. Introduction to quality management in ART clinics. In: Bento F, Esteves S, and Agarwal A (eds.), *Quality Management in ART Clinics: A Practical Guide.* 1st ed., Springer Science+Business Media, New York, pp. 3–6, 2013.
2. Commission of the European Parliament, 2004. Directive 2004/23/EC of the European Parliament and of the Council of 31 March 2004 on setting standards of quality and safety for the donation, procurement, testing, processing, preservation, storage and distribution of human tissues and cells.
3. ANVISA. Brazilian National Agency for Sanitary Surveillance, 2006. Resolução no. 33 da Diretoria colegiada da Agência Nacional de Vigilância Sanitária (amended by RDC23 of 27 May 2011 on setting standards of quality and safety for the donation, procurement, testing, processing, preservation, storage and distribution of human tissues and cells).
4. Gluck PA. Medical error theory. *Obstet Gynecol Clin North Am.* 2008; 35: 11–7.
5. Bento F. How to get information. In: Bento F, Esteves S, and Agarwal A (eds.), *Quality Management in ART Clinics: A Practical Guide.* 1st ed., Springer Science+Business Media, New York, pp. 59–68, 2013.
6. Ziegler D, Gambone JC, Meldrum DR, and Chapron C. Risk and safety management in infertility and assisted reproductive technology (ART): From the doctor's office to the ART procedure. *Fertil Steril.* 2013; 100: 1509:17.
7. Reason J. Human error: Models and management. *BMJ* 2000; 320: 768.
8. The Association of Clinical Embryologists (ACE). https://www.embryologists.org.uk/.

section five

Clinical outcome and new developments

chapter twenty-two

Summary evidence for the effect of laboratory air quality on pregnancy outcome in in vitro fertilization

Sandro C. Esteves and Fabiola C. Bento

Contents

Abstract

This chapter discusses the importance of air quality control in assisted reproductive technology (ART) laboratories. We systematically reviewed the published evidence and critically analyzed the impact of controlling air quality control in the laboratory environment. Fair evidence derived from both animal and human studies indicates that controlling laboratory air contamination positively impact in vitro fertilization outcomes.

22.1 *Introduction*

Human gametes and embryos cultured in vitro are extremely sensitive to oscillations in temperature, humidity, light exposure, contaminants, and physical trauma. Toxic agents, including bacteria, particulate matter, dust, and chemicals (volatile organic compounds [VOCs]), have been implicated in impaired fertilization and embryo development, and consequently, live birth.[1–10] These effects can be counteracted to some extent by controlling laboratory air quality, as indicated by improvements in embryo development and implantation potential in both animal and human studies.[4,6,9–16] As a matter of fact, attention to laboratory air filtration has been one of the key elements in some high-performing in vitro fertilization programs, thus suggesting that laboratory environment and air quality are among the many factors contributing to the success of ART.[17]

In this chapter, we conducted an extensive search using the Medline/Pubmed, SJU discover, and Google Scholar databases to identify all relevant studies focusing on both animal and human studies evaluating the effects of laboratory air quality on the reproductive outcome of in vitro cultured embryos. There were no limits placed on the year of publication, but we restricted the search to articles published in English. We also searched among the references of the identified articles and included abstracts published in international conferences. The search combined relevant terms and descriptors related to air quality, clean room, VOCs, embryo development, in vitro fertilization (IVF), intracytoplasmic sperm injection (ICSI), and assisted reproductive technology (ART).

Our electronic search retrieved 357 articles. An additional 47 articles were identified by hand searches among the references of published articles. After screening the titles and abstracts, we determined that 47 articles were potentially eligible for inclusion. Among these, 28 articles were excluded. Sixteen of them comprised reviews, letters, or commentaries. Twelve articles involved ambient air quality and pregnancy rates, but they did not specifically evaluate in vitro fertilization settings. Nineteen articles were included in the qualitative analysis, as shown in Table 22.1.

22.2 *Effect of laboratory air quality to embryo development in vitro*

An early study conducted in seven ART clinics showed that air quality deteriorated with regard to VOC contamination as it passed from the exterior of the buildings into the embryology laboratory, and deteriorated further inside incubators. The numbers ranged from an average of 533 μg/m^3 outside air VOCs to an average of 2769 μg/m^3 in the incubators, representing a fivefold increase in VOC concentration.[2] VOCs have been linked to impaired outcomes in ART.[1,2,5,7,18] VOCs may induce depletion of intracellular antioxidants, such as glutathione, thus suggesting that VOC exposure may decrease embryo ability to defend against oxidative damage.[3] Exposure of mouse embryos to acrolein (an unsaturated aldehyde) in the early cleavage period decreased the numbers of blastocysts formed.[3] One bovine breeding program reported a 5% increase in pregnancy rate with use of an intra-incubator air filter system.[19] The authors utilized an intra-incubator air purification unit containing activated carbon and high efficiency particulate air (HEPA) filtration. However, intra-incubator carbon-impregnated filters may lack enough activated carbon to scrub a large and variable VOC load in the presence of high humidity.

In an early retrospective cohort study involving infertile couples undergoing IVF, Boone et al. observed that the construction of a class 100 clean room improved air quality and IVF rate, and increased the number of high-quality embryos available for transfer.[6] On the contrary, similar embryo development and pregnancy outcome have been reported by culturing human embryos in incubators with and without HEPA air filtration.[20] Of note, while Boone et al. implemented a highly efficient built-in centralized filtration system to their IVF laboratory and adjacent critical areas, Souza et al. used intra-incubator HEPA filters lacking VOC filtration.[6,20]

More recently, several investigators have shown that sperm injection cycles performed in clean room laboratories equipped with air filtration for particulates and VOC were associated with better outcomes. In one study, Knaggs et al. rebuilt their IVF facilities as clean rooms in accordance with the European Union directive, and reported that the overall clinical pregnancy rate for the six-month period after moving into the new laboratory was significantly higher than the six-month period in the old laboratory (42.6% vs. 30.6%).[11]

Table 22.1 Summary of evidence assessing the impact of laboratory air quality in IVF outcomes

First author and reference	Year	Study design	Study population	Method	Outcome
Little[1]	1990	Observational analytic cohort study	In vitro cultured rat embryos	Cellular protein and DNA damage analysis	Aldehyde (acrolein) was incorporated to the yolk sac and caused embryotoxicity
Cohen[2]	1997	Descriptive qualitative study	None	Air sampling and VOC determination in human IVF laboratories	Higher levels of VOC (mainly toluene and isopropyl alcohol) in HEPA-filtered laboratory ambient air and incubators compared to outside unfiltered ambient air
Schimmel[18]	1997	Descriptive qualitative study	None	Air sampling and VOC determination in human IVF laboratories	Higher levels of VOC found in CO_2 tanks and incubators compared to outside air; air filtration using carbon activated and potassium permanganate reduced VOC levels
Hall[3]	1998	Combination of descriptive qualitative and observational analytic cohort studies	In vitro cultured mouse embryos	Air sampling and VOC determination in human IVF laboratories; acrolein bioassay using 2-cell mouse embryos	Increased levels of VOC observed in ambient air of human IVF laboratories. Reduction in aldehyde levels by air filtration using carbon-activated and permanganate. In vitro mouse embryo development, implantation and post-implantation development inversely correlated with acrolein concentration
Mayer[4]	1999	Prospective randomized crossover study	129 IVF and ICSI cycles; humans	Assessment of IVF outcomes after embryo culture in incubators with and without VOC filtration	Higher pregnancy rates in couples whose embryos were cultured in incubators equipped with VOC air filters
Racowsky[5]	1999	Observational analytic cohort study	467 IVF and ICSI cycles; humans	Assessment of IVF outcomes after embryo culture in laboratories and incubators with and without VOC filtration	Reduction in miscarriage rates in IVF cycles performed in laboratory and incubators equipped with carbon-activated filters

(Continued)

Table 22.1 (Continued) Summary of evidence assessing the impact of laboratory air quality in IVF outcomes

First author and reference	Year	Study design	Study population	Method	Outcome
Boone[6]	1999	Observational analytic cohort study	275 infertile couples undergoing IVF; humans	Air sampling and IVF outcomes after construction of a clean room with centralized particle filtration for IVF, oocyte retrieval, and embryo transfer	Reduction in air particles and increase in the number of high-quality embryos for uterine transfer
Worrilow[7]	2000	Descriptive qualitative study	None	Air sampling in a newly designed IVF laboratory equipped with a centralized heating, ventilation, and air conditioning (HVAC) system and VOC filtration	All areas within the IVF laboratory and accompanying procedure rooms qualified as class 100 areas. No VOCs were found at concentrations above detectable limits or greater than 0.1 parts per billion
Worrilow[8]	2002	Observational analytic cross-sectional study	IVF cycles[a]; humans	Outside ambient air and indoors (IVF lab) air sampling for particles and VOCs over a 2-year period. Assessment of IVF outcomes performed in a clean room laboratory with VOC filtration	Levels of outside air VOCs serving the IVF lab air control system varied according to seasonal humidity and temperature, which affected implantation rates
Esteves[9]	2004	Observational analytic cohort study	468 ICSI cycles in an unselected IVF population; humans	ICSI outcomes in clean room facilities (equipped with centralized particle and VOC air filtration for embryo culture, gamete retrieval and embryo transfer) compared with an IVF lab equipped with stand-alone air filtration system	Increase in high-quality embryos and clinical pregnancy rates, and reduction in miscarriage rates in cycles performed in clean room facilities compared with conventional IVF lab with portable air filtration system
von Wyl[12]	2004	Descriptive qualitative study	None	VOC and air particle determination in an old IVF laboratory and in a newly built facility with positive-pressure air filtration for particles	Air concentrations of the measured compounds were lower in the new over pressurized IVF laboratory

(*Continued*)

Table 22.1 (Continued) Summary of evidence assessing the impact of laboratory air quality in IVF outcomes

First author and reference	Year	Study design	Study population	Method	Outcome
Esteves[10]	2006	Observational analytic cohort study	399 ICSI cycles in couples whose male partners had severe male factor infertility; humans	ICSI outcomes in clean room facilities (equipped with centralized particle and VOC air filtration for embryo culture, gamete retrieval, and embryo transfer) compared with a conventional IVF lab equipped with portable air filtration system	Increase in high-quality embryos and clinical pregnancy rates, and reduction in miscarriage rates after oocyte/sperm retrievals, ICSI, and embryo transfers performed in clean room facilities compared with conventional IVF lab
Knaggs[11]	2007	Observational analytic cohort study	Infertile couples undergoing IVF/ICSI cycles[a]; humans	IVF/ICSI outcomes in a newly designed and constructed laboratory facility meeting the European Union tissues and cell directive. Analysis of key performance indicators in a period prior to and after the move into the new embryology facility	Implantation and pregnancy rates increased after the move into the clean room
Merton[19]	2007	Randomized controlled study	Bovine zygotes	Zygotes were placed either in a conventional incubator (control group) or in an identical incubator with an intra-incubator air purification unit (HEPA + activated carbon) for in vitro culture	The embryo production rate at Day 7 was not affected by the air purification unit (23.4 and 24.7% morulae and blastocysts per oocyte for control and study groups, respectively) nor was there any significant effect on embryo stage or quality. However, the pregnancy rate was improved (P = 0.043) for both fresh (46.3% vs. 41.0%) and frozen/thawed embryos cultured in incubators with air purification (40.8% vs. 35.6%)

(Continued)

Table 22.1 (Continued) Summary of evidence assessing the impact of laboratory air quality in IVF outcomes

First author and reference	Year	Study design	Study population	Method	Outcome
Souza[20]	2009	Observational analytic cohort study	123 ICSI cycles in unselected IVF population; humans	Cycles were divided into two groups: in group 1 (n = 60) embryo culture was performed in a ISO class 8 air quality incubator; in group 2 (n = 63) embryo culture was performed in ISO class 5 air quality incubator (HEPA filtration)	Number of embryos available for transfer, number of good quality embryos transferred, implantation rate, and clinical pregnancy were not statistically different between groups
Khoudja[13]	2012	Combination of descriptive qualitative and observational analytic cohort studies	1403 infertile couples undergoing IVF/ICSI cycles; humans	IVF outcomes in laboratories equipped with stand-alone and centralized particle and VOC air filtration systems. The latter was designed and constructed by incorporating a novel air purification method involving specially treated honeycomb matrix media with a Landson™ system	VOC levels decreased and overall air quality improved after installation of a novel air purification method. Significantly better fertilization, cleavage, blastulation, pregnancy, and implantation rates were observed with this new technology
Esteves[14]	2013	Combination of descriptive qualitative and observational analytic cohort studies	2315 ICSI cycles in unselected IVF population; humans	ICSI outcomes in newly designed clean room facilities (equipped with centralized particle and VOC air filtration) for embryo culture, gamete retrieval, and embryo transfer. A historical cohort in which IVF cycles were carried out in a conventional IVF lab equipped with a portable air filtration system was included for comparison	Negligible levels of VOCs in the clean room IVF lab; clean room facilities were classified as ISO 5 (IVF lab), ISO 7 (operating theater), and ISO 8 (embryo transfer room). Significantly higher rates of high-quality embryos and live birth rates, and lower miscarriage rates, in cycles carried out in clean room facilities

(*Continued*)

Table 22.1 (Continued) Summary of evidence assessing the impact of laboratory air quality in IVF outcomes

First author and reference	Year	Study design	Study population	Method	Outcome
Munch[16]	2015	Observational analytic cohort study	524 fresh and 156 cryopreserved IVF cycles; humans	IVF outcomes in a lab equipped with carbon filtration	Fertilization, cleavage, and blastulation rates for fresh cycles declined during the period of absent carbon filtration and restored after reintroduction of carbon filtration
Heitmann[15]	2015	Combination of descriptive qualitative and observational analytic cohort studies	820 IVF/ICSI cycles in unselected IVF population; humans	IVF/ICSI outcomes in a clean room IVF lab (equipped with centralized particle and VOC air filtration) compared with an IVF lab equipped with a stand-alone air filtration system	Air quality testing demonstrated decrease in total VOC concentrations in the new IVF lab compared with the previous facility, which was associated with significantly higher implantation and live birth rates

Source: Adapted from Esteves SC and Bento FC. *Asian Journal of Andrology* 2015 Nov 10 [ahead of print].

Note: HEPA: high efficiency particulate air; ICSI: intracytoplasmic sperm injection; ISO: International Organization for Standardization; IVF: in vitro fertilization; VOC: volatile organic compound.

[a] Number of cycles not described.

Our IVF facilities were also built as clean rooms in full compliance with the Brazilian Cells and Tissues Directive. We observed that there was no detrimental effect of operating under clean room and good manufacturing practice (GMP) conditions. On the contrary, we have noted that operating under such stringent air quality standards was not only feasible but also associated with better embryo development and pregnancy outcomes after moving to the new clean room facilities.[14] Live birth rates increased (35.6% vs. 25.8%, $p = 0.02$) while miscarriage rates decreased (28.7% vs. 20.0%, $p = 0.04$) in the first triennium after clean room implementation. Heitmann et al. have also described how they have implemented a highly efficient air filtration by installing a centered system supplying filtered air to the IVF lab and adjacent areas (operating room and embryo transfer room), combining a mixture of fresh outside air and recirculated air. By analyzing retrospective data, live birth rates were increased by improvements in air quality and laboratory environment.[15] Last, Munch et al. reported poor embryo development after inadvertent removal of carbon filters.[16] The authors observed that the key performance indicators for laboratory variables returned to normal levels after reinstallation of carbon filters.

A summary evidence of the studies evaluating the effect of laboratory air quality to embryo development in vitro and pregnancy outcome by ART are provided in Table 22.1. Collectively, fair evidence from both animal and human studies indicates an association between poor laboratory air quality conditions and impaired embryo development, with overall decreased implantation and pregnancy rates. On the contrary, implementation of measures to improve laboratory air quality has been associated with increased IVF success.

22.3 *Impact of air quality control to clinical practice in the IVF setting*

The impact of applying clean room air quality standards to assisted conception facilities has been debated with regard to its feasibility and effectiveness. While some authors argue that implementation of strict air quality control, as required by some regulatory agencies, is likely to have negligible impact on the risks of culture contamination and operator infection and could even compromise the ability to maintain gametes and embryos under optimum environmental conditions,[21,22] others suggest that compliance with air quality standards is not only feasible but also has a positive impact on IVF clinical results.[11,14,15,23]

22.4 *Why air quality is a major determinant of IVF success*

In reproductive laboratories, indoor particles of interest measure between 0.1 and 10 μm. Because bacteria, fungi, and spores can attach themselves to particles, an important goal of air filtration in the IVF environment is to decrease the number of air particles in suspension through the use of high efficiency filtration systems. Removal of airborne particulates by forced movement of air using positive air pressurization through a series of filters of increasing efficiency, achieved by decreasing the diameter of the membrane pores, therefore equates to an increase in air quality.[24] Because bacteria and other contaminants can attach themselves to particles, a decrease in particles equates to an increase in air quality. First, air filtration eliminates larger particles such as dust, and subsequently, HEPA or ultra low penetration air (ULPA) filters trap small particulates, fungi, spores, and bacteria, thus decreasing microbiological contamination.[24] HEPA air filters have 99.97% minimum particle-collective efficiency for particles as small as 0.3 μ.

Although air particle filtration is a logical concept, other filtration mechanisms rather than particle elimination are needed to control contamination in the reproductive laboratory environment. For instance, VOCs that are constantly generated by laboratory materials and cleaning agents are 100 to 1000 times smaller than the effective pore size of HEPA filters, and cannot be trapped by such filters.[2,3,25] VOCs are organic chemical compounds whose composition allows them to evaporate under normal indoor atmospheric conditions of temperature and pressure. Indoor VOCs react with the indoor ozone, and the chemical reactions produce submicron-sized particles and harmful by-products that may be associated with adverse health effects in some sensitive populations.

In ART setting, VOCs including benzene can be found in CO_2 gas cylinders, while ethylbenzene and benzaldehyde are emitted from plastic ware. Elevated levels of other VOCs, including toluene and formaldehyde coming from insulation used in air handling systems, refrigerant gases, isopropyl alcohol fumes, and aliphatic hydrocarbons, have been described in ART laboratories. Laboratory cleaning agents and writing instruments generally produce VOC.

Removal of volatile organic compounds is achieved by potassium permanganate impregnated pelletized coal or coconut shell-based activated carbon filters. The spaces between the carbon particles contain a cloud of delocalized electrons that acts as electronic glue, thus forcing the chemical contaminants to bind to the carbon. Coconut shell activated carbon is now preferred over coal-based activated carbon because it has higher density and purity and is virtually dust-free. Also, the pore structure of coconut shell-based carbons is thinner thus resulting in a higher retention rate.[26] However, alcohols and ketones are not easily removed by carbon, but they can be oxidized, and thereby detoxified, by potassium permanganate.[2,3,27]

VOCs can be measured by adsorption from air on Tenax TA, thermal desorption, gas chromatographic separation over a 100% nonpolar column (dimethylpolysiloxane) or mass spectrometry.[3] A common method is the use of Summa canisters to capture air samples for VOC followed by a gas chromatography/mass spectrometry (GC/MS). While the cost is relatively high, the sampling is simple and captures the common VOCs at a level of unit micrograms/cubic meter.[2] However, GC/MS requires sophisticated equipment and lacks the prospect for rapid real-time monitoring. Alternatively, VOCs can be detected based on different principles and interactions between organic compounds and sensor components. There are electronic devices that can detect parts per million (ppm) concentrations and predict with reasonable accuracy the molecular structure of the volatile organic compounds in the environment or enclosed atmospheres.[28] Holographic sensors, for example, can give a direct reading of the analytic concentration as a color change. The main limitation of using sensors to measure VOC levels is related to their lower detection limits. Devices usually detect VOCs as ppm, which may be inadequate to measure individual harmful VOCs present in much lower concentrations in the IVF setting. Measurement devices with lower detection limits as parts per billion would be more adequate for monitoring VOC levels in reproductive laboratories.[3] As such, it is important to understand that measurement for VOCs in indoor air is highly dependent on how they are measured. All available measurement methods are selective in what they can measure and quantify accurately, and none are capable of measuring all VOCs that are present. For example, benzene and toluene are measured by a different method than formaldehyde and other similar compounds. The range of measurement methods and analytical instruments is large and will determine the sensitivity of the measurements as well as their selectivity or biases. It has been shown that incorporating commercial filters imbedded with activated carbon and potassium permanganate in the air ventilation system offers a more practical solution compared to the expensive and labor-intensive VOC testing as currently performed.[2,3,14,15,27]

Equally important to the systems applied to control air quality are the methods for training laboratory personnel and validating/monitoring the installations while in operation, that is, during normal routine workload. Personnel should understand the principles of a clean room, including the function of airflows and airlocks, hygiene, dress code, and use of cleaning agents. Expensive filters such as HEPA are not replaced unless they show nonconformance during periodic inspections. Although direct VOC measurements are not routinely undertaken in our facility, VOC filter efficiency is monitored periodically by sending chemical module samples to the manufacturer to determine remaining chemical bed activity, thus guiding how often filters should be replaced. Filter saturation levels depend on outside air quality and levels of indoor VOC generation, and replacement of filters by analyzing objective data helps minimize operational costs.

22.5 *Clean room technology in reproductive laboratories: The question is not why but how*

Although practitioners and specialty societies have acknowledged the importance of the laboratory environment, many of us remain undecided on how air filtration should be carried out.[12,17,21,23,29] We have discussed this critical issue in a recent commentary, by posing the following questions: Is air particle filtration enough or do we have to combine VOC filtration? Are commercially available freestanding units sufficient or is it necessary to implement more sophisticated built-in systems? How often do we have to replace the filters? What periodic testing is needed to ensure conformity? Will the implementation of air filtration change results in terms of pregnancy? With so many uncertainties, many of us have opted to install commercially available filtration systems without proper risk assessment and validation procedures.[30] Little attention is paid, for instance, to other critical issues that affect indoor air quality, such as laboratory premises (age and size of laboratory, off-gassing of equipment/furniture and construction materials, atmospheric air pollution, proximity to anesthetic gases), humidity and room temperature, disposable materials and cleaning agents utilized in the laboratory, and personnel (number per workspace, use of protective clothing, cosmetics). Ideally, a risk management analysis with regard to laboratory air quality should take all the aforementioned into consideration not only to reduce but also to avoid the risks associated with poor air quality conditions, and can be applied to both existing and new facilities.[30]

Given the importance of both particulate matter and VOCs in the ART setting, we have proposed that a better definition for ART clean rooms would be "a room in which the concentration of airborne particles and VOCs is controlled, and which is constructed and used in a manner to minimize the introduction, generation, and retention of particles and VOCs inside the room, and in which temperature, humidity, and pressure are controlled."[13,31] Ideally, an air filtration system controlling indoor particulates and VOCs should be implemented using a centralized system supplying filtered air not only in the IVF lab but also in the adjacent areas where important IVF processes take place, namely, the operating room and the embryo transfer room. Humidity and temperature should be controlled to ensure optimal desorption efficiency of VOC filtration. In addition, construction materials and laboratory furniture that emitted low VOCs should be carefully selected. It is unlikely that portable units would provide the same air quality than a robust, centralized air filtration system. A detailed description about how we implemented clean room technology using the aforesaid definition to our facility is presented in Chapter 26.

22.6 Conclusions

Fair evidence indicates that laboratory air quality is associated with IVF outcome. Air quality control should combine filtration of particulates and VOC, but target limits are still unknown. Built-in systems supplying filtered air to the IVF lab and adjacent areas, combining a mixture of fresh outside air and recirculated air, seems to be the optimal approach. Irrespective of whether it is a new facility or an existing one, ideal environments can be set up by equipping laboratory and associated premises with properly dimensioned filtration systems in combination with preventive measures to avoid contamination. A risk management analysis taking into consideration all variables that play a role in air contamination, as described earlier, is paramount for the reduction of the risk of poor IVF outcomes due to improper air quality conditions. Implementation of clean room standards to reproductive laboratories, which include air quality control through filtration of airborne particles and VOCs and the adoption of good laboratory practices, offers adequate conditions for contamination control and risk management. We and others have demonstrated that it is feasible to handle human gametes and to culture embryos in clean room environments in full compliance with air quality standards directives. Current evidence indicates that performing IVF in controlled environments optimize success.

References

1. Little SA and Mirkes PE. Relationship of DNA damage and embryotoxicity induced by 4-hydroperoxydechosphamine in postimplantation rat embryos. *Teratology* 1990; 41: 223–31.
2. Cohen J, Gilligan A, Esposito W, Schimmel T, and Dale B. Ambient air and its potential effects on conception in vitro. *Hum Reprod* 1997; 12: 1742–9.
3. Hall J, Gilligan A, Schimmel T, Cecchi M, and Cohen J. The origin, effects and control of air pollution in laboratories used for human embryo culture. *Hum Reprod* 1998; 13: 146–55.
4. Mayer JF, Nehchiri F, Weedon VM, Jones EL, Kalin HL, Oehninger SC et al. Prospective randomized crossover analysis of the impact of an incubator air filtration on IVF outcomes. *Fertil Steril* 1999; 72: S42.
5. Racowsky C, Jackson KV, Nureddin A, de los Santos MJ, Kelley JR, and Pan, Y. Carbon-activated air filtration results in reduced spontaneous abortion rates following IVF. Proceedings of the 11th World Congress on In Vitro Fertilization and Human Reproductive Genetics. Sydney, Australia.
6. Boone WR, Johnson JE, Locke A-J, Crane MM, and Price TM. Control of air quality in an assisted reproductive technology laboratory. *Fertil Steril* 1997; 71: 150–4.
7. Worrilow KC, Huynh HT, Gwozdziewicz JB, Schillings W, Peters AJ. A retrospective analysis: The examination of a potential relationship between particulate (P) and volatile organic compound (VOC) levels in a class 100 IVF laboratory cleanroom (CR) and specific parameters of embryogenesis and rates of implantation (IR). *Fertil Steril* 2001; 76: S15–6.
8. Worrilow KC, Huynh HT, Bower JB, Schillings W, and Peters AJ. A retrospective analysis: Seasonal decline in implantation rates (IR) and its correlation with increased levels of volatile organic compounds (VOC). *Fertil Steril* 2002; 78: S39.
9. Esteves SC, Gomes AP, and Verza S Jr. Control of air pollution in assisted reproductive technology laboratory and adjacent areas improves embryo formation, cleavage and pregnancy rates and decreases abortion rate: Comparison between a class 100 (ISO 5) and a class 1000 (ISO 6) cleanroom for micromanipulation and embryo culture. *Fertil Steril* 2004; 82: S259–60.
10. Esteves SC, Verza S Jr, and Gomes AP. Comparison between International Standard Organization (ISO) type 5 and type 6 cleanrooms combined with volatile organic compounds filtration system for micromanipulation and embryo culture in severe male factor infertility. *Fertil Steril* 2006; 86: S353–4.

11. Knaggs P, Birch D, Drury S, Morgan M, Kumari S, Sriskandakumar R et al. Full compliance with the EU directive air quality standards does not compromise IVF outcome. *Hum Reprod* 2007; 22: i164–5.
12. Von Wyl S and Bersinger NA. Air quality in the IVF laboratory: Results and survey. *J Assist Reprod Genet* 2004; 21: 283–4.
13. Khoudja RY, Xu Y, Li T, and Zhou C. Better IVF outcomes following improvements in laboratory air quality. *J Assist Reprod Genet* 2013; 30: 69–76.
14. Esteves SC and Bento FC. Implementation of air quality control in reproductive laboratories in full compliance with the Brazilian Cells and Germinative Tissue Directive. *Reprod Biomed Online* 2013; 26: 9–21.
15. Heitmann RJ, Hill MJ, James AN, Schimmel T, Segars JH, Csokmay JM, Cohen J, and Payson MD. Live births achieved via IVF are increased by improvements in air quality and laboratory environment. *Reprod Biomed Online* 2015; 31: 364–71.
16. Munch EM, Sparks AE, Duran HE, and Van Voorhis BJ. Lack of carbon air filtration impacts early embryo development. *J Assist Reprod Genet* 2015; 32: 1009–17.
17. Van Voorhis BJ, Thomas M, Surrey ES, and Sparks A. What do consistently high-performing in vitro fertilization programs in the U.S. do? *Fertil Steril* 2010; 94: 1346–9.
18. Schimmel T, Gilligan A, Garrisi GJ, Esposito B Jr, Cecchi M, Dale B, and Cohen J. Removal of volatile organic compounds from incubators used for gamete and embryo culture. *Fertil Steril* 1997; 67: S165.
19. Merton JS, Vermeulen ZL, Otter T, Mullaart E, de Ruigh L, and Hasler JF. Carbon-activated gas filtration during in vitro culture increased pregnancy rate following transfer of in vitro-produced bovine embryos. *Theriogenology* 2007; 67: 1233–8.
20. Souza Mdo C, Mancebo AC, da Rocha Cde A, Henriques CA, Souza MM, and Cardoso FF. Evaluation of two incubation environments—ISO class 8 versus ISO class 5—On intracytoplasmic sperm injection cycle outcome. *Fertil Steril* 2009 May; 91(5): 1780–4.
21. Mortimer D. A critical assessment of the impact of the European Union Tissues and Cells Directive (2004) on laboratory practices in assisted conception. *Reprod Biomed Online* 2005; 11: 162–76.
22. Bhargava PM. Commentary on the critical assessment of the impact of the recent European Union Tissues and Cells Directive. *Reprod Biomed Online* 2005; 11: 161.
23. Hartshorne GM. Challenges of the EU 'tissues and cells' directive. *Reprod Biomed Online* 2005; 11: 404–7.
24. National Environmental Balancing Bureau, 1998. Procedural Standards for Certified Testing of Cleanrooms, Vienna, VA. http.www.nebb.org (accessed February 14, 2015).
25. Esteves SC and Agarwal A. Explaining how reproductive laboratories work. In: Bento F, Esteves S, and Agarwal A. (eds.), *Quality Management in ART Clinics: A Practical Guide*. 1st ed., Springer Science+Business Media, New York, pp. 79–127, 2013.
26. Chiang YC, Chiang PC, and Huang CP. Effects of pore structure and temperature on VOC adsorption on activated carbon. *Carbon* 2001; 39: 523–34.
27. Morbeck DE. Air quality in the assisted reproduction laboratory: A mini-review. *J Assist Reprod Genet* 2015; 32: 1019–24.
28. Martinez-Hurtado JL, Davidson CAB, Blyth J, and Lowe CR. Holographic detection of hydrocarbon gases and other volatile organic compounds. *Langmuir* 2010; 26: 15694–99.
29. Kastrop P. Quality management in the ART laboratory. *Reprod Biomed Online* 2003; 7: 691–4.
30. Esteves SC and Bento FC. Air quality control in the ART laboratory is a major determinant of IVF success. *Asian J Androl* 2015 Nov 10 [ahead of print].
31. Esteves SC and Bento FC. Implementation of cleanroom technology in reproductive laboratories: The question is not why but how. *Reprod Biomed Online* 2016; 32: 9–11.

chapter twenty-three

Clean room technology for low resource IVF units

Alex C. Varghese and Giles Palmer

Contents

Abstract

Recently nongovernmental and governmental organizations have initiated IVF units as part of public health programs. Even smaller units performing only classical in vitro fertilization (IVF) or with the provision for intracytoplasmic sperm injection (ICSI) have come up in many suburban and rural settings of developing countries. Despite offering affordable IVF to the patient population, the success rates of these units vary considerably from batch to batch of IVF cycles. The last three decades also witnessed a spur of research on reproductive cells both in vivo and in vitro that shed light on the complex nature and homeostasis required for culturing pre-implantation embryos in vitro. Any compromise on these physiological requirements for the health and well-being of oocytes and sperm or embryos can culminate in lower implantation rates or long-term consequences in the resulting offspring by epigenetic perturbations. Hence, the task of establishing an IVF unit as a service to society needs to be planned with the utmost care and scientific inputs, including laboratory air quality control.

23.1 Introduction

Multiple factors such as infectious, environmental, genetic, and even dietary in origin can contribute to infertility. An estimated 48.5 million couples worldwide in 2010 were unable to have a child despite active trying. With the advent of assisted reproductive technology (ART) many of these couples could achieve a pregnancy through various in vitro fertilization methods. Since the inception of successful human IVF programs in the United Kingdom in 1978, the technology became popular in many developed countries. In time patients from developing countries also started reaping the benefits of IVF technologies as many IVF units were established in urbane cities and many countries introduced specialist training for reproductive medicine. Gynecologists received training in reproductive medicine and clinical embryology from established IVF units. However, the truth is that the technology is available only to those few privileged couples that can afford the high cost of the treatments. Public funding and the provision of health insurance for IVF treatment differ widely between countries; there is no uniformity in the provision of this treatment even in the developed world.

However, recently many nongovernmental (NGO) and governmental organizations have initiated IVF units as part of public health programs. Even smaller units performing only classical IVF or with provision of ICSI have come up in many suburban and rural settings of developing countries. However, the success rates of these units vary considerably from batch to batch of IVF cycles. Many of these units offer affordable IVF to the patient population.

The last three decades also witnessed a spur of research on reproductive cells both in vivo and in vitro that has shed light on the complex nature and homeostasis required for culturing pre-implantation embryos in vitro. Any compromise on these physiological requirements for the health and wellbeing of oocytes and sperm or embryos can culminate in lower implantation rates or long-term consequences in the resulting offspring by epigenetic perturbations. Hence, the task of establishing an IVF unit as a service to society needs to be planned with the utmost care and scientific inputs, including laboratory air quality control.

It is true that setting up an IVF unit is not only an economical task. Until a few years ago many developing countries used to import all the equipment for an IVF unit. Although such countries still need to import vital equipment like CO_2 incubators and ICSI workstations along with the culture media for the routine use, many developing countries have started manufacturing essential equipment locally thereby reducing the cost. For example, in India, out of approximately 1200 IVF units, more than 50% are in suburban or rural settings. Many of these cater to 50–300 patients per year through batching in IVF programs. The actual cost of setting up an IVF unit may vary from country to country and also depends on the services they offer (Table 23.1).

Table 23.1 Comparison of costs of IVF equipment being imported in developing countries versus locally manufactured ones

Equipment	Cost (approx.) for imported equipment[a]	Cost (approx.) for locally manufactured equipment[a]
CO_2 incubator (box type)	US$ 9,000	NA
IVF workstation (heated stage) with stereomicroscope (trinocular)	US$ 30,000	US$ 10,000
ICSI workstation	US$ 30,000	NA
Warming incubator	US$ 2,000	US$ 500
Heating blocks	US$ 1,000	US$ 500
Centrifuge	US$ 2,000	US$ 600
Andrology optical microscope (binocular)	US$ 2,000	US$ 500
Modular lab with dedicated AHU with particle and VOC air filtration	US$ 50,000 to 100,000	US$ 40,000
AHU stand-alone tower with HEPA and carbon filters	US$ 8,000 to 10,000	US$ 5,000

Note: AHU: air handling unit; HEPA: high efficiency particulate air filtration; NA: local manufacturer not available; VOC: volatile organic compound.

[a] Costs are approximate, considering the current market in India for the year 2015.

23.2 Current scenario of low resource IVF units

When we speak about low cost IVF units in developing countries, we come across basically two categories, namely (1) IVF units set up by specialists or NGOs with an intention to offer a medical service at an affordable cost to a society that cannot afford the same, and (2) IVF units set up by gynecologists in suburban/rural areas as part of the established hospitals where they serve or own the shares. These types of units may or may not be capable of establishing state-of-the-art laboratory facilities. The situation might become more complicated as to the difficulty of having financial resources to keep on adding newer gadgets as the technology progresses due to financial constraints. Moreover, many of them start the unit with a passion to offer infertility services without extensive training in reproductive medicine. These groups used to depend on the IVF vendors for designing and establishing IVF laboratories and many times without much input/consultation from senior embryologists. These units in fact serve a section of infertile couples from rural settings who find it difficult to travel to major cities to avail the services from larger and well-established units.

As mentioned above, the process of in vitro fertilization comprises a multitude of processes that need to be carried out diligently and with appropriate culture systems to minimize stress for the gametes and embryos being manipulated or handled in vitro. But when we examine the low resource units, they happen to be compromised with regard to design, processes, equipment, technical competence, and total quality management.

Since most units of that sort are established in existing hospital complexes, the first compromise is in selecting the right space. It happens sometimes that the location is in unacceptable sites as per strict clean room disciplines. Moreover, in such units there is no control over the procedures that are being carried out in adjacent areas and also in the noxious chemical disinfectants being used elsewhere whose vapors might sweep into the laboratory air. Also, nonmedical grade gases are often used for CO_2 incubators, as there is no regulatory certification for CO_2 gases in many developing countries. Many of the units depend on the food-grade CO_2 gas and the quality of the gas in each batch of cylinder is inconsistent. This in turn may affect the embryo development environment and result in variable outcomes in pregnancy rates and early miscarriages. The gaseous atmosphere in incubators often is a combination of room air, CO_2, and sometimes also N_2 from compressed gas tanks. All of these sources may contain contaminants. Schimmel and colleagues, in 1997, showed that among the various organic compounds found in laboratory gases, benzene was derived specifically from the CO_2 tanks.[1] In some IVF systems, a high percentage (>90%) of ambient air in the incubator is obtained directly from the laboratory room through an opened door or the inlet port at the back of the incubator. Surprisingly, Cohen and colleagues found that unfiltered outside air was cleaner than both the laboratory air and incubators' air.[2] This can result from the accumulation of volatile organic compounds (VOCs) from the laboratory complex and from laboratory products such as plastic dishes. Refrigerant gases, isopropyl alcohol fumes, various aliphatic hydrocarbons, and select aromatic compounds were found to be at higher levels in the laboratory air and inside the incubators compared to outside air. Cohen et al. also determined that a large number of VOCs were detectable in compressed CO_2 used for in vitro culture.[2]

Many smaller units have started using air-handling units (AHUs) to give a positive pressure air supply in the IVF laboratories in comparison to the adjacent rooms. However, the vendors who supply such AHUs are those who design and install clean room facilities mainly for pharmaceutical production houses and hospital theatre complexes. Hence, their main concern is reduction in particle count and putting systems for elimination of any microbial growth. It has been found that many of these AHU units are without any activated

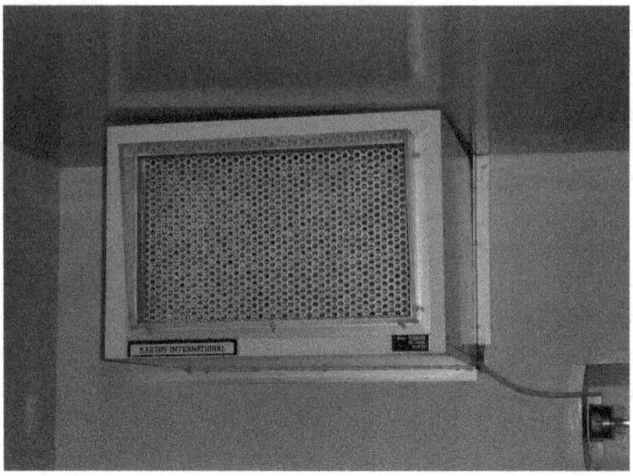

Figure 23.1 A wall-mounted diffuser with high efficiency particulate air (HEPA) filtration.

carbon filters to deal with VOCs, which represent a major concern for pre-implantation embryo growth. The ambient air of IVF laboratories may contain harmful VOCs (e.g., styrene, formaldehyde, aldehydes, toluene, etc.), microbes and their spores, and perfumes, all of which affect embryonic development.[3] Air contaminants, such as chemical air contaminants (CACs) and VOCs, which are introduced from various sources, may interact with samples, tissues, media, and oil, and consequently, have serious effects on IVF outcome.

A sole wall-mount AHU (Figure 23.1) equipped with a pre-filter and high efficiency particulate air (HEPA) filter may give positive pressure to the IVF lab and also bring in clean air without much particle count. However, such units are unable to handle chemical contaminants that may arise both from the laboratory itself and from the surrounding environment unless VOC filters are included. This is more alarming when the lab is situated in a hospital complex and in areas where diesel power generators are in regular use especially in summer months in some developing countries due to frequent power cuts.

Even today many laboratories use alcohols for cleaning benches and work surfaces. It is well documented that alcohol vapors used in the adjacent operating theaters or lab itself can accumulate inside the big box incubators. In those cases, the worst scenario occurs in laboratories that do not have any positive air pressure units. In this context, laminar air flow (LAF) hoods and portable stand alone air filtration units devoid of VOC filtration will not be effective because air with high VOC levels will be simply recirculated.

23.3 Clean room systems

A detailed description of clean room systems applicable for IVF units is presented elsewhere in this book (Chapters 1, 5, 7, and 12). Notwithstanding, it is important to discuss how low cost IVF centers can incorporate such systems. Ideally, a risk management analysis should be done once the unit design is initiated. For existing facilities, it is still possible to modify or integrate clean room systems so as to offer a safe microenvironment for embryo development.

Low resource IVF units are usually located in compromised surroundings with regard to air quality. There is little or no control over the air quality of hospital complexes in which IVF takes place. Moreover, IVF unit managers/directors usually have little information about how compromised the hospital air quality is. It is therefore ideal to construct the unit in an isolated area of the hospital where traffic is considerably less. IVF units should be away from general operating theater complexes. This can be achieved by selecting areas located in upper floors. Some anecdotal evidence rules out setting up the units in the basement. Though the latter might seem to be an ideal place due to its isolation, contaminated and chemically noxious air can settle down to the bottom floors. Nonetheless, basements can be made suitable by applying properly designed and installed clean room systems. Importantly, an integrated team comprising the unit's manager, embryologists, technicians, and engineers should work together to maintain a healthy laboratory environment. Unfortunately, this is not the case in low cost IVF units in which personnel and resources are often limited.

23.3.1 *Things to ponder when constructing a new IVF lab*

1. It is ideal to ask clean room vendors to conduct an analysis on the air quality of the planned room itself and surroundings. This might involve checking air samples for particle counts, VOCs, and microbes. If the unit is planned in tropical countries, the mold growth on walls/ceilings and ventilation ducts needs to be thoroughly checked before the installation of required clean room systems.
2. Laboratory and operating room (OR) walls and ceilings need microbial resistant panels that can be easily cleaned. Although VOC-free epoxy paints have been traditionally used for the walls, many labs nowadays opt for modular panels that are easy to be fitted on the walls and ceiling (e.g., Bioclad panels). These panels offer a false ceiling option where the air handling ducts can be brought in and LED/incandescent lights can be placed in concealed shields to provide an aesthetic and clean surface. Even jointless tiles are an option for the walls and a false ceiling can be constructed with VOC-free materials (e.g., stainless steel, anodized/aluminum, PVC, etc.).
3. Outside air is always cleaner than the IVF lab air with regard to VOC content unless VOC filtration is built in. Ideally, laboratory air handling units should take up 20–30% outside air along with recirculated air. This provides an efficient mechanism to supply clean air to the lab environment. The rule of the thumb is that the IVF lab should always be over-pressured or positively pressured compared to the adjacent rooms (OR, corridors, and other adjacent dirty areas).[4] In recent years, a few standalone air-handling units (AHU) have come up specifically for IVF units (Figure 23.2). These units can be placed in a utility room adjacent to the IVF lab. The ducts from these AHUs are opened to the walls/ceiling of the IVF lab with a dispenser. These are economical systems and may contain pre-filters, alumina filters, activated charcoal filters, and HEPA/ULPA filters (see Chapter 5). Since these units operate with small blowers, the actual air exchange rate to the room and thereby a positive pressure might be minimal compared to the dedicated air-handling units. Moreover, if the opening of the air ducts is placed in the false ceiling with a diffuser, one should get high power blowers for these units; otherwise, multiple units need to be installed.
4. For dedicated clean room facilities, the HVAC system takes care of the temperature and other physical parameters. In the case of low cost systems, some alternative options are required. If the unit were installing systems as shown in Figures 23.1 and 23.2, an option would be to install one or two split air conditioners in the utility room. The cooled air in this small room is taken up by the AHU so as to cool the room to the required temperature. But these may not be efficient air conditioning systems for the lab as the air conditioner is not directly connected to the AHU. This is more problematic in tropical countries where the summer temperature goes beyond 40°C. In such localities, one may consider installing a split air conditioner, or a cassette air conditioner (ceiling mounted) in the IVF lab to bring down the temperature to the required range. The higher the lab

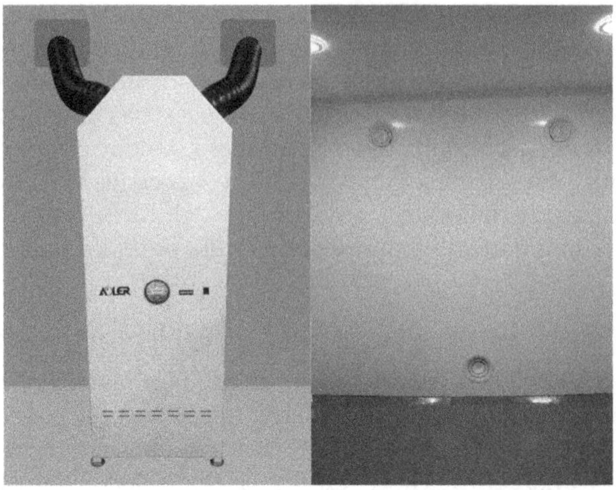

Figure 23.2 Stand-alone air-handling unit with multi-stage filtration including activated carbon. (Courtesy of Adler Systems Inc., India.)

temperature, the higher is the VOC generation in the lab environment. Hence, during the resting phase of the lab, especially at nighttime, it is better to bring down the lab temperature to around 20°C. Low cost PED-based VOC meters are available nowadays, which measure VOC in parts per million (ppm). Continuous VOC monitoring in the lab using such devices will give the user an idea of alarming VOC levels. And occasional validation by external agencies on the physical parameters such as VOC measurement in parts per billion (ppb), microbial count, particle count, filter efficiency testing, etc., will help in maintaining consistency of the lab environment and thereby pregnancy outcome. Activated carbon filters used to trap VOCs can be double-edged swords. There is a threshold level beyond which these filters become inefficient in adsorbing chemically active compounds. Once the filter is saturated, VOCs will get across these filters and reach the lab environment. Hence, it is critical to change the activated carbon filters at regular intervals or based on VOC concentrations in the environment. It is advised not to depend on any light indicator function on the AHU unit to change the activated carbon filters. It is better to guide filter changes based on lab VOC level monitoring.

5. Laminar airflow (LAF) cabinets protect the specimen placed in the working bench through a clean flow of HEPA/ULPA filtered air. Hence, LAF cabinets also act as air-cleaning devices. Some manufactures install a pelletized activated carbon filter after the pre-filter. This is also a cost-effective system that can be incorporated along with the above-mentioned options.
6. There is no single solution to totally curb the VOC levels from the lab environment. The combination of good laboratory practices along with clean room systems and proper laboratory infrastructure including furniture is likely to yield an optimal air quality in terms of chemical contamination. In addition to the positive pressure modules equipped with carbon filters, it may be advisable in low-budget units to place a stand-alone VOC filtration unit inside the lab. Recently, more emphasis has been given on photo catalytic oxidation to remove VOC from lab air. These units can be either wall-mounted (Airocide, Brisk Innovations) or installed in the lab floor. Some models combine HEPA filters along with activated carbon and photocatalytic oxidation in their AHUs (see Chapter 11). Our personal experience with batch IVF centers

is that the above-mentioned systems, if placed inside the lab, work well along with a positive pressure module having activated carbon filters.

7. The air/gas mixture inside a box incubator comes from two sources, namely (1) CO_2/N_2 cylinder and (2) ambient air. Chemical contamination of both can result in high VOC levels inside the culture chamber. A new incubator can release VOCs as high as >100 times up to six months after its installation compared to the old ones.[5] As discussed in Chapter 9, it is mandatory to connect an activated carbon filter in the gas lines. These filters need to be changed periodically or with each cylinder change. It is of utmost importance to obtain the gas cylinders only from reliable vendors that maintain good quality in the production/filling and transportation process. The gas cylinders should be clean, and it is also important to ask the vendors to clean them once in a while. The regulators must be stainless steel and it is advisable to have a gas cylinder change-over level so that once one cylinder is empty it gets switched over to the next one without any human intervention. It is our personal experience that low implantation rates or high early miscarriage rates many times can be boiled down to low quality gases used in some ART clinics, particularly in some developing countries where gases of medical grade are not available.
8. Some models of box incubators have the option of HEPA VOC filters inside the chambers (FORMA Steri-Cult). Many bench top incubators (K-System, ESCO, etc.) have a built-in activated carbon inline filter on its gas line. Some embryologists keep activated carbon pellets (Purafil, USA) in 100 mm dishes inside the incubators and replace it every 6–8 days. This looks like a simplified method to absorb the VOCs inside the box incubator. On the contrary, such systems can be quite dangerous as high incubator humidity not only decreases VOC adsorption efficiency but also increases VOC de-adsorption. Additionally, these activated carbon pellets may also absorb CO_2 and therefore incubators might need to be recalibrated. Another option is to place smaller VOC filtration units inside the box incubator (Incubator Filter Box, Labotect, Germany) (Figure 23.3).

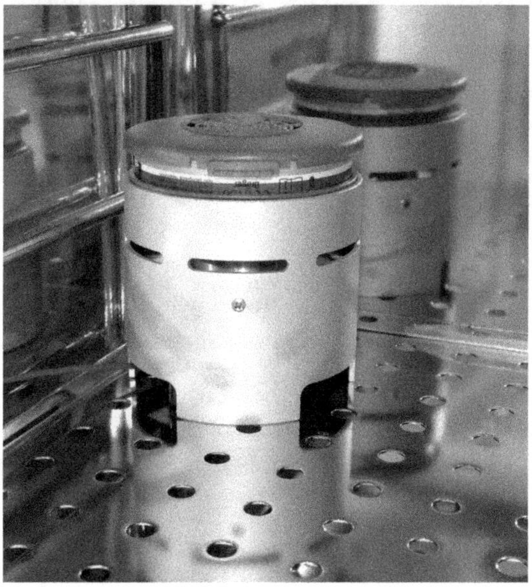

Figure 23.3 Incubator's air filtration unit. (Labotect, Germany.)

23.3.2 Clean room maintenance and discipline

Maintaining a clean room facility is not an easy task and does not comprise just installing some air-cleaning units. Continuous monitoring, maintenance, and discipline are equally important to achieve a desirable outcome. Personnel working in the unit must be educated from the beginning about the operational standard in a clean room facility.

One major problem encountered in low cost IVF units is that the majority of them have no full time trained embryologist to take care of the laboratory on a regular basis. This is exemplified by the fact that many developing countries still do not have any strict government regulations on how ART is practiced. It is the clinical director who performs both the clinical management and the organizational and managerial issues in the laboratory. This definitely has its own pitfalls. Ideally, units should appoint an IVF technician for the maintenance of the laboratory activities and keeping track of the processes performed. It has also been noticed that units performing IVF in batches of say three to five days once a month or two, shut down all the laboratory equipment and AHU units until the next batch commences. This does not seem to be a good practice. The lab air at resting phase can bring in more contaminants and it will require great effort to clean the facility to make it conductive for embryo culture. Similarly, CO_2 incubators that are shut down after every batch will require calibration of CO_2 by an external analyzer (ideally by a company engineer) each time it starts again.

23.4 Conclusion

The smaller the units and the lesser the number of cases, the more emphasis can be dedicated on the quality and data management systems in place without much effort. As described in previous sections, the clinical director should have a fair understanding of the clean room technology and its direct correlation with ART outcome. Before setting up an IVF unit, it is advisable for the clinical director to undergo a short-term training in clinical embryology and to understand the fundamentals of the discipline so as to invest in the right equipment and processes. Life becomes much easier for management if the unit has a good vendor with skilled engineers. If the unit cannot afford to appoint a full time embryologist, the option should be to hire a technician. He or she should be properly trained on laboratory maintenance, record keeping, quality checks and auditing, ordering, etc. He or she can be trained and get proficient in andrology laboratory procedures, dish preparation, sperm preparation during IVF/ICSI, etc. There should be standard operating procedures (SOPs) in place for the equipment operations and procedures performed and clear instructions on the practices/disciplines to be carried out in a clean room facility.

References

1. Schimmel T, Gilligan A, Garrisi GJ, Esposito B, Cecci M, Dale B et al. Removal of volatile organic compounds from incubators used for gamete and embryo culture. *Reprod Fertil.* 1997; 68(Suppl 1): S165.
2. Cohen J, Gilligan A, Esposito W, Schimmel T, and Dale B. Ambient air and its potential effects on conception in vitro. *Hum Reprod.* 1997; 12: 1742–9.
3. Hall J, Gilligan A, Schimmel T, Cecchi M, and Cohen J. The origin, effects and control of air pollution in laboratories used for human embryo culture. *Hum Reprod.* 1998; 13(Suppl. 4): 146–55.
4. Esteves SC and Bento FC. Implementation of air quality control in reproductive laboratories in full compliance with the Brazilian Cells and Germinative Tissue Directive. *Reprod Biomed Online.* 2013; 26: 9–21.
5. Cohen J, Gilligan A, and Willadsen S. Culture and quality control of embryos. *Hum Reprod.* 1998; 13(Suppl 3): 137–47.

chapter twenty-four

Sealed culture systems with time-lapse video monitoring

Kelly Athayde Wirka and Dean E. Morbeck

Contents

Abstract

The introduction of time-lapse video monitoring into the in vitro fertilization laboratory has ushered in another level of embryo assessment and provided additional insight into early embryo development. By allowing real-time observations based on frequent image capture and by limiting the need to remove embryos from the incubator, time-lapse video monitoring technology has enabled the concept of a "sealed culture system" or "less-disturbed culture system." This chapter will focus on the many aspects of these culture systems enabled by time-lapse video monitoring, beginning with the potential benefits of time-lapse imaging and "sealed culture" in terms of air quality, and then expanding the discussion to include other potential challenges and benefits, in particular the role of time-lapse for embryo selection.

24.1 Introduction

Creating and maintaining optimal in vitro conditions that mimic the natural, in vivo environment and facilitate optimal development of viable embryos is of paramount importance to any in vitro fertilization (IVF) laboratory. Thus, laboratory air quality and optimal culture conditions have been the subject of intense research during the past decades. Laboratory air quality can impact the atmospheric environment within the incubator, which is a key element of the culture system and functions to maintain stable and appropriate conditions for embryo culture.[1] Introduction of extended culture to the blastocyst stage has added additional pressure to these culture systems,[2] thus increasing even further the importance of a quality stable culture environment.

The culture system plays an important role in the success rates of an IVF clinic. A "culture system" defines all aspects of embryo culture in a laboratory—the type of media and culture vessels, volume per drop/well, embryo density, CO_2 and O_2 tension, pH, temperature, and type of incubation (i.e., box or benchtop incubators, use of desiccator jars, etc.). The culture system also defines workflow and drives much of the laboratory routine. Although embryologists may have different opinions regarding which is the best culture system, there is overall agreement that such a system should be disturbed as little as possible in order to optimize embryo culture conditions. The desire to minimize disruptions of the culture environment resulted in the practice of limiting embryo assessment to specific time points during embryo growth,[3] therefore defining embryo grading on static snapshots based on certain milestones of embryo development.

The introduction of time-lapse video monitoring into the IVF laboratory has ushered in another level of embryo assessment and provided additional insight into early embryo development. By allowing real-time observations based on frequent image capture and by limiting the need to remove embryos from the incubator, time-lapse video monitoring technology has enabled the concept of a "sealed culture system." Although the term "sealed culture" implies no disturbance during the embryo culture process, it is still common for laboratories using time-lapse video monitoring to change or refresh media on day 3 independent of the medium choice, sequential or single step. This lab practice is mostly related to the concern regarding degradation of medium components and ammonium production.[4,5] Nevertheless, there is evidence that successful embryo development and clinical outcomes can be obtained with continuous uninterrupted single medium used throughout the blastocyst culture.[6]

This chapter will focus on the many aspects of "sealed culture systems" or "less-disturbed culture systems" enabled by time-lapse video monitoring, beginning with the potential benefits of time-lapse imaging and "sealed culture" in terms of air quality, then expanding the discussion to include other potential challenges and benefits, in particular the role of time-lapse for embryo selection.

24.2 Culture systems with time-lapse monitoring

The "sealed" or "less-disturbed" nature of embryo culture using time-lapse imaging presents many exciting opportunities for improving the quality of the culture environment. In addition, there are several other facets of time-lapse monitoring that hold potential for improving the IVF process. These include improved workflow/laboratory efficiency, robust quality assurance, patient education, quality control testing, new information on embryo development and selection, and utility as a platform for future innovation.

The core principle of time-lapse monitoring in embryo culture is to obtain more information with fewer disturbances. In principle, time-lapse monitoring can provide key elements necessary to control the quality of the air that has the longest contact time with gametes and embryos. Though it is possible to obtain complete control of the air during culture by performing blastocyst culture with continuous, single step medium in a "sealed" environment, such as a desiccator jar[6] or sealed plastic bag,[7] the inability to obtain developmental data is a significant limitation. Time-lapse offers the ability to monitor embryo development while limiting the number of times room air is introduced into the incubator chamber, thus maintaining optimal recirculation of incubator air, preferably with continual "scrubbing" with carbon filtration for volatile organic compounds (VOCs).

Time-lapse monitoring also offers a consistent means to obtain air quality indicators without disturbing embryos. In standard practice, embryo quality is used as an indicator of the quality of the culture environment. For example, following the implementation of clean room technology to improve air quality in the laboratory, fertilization rates,[8] day 3 cell number,[9] high quality embryos,[10] and blastocyst rates[8] increased. Time-lapse monitoring, however, not only provides access to embryo quality, but also includes a built-in system for recording data that allow routine quality indicator analysis using control charts.[11–13]

The stability of temperature and gas concentrations (CO_2 and O_2) can vary widely with incubator design and it is an important consideration for air quality. The MINC incubator[14] was the first purpose-built incubator for embryo culture and has led a revolution in embryo culture methods including several benchtop incubators on the market. In essence, either benchtop or box incubators could be used as "sealed" or "less-disturbed" culture systems, although neither provide the benefits of time-lapse inherently. The main attraction of benchtop incubators is that they provide a small chamber that can be dedicated to one patient and deliver a steady flow of filtered air, resulting in improved temperature maintenance[14] and gas recovery,[15] and therefore improved embryo development.[15]

However, a detailed comparative analysis of embryo culture incubators concluded that different types of incubators, including benchtop and box incubators, can have the same performance if managed properly.[1] The importance of limiting the number of disturbances to the culture environment should not be underestimated, since the frequency of door openings adversely affects embryo development, independently of the type of incubator being used.[16–19] Coupling this decreased frequency of door openings with a carbon-activated inline filter for gas delivery or recirculation provides an additional reduction of harmful VOCs. The optimal combination of less door openings and improved VOC filtration can ultimately provide embryos with a stable environment with excellent air quality.

In principle, a sealed or less-disturbed culture system using time-lapse imaging that results in fewer disruptions and high quality air should result in better embryo development and outcomes, yet available evidence does not show a consistent benefit. Cruz and colleagues performed a prospective cohort study with donor oocytes showing comparable development of embryos cultured in a time-lapse versus a conventional cell culture incubator.[20] These results were later confirmed in a randomized control trial (RCT) with sibling embryos.[21] In contrast, a large retrospective, multicenter study noted a 15.7% increase in clinical pregnancy rate comparing time-lapse to a conventional cell culture incubator.[22] A recent prospective RCT confirmed these results and demonstrated an increase in the number of optimal embryos on day 3 and day 5 in the time-lapse group.[23] However, limitations of these studies make it difficult to assess the impact of sealed or less-disturbed culture on improved clinical outcome. For example, an uninterrupted culture was not used in the first two studies[20,21]; these groups removed embryos from both the conventional and the time-lapse incubators for manual scoring on days 2, 3, and 5 (when embryos were cultured to blastocyst stage). Rubio and colleagues showed improved embryo development with uninterrupted (embryos transferred on day 3) and a less-disturbed culture (medium was changed for embryos cultured to blastocyst stage); however, the impact of these improvements on clinical pregnancy rates is not known because the incubation method was confounded by the use of time-lapse-based embryo selection methods.[23] While the idea that sealed culture can improve outcomes is attractive, further studies are needed to effectively answer this question.

24.3 *Potential challenges of culture systems with time-lapse monitoring*

Time-lapse monitoring systems present unique challenges that require special attention. These include issues of safety, efficiency and workflow, cost-benefit, redundancy, dependence on technology, and a learning curve for working with new technology and supplies. Individually, these factors are reasonable—combined, they can represent a major shift in patient care and how a laboratory works.

While many of these factors do not impact air quality, some of them can impact the culture environment and therefore its safety. All culture systems have limitations and risks of failure. In the case of time-lapse culture systems, there could be risks to embryo development from a variety of sources: VOCs, mentioned previously, heat due to motion and friction of moving parts, presence of magnetic fields, shear stress of moving culture dishes, and presence of lubricants.[24] VOC filtration is a critical component that is particularly important when a time-lapse system has electronics or moving components that can fail and begin to produce VOCs within the incubator. Any change to the materials used in the chamber can also increase VOC levels, though this is the case with virtually every incubation system. In contrast to desiccator jars and benchtop incubators that do not contain moving parts, time-lapse systems and even traditional water or air-jacketed incubators often have fans and other components that could fail and produce VOCs. While highly unlikely and mostly theoretical, the possibility is germane for a discussion on air quality.

Embryos monitored by time-lapse systems are subjected to frequent image capture, which raises another concern regarding safety: light exposure. Studies have shown that extensive light exposure may be detrimental to mammalian embryo development.[25,26] Image capture, which usually varies from 5- to 20-minute intervals, requires illumination and exposure to camera light. Although the light exposure is brief, it is much more frequent compared to standard embryo assessment which usually takes place once a day. A few studies have focused on evaluating the safety aspects of time-lapse, including light exposure. Nakahara and colleagues found that embryo development through day 3 was similar between embryos that were cultured in an incubator with an integrated time-lapse system (observations every 15 minutes) compared to embryos cultured in a conventional incubator (observations once a day).[27] Other groups have also shown comparable[24,28] or improved[23,29] development for embryos cultured in a time-lapse incubator versus a conventional incubator. Although few studies were designed to specifically address individual safety aspects of time-lapse monitoring—such as the individual contributions of heat production, light exposure, and VOC generation—published literature support the overall safety of time-lapse technology based on the reported developmental outcome of embryos monitored by different time-lapse systems.[28,30–35]

Another challenge inherent to culture systems with time-lapse monitoring is related to efficiency and workflow. Time-lapse imaging generates a vast amount of images per embryo, which can provide useful information regarding embryo development. Nevertheless, how these images are analyzed and how the information obtained from such analysis can be clinically used remains a challenge. The process for image data analysis, including video review and manual annotations, can be extremely time-consuming and can therefore impact workflow and efficiency. Further, this manual analysis is laborious and requires extensive training and practice for each time-lapse user,[36] thus imposing learning curve and adoption challenges. A recent study suggested that intra- and inter-observer variability impact the precision of time-lapse annotations, particularly those focused on later stage events of embryo development.[37] The inability to confidently and efficiently review and interpret time-lapse videos can lead to significant challenges in the standardization and clinical use of time-lapse information.

Cost is another aspect that poses a great challenge for laboratories interested in culture systems with time-lapse technology. Like any new technology introduced into the clinical setting, its implementation can add significant costs to the clinical procedure, which may bring additional expenses to patient treatment. Cost may also define how many systems can be implemented and therefore dictates capacity. Capacity can impact efficiency and workflow if there are not enough systems available to patients/embryos. Although these are currently considered additional challenges, they may be overcome once time-lapse monitoring technology becomes more affordable and scalable.

24.4 The use of time-lapse monitoring for embryo selection

In addition to the concept of sealed culture systems, time-lapse video monitoring provides a new level of insight regarding in vitro human embryogenesis that holds promise for improving embryologists' ability to select the most viable embryo for transfer. Embryo development can be observed in real time, allowing identification of important milestones in early embryo development. The additional information available using time-lapse monitoring offers an attractive, non-invasive tool for embryo selection.

Time-lapse technology is not new—it has been applied to observe the development of mammalian embryos for decades. Studies using rabbits started as early as 1929 and were followed by others using mice and cattle.[38] In the late 1990s, Payne and collaborators used the technology to observe and describe the fertilization process of 50 human oocytes after intracytoplasmic sperm injection.[3] Other studies also described exciting observations that contributed to a better understanding of the morphological changes throughout human embryogenesis[39–42] and further stimulated an interest in the clinical significance of specific milestones of embryo development. Only recently, however, did the concept arise of applying time-lapse video monitoring for routine screening in order to determine developmental potential. Wong and colleagues were the first group to show scientific evidence that time-lapse technology could be used to predict human blastocyst development.[43] Specifically, this group of researchers discovered that cell division time intervals within the first two cleavages could predict development to the blastocyst stage, and, further, that the time intervals were correlated with distinct gene expression profiles. These findings contributed to a shift: time-lapse moved from being an "observational" technology to a potentially "predictive" one. The ability to predict blastocyst formation has since been confirmed in a prospective, multicenter study,[44] which contributed to the development of a noninvasive test—the Eeva™ Test, which combines time-lapse image data with cell-tracking analysis software. The authors showed that adding specific time-lapse markers to traditional morphology not only significantly improved the specificity and positive predictive value for accurate prediction of blastocyst development but also reduced inter-observer variability.[32]

Time-lapse imaging as a noninvasive test of embryo viability has been an area of intense scientific investigation. Several time-lapse markers have been reported to correlate with human embryo developmental outcomes, including implantation and clinical pregnancy.[28,31–35,45] Although extremely promising, the number of robust prospective studies is limited, particularly for clinical outcomes such as implantation, clinical pregnancy, and live birth.[46] Various clinics have reported improved clinical pregnancy rates after implementing sealed or less-disturbed culture and the use of time-lapse markers for embryo selection.[23,29] However, to truly evaluate the impact of time-lapse markers on clinical outcomes, it is necessary to control for the confounding effect of the undisturbed or less-disturbed culture inherent in the time-lapse systems. Otherwise, it is not possible to distinguish if improvements are related to the culture environment (less-disturbed culture) or to the actual time-lapse markers being used to screen and select embryos. As of this writing, there have been no robust clinical trials addressing how much of the improvement in clinical outcome can be attributed to the "sealed culture" conditions or to the use of time-lapse markers being applied to embryo selection.

Although there are limited data to suggest that time-lapse markers can effectively select embryos that have a which have higher potential of implantation, the technology could potentially help to deselect embryos with a lower chance to implant. Time-lapse video monitoring permits the identification of certain unusual embryo behaviors during early embryo development, also called atypical phenotypes. Four novel atypical phenotypes have been recently associated with poor embryo development.[30] One of these reported atypical phenotypes associated with poorer developmental potential is abnormal cleavage (AC), which occurs when more than two cells originate from a single cell division event. Another related example is direct cleavage (DC), which occurs when division from two to three cells happens in less than five hours.[47] Both AC and DC are quite prevalent, 18% and 13.7%, respectively, and embryos with these phenotypes have been described to exhibit extremely low implantation, 3.7% and 1.2%, respectively.[30,47] Importantly, standard morphological evaluation is not able to identify such embryos as most of them exhibit good morphology and are therefore considered top candidates for embryo transfer and/or freezing.[30] While there is evidence that AC and DC embryos have limited capability to implant, no study has yet evaluated the live birth rates of such embryos that have successfully implanted. Further studies are needed to elucidate the etiology of AC, DC, and other abnormal phenotypes and to continue to evaluate their association with clinical outcomes.

24.5 Conclusion

Time-lapse video monitoring is changing the practice of embryology and the field of human assisted reproduction. While the IVF community waits for randomized clinical trials designed to investigate the true value of time-lapse markers in improving implantation, clinical pregnancy, and live birth rates, other potential improvements described in this chapter including the benefits of sealed or less-disturbed culture present a new paradigm for the assisted reproduction laboratory that is a reality today.

References

1. Swain JE. Decisions for the IVF laboratory: Comparative analysis of embryo culture incubators. *Reprod Biomed Online.* 2014; **28**(5): 535–47.
2. Gardner DK and Lane, M. Extended culture in IVF. In: Nagy ZP, Varguese A, and Agarwal A, eds. *Clinical Embryology: A Practical Guide.* New York: Springer; 2013, pp. 99–113.
3. Payne D, Flaherty SP, Barry MF, and Matthews CD. Preliminary observations on polar body extrusion and pronuclear formation in human oocytes using time-lapse video cinematography. *Hum Reprod.* 1997; **12**(3): 532–41.
4. Gruber I and Klein M. Embryo culture media for human IVF: Which possibilities exist? *J Turk Ger Gynecol Assoc.* 2011; **12**(2): 110–7.
5. Gardner DK, Lane M, Stevens J, and Schoolcraft WB. Noninvasive assessment of human embryo nutrient consumption as a measure of developmental potential. *Fertil Steril.* 2001; **76**(6): 1175–80.

6. Reed ML, Hamic A, Thompson DJ, and Caperton CL. Continuous uninterrupted single medium culture without medium renewal versus sequential media culture: A sibling embryo study. *Fertil Steril.* 2009; **92**(5): 1783–6.
7. Bavister BD and Poole KA. Duration and temperature of culture medium equilibration affect frequency of blastocyst development. *Reprod Biomed Online.* 2005; **10**(1): 124–9.
8. Khoudja RY, Xu Y, Li T, and Zhou C. Better IVF outcomes following improvements in laboratory air quality. *J Assist Reprod Genet.* 2013; **30**(1): 69–76.
9. Boone WR, Johnson JE, Locke AJ, Crane MMt, and Price TM. Control of air quality in an assisted reproductive technology laboratory. *Fertil Steril.* 1999; **71**(1): 150–4.
10. Esteves SC and Bento FC. Implementation of air quality control in reproductive laboratories in full compliance with the Brazilian Cells and Germinative Tissue Directive. *Reprod Biomed Online.* 2013; **26**(1): 9–21.
11. Kennedy CR and Mortimer D. Risk management in IVF. *Best Pract Res Clin Obstet Gynaecol.* 2007; **21**(4): 691–712.
12. Mortimer D. Quality management in the IVF laboratory. In: Jansen R and Mortimer D, eds. Towards Reproductive Certainty: Fertility & Genetics Beyond 1999: The Plenary Proceedings of the 11th World Congress on In Vitro Fertilization & Human Reproductive Genetics. Pearl River, NY: Parthenon; 1999, p. xv.
13. Mortimer D and Mortimer S. *Quality and Risk Management in the IVF Laboratory.* Cambridge, UK: Cambridge University Press; 2005.
14. Cooke S, Tyler JPP, and Driscoll G. Objective assessments of temperature maintenance using in vitro culture techniques. *J Assist Reprod Genet.* 2002; **19**(8): 368–75.
15. Fujiwara M, Takahashi K, Izuno M, Duan YR, Kazono M, Kimura F et al. Effect of micro-environment maintenance on embryo culture after in-vitro fertilization: Comparison of top-load mini incubator and conventional front-load incubator. *J Assist Reprod Genet.* 2007; **24**(1): 5–9.
16. Scott LF, Sundaram SG, and Smith S. The relevance and use of mouse embryo bioassays for quality control in an assisted reproductive technology program. *Fertil Steril.* 1993; **60**(3): 559–68.
17. Gardner DK and Lane M. Alleviation of the '2-cell block' and development to the blastocyst of CF1 mouse embryos: Role of amino acids, EDTA and physical parameters. *Hum Reprod.* 1996; **11**(12): 2703–12.
18. Avery B, Melsted JK, and Greve T. A novel approach for in vitro production of bovine embryos: Use of the Oxoid atmosphere generating system. *Theriogenology.* 2000; **54**(8): 1259–68.
19. Zhang JQ, Li XL, Peng Y, Guo X, Heng BC, and Tong GQ. Reduction in exposure of human embryos outside the incubator enhances embryo quality and blastulation rate. *Reprod Biomed Online.* 2010; **20**(4): 510–5.
20. Cruz M, Gadea B, Garrido N, Pedersen KS, Martinez M, Perez-Cano I et al. Embryo quality, blastocyst and ongoing pregnancy rates in oocyte donation patients whose embryos were monitored by time-lapse imaging. *J Assist Reprod Genet.* 2011; **28**(7): 569–73.
21. Kirkegaard K, Hindkjaer JJ, Grondahl ML, Kesmodel US, and Ingerslev HJ. A randomized clinical trial comparing embryo culture in a conventional incubator with a time-lapse incubator. *J Assist Reprod Genet.* 2012; **29**(6): 565–72.
22. Meseguer M, Rubio I, Cruz M, Basile N, Marcos J, and Requena A. Embryo incubation and selection in a time-lapse monitoring system improves pregnancy outcome compared with a standard incubator: A retrospective cohort study. *Fertil Steril.* 2012; **98**(6): 1481–9.
23. Rubio I, Galan A, Larreategui Z, Ayerdi F, Bellver J, Herrero J et al. Clinical validation of embryo culture and selection by morphokinetic analysis: A randomized, controlled trial of the EmbryoScope. *Fertil Steril.* 2014; **102**(5): 1287–1294 e5.
24. Kirkegaard K, Hindkjaer JJ, Grondahl ML, Kesmodel US, Ingerslev HJ. A randomized clinical trial comparing embryo culture in a conventional incubator with a time-lapse incubator. *J Assist Reprod Genet.* 2012; **29**(6): 565–72.
25. Oh SJ, Gong SP, Lee ST, Lee EJ, and Lim JM. Light intensity and wavelength during embryo manipulation are important factors for maintaining viability of preimplantation embryos in vitro. *Fertil Steril.* 2007; **88**(4 Suppl): 1150–7.
26. Takenaka M, Horiuchi T, Yanagimachi R. Effects of light on development of mammalian zygotes. *Proc Natl Acad Sci USA.* 2007; **104**(36): 14289–93.

27. Nakahara T, Iwase A, Goto M, Harata T, Suzuki M, Ienaga M et al. Evaluation of the safety of time-lapse observations for human embryos. *J Assist Reprod Genet.* 2010; **27**(2–3): 93–6.
28. Cruz M, Gadea B, Garrido N, Pedersen KS, Martinez M, Perez-Cano I et al. Embryo quality, blastocyst and ongoing pregnancy rates in oocyte donation patients whose embryos were monitored by time-lapse imaging. *J Assist Reprod Genet.* 2011; **28**(7): 569–73.
29. Meseguer M, Rubio I, Cruz M, Basile N, Marcos J, and Requena A. Embryo incubation and selection in a time-lapse monitoring system improves pregnancy outcome compared with a standard incubator: A retrospective cohort study. *Fertil Steril.* 2012; **98**(6): 1481–9 e10.
30. Athayde Wirka K, Chen AA, Conaghan J, Ivani K, Gvakharia M, Behr B et al. Atypical embryo phenotypes identified by time-lapse microscopy: High prevalence and association with embryo development. *Fertil Steril.* 2014; **101**(6): 1637–48 e1–5.
31. Desai N, Ploskonka S, Goodman LR, Austin C, Goldberg J, and Falcone T. Analysis of embryo morphokinetics, multinucleation and cleavage anomalies using continuous time-lapse monitoring in blastocyst transfer cycles. *Reprod Biol Endocrinol.* 2014; **12**: 54.
32. Conaghan J, Chen AA, Willman SP, Ivani K, Chenette PE, Boostanfar R et al. Improving embryo selection using a computer-automated time-lapse image analysis test plus day 3 morphology: Results from a prospective multicenter trial. *Fertil Steril.* 2013; **100**(2): 412–9.
33. Azzarello A, Hoest T, and Mikkelsen AL. The impact of pronuclei morphology and dynamicity on live birth outcome after time-lapse culture. *Hum Reprod.* 2012; **27**(9): 2649–57.
34. Hlinka D, Kalatova B, Uhrinova I, Dolinska S, Rutarova J, Rezacova J et al. Time-lapse cleavage rating predicts human embryo viability. *Physiol Res.* 2012; **61**(5): 513–25.
35. Meseguer M, Herrero J, Tejera A, Hilligsoe KM, Ramsing NB, and Remohi J. The use of morphokinetics as a predictor of embryo implantation. *Hum Reprod.* 2011; **26**(10): 2658–71.
36. Chen AA, Tan L, Suraj V, Reijo Pera R, and Shen S. Biomarkers identified with time-lapse imaging: Discovery, validation, and practical application. *Fertil Steril.* 2013; **99**(4): 1035–43.
37. Sundvall L, Ingerslev HJ, Breth Knudsen U, and Kirkegaard K. Inter- and intra-observer variability of time-lapse annotations. *Hum Reprod.* 2013; **28**(12): 3215–21.
38. Vajta G and Hardarson T. Real-time embryo monitoring device for embryo selection. In: Nagy P, Varguese A, and Agarwal, A, eds. *Clinical Embryology: A Practical Guide.* New York: Springer; 2013, pp. 367–75.
39. Pribenszky C, Losonczi E, Molnar M, Lang Z, Matyas S, Rajczy K et al. Prediction of in-vitro developmental competence of early cleavage-stage mouse embryos with compact time-lapse equipment. *Reprod Biomed Online.* 2010; **20**(3): 371–9.
40. Mio Y and Maeda K. Time-lapse cinematography of dynamic changes occurring during in vitro development of human embryos. *Am J Obstet Gynecol.* 2008; **199**(6): 660 e1–5.
41. Lemmen JG, Agerholm I, and Ziebe S. Kinetic markers of human embryo quality using time-lapse recordings of IVF/ICSI-fertilized oocytes. *Reprod Biomed Online.* 2008; **17**(3): 385–91.
42. Hardarson T, Lofman C, Coull G, Sjogren A, Hamberger L, and Edwards RG. Internalization of cellular fragments in a human embryo: Time-lapse recordings. *Reprod Biomed Online.* 2002; **5**(1): 36–8.
43. Wong CC, Loewke KE, Bossert NL, Behr B, De Jonge CJ, Baer TM et al. Non-invasive imaging of human embryos before embryonic genome activation predicts development to the blastocyst stage. *Nature Biotechnology.* 2010; **28**(10): 1115–21.
44. Conaghan J, Chen AA, Willman SP, Ivani K, Chenette PE, Boostanfar R et al. Improving embryo selection using a computer-automated time-lapse image analysis test plus day 3 morphology: Results from a prospective multicenter trial. *Fertil Steril.* 2013; **100**(2): 412–9 e5.
45. Chavez SL, Loewke KE, Han J, Moussavi F, Colls P, Munne S et al. Dynamic blastomere behaviour reflects human embryo ploidy by the four-cell stage. *Nat Commun.* 2012; **3**: 1251.
46. Kaser DJ and Racowsky C. Clinical outcomes following selection of human preimplantation embryos with time-lapse monitoring: A systematic review. *Hum Reprod Update.* 2014; **20**(5): 617–31.
47. Rubio I, Kuhlmann R, Agerholm I, Kirk J, Herrero J, Escribá M-J et al. Limited implantation success of direct-cleaved human zygotes: A time-lapse study. *Fertil Steril.* 2012; **98**(6): 1458–63.

section six

International experience

Case studies

chapter twenty-five

Clean room technology and IVF outcomes: United States

Terrence D. Lewis, Aidita N. James, Micah J. Hill, and Ryan J. Heitmann

Contents

Abstract

Infertility is a common disease, affecting 10–15% of couples, causing many to seek treatment with assisted reproductive techniques (ARTs). Numerous factors have been attributed to successful ART cycles. One commonly understood, but less emphasized factor is the laboratory environment and air quality. Our facility had the unique opportunity to compare separate ART laboratories, as a result of a required move. Environmental and laboratory conditions were specifically focused on the design and planning of the new laboratory. As a result, we noted significant improvements in embryo implantations and live births. Embryo quality improved leading to more single blastocyst embryo transfers, which secondarily decreased multiple gestations and increased available supernumerary embryos for vitrification. Profound positive effects on laboratory measures and patient outcomes can be achieved with improvements in ART laboratory conditions and air quality and reemphasized their importance in the success of an ART program.

25.1 Introduction

Infertility is a disease in which conception has not occurred after 12 months of regular intercourse in patients under the age of 35, or after six months in patients over 35 years old.[1,2] This disease is highly prevalent, occurring in approximately 10–15% of all reproductive age couples.[3,4] Recent studies suggest the incidence of infertility has markedly increased over the past decade.[5,6] A complete infertility evaluation includes a thorough history and physical examination, assessment of ovarian reserve and ovulation, assessment of the uterus and fallopian tubes typically with a hysterosalpingogram (HSG), and assessment of male sperm with a semen analysis.[1,2]

Etiologies of infertility are divided into subcategories including ovulatory dysfunction, tubal factor, endometriosis, uterine factor, male factor, and unexplained.[7] Conditions including severe male factor, complete tubal obstruction, and multifactor infertility often require the utilization of assisted reproductive technologies (ARTs), which encompass all techniques involving direct manipulation of oocytes outside of the human body. The use of ART has increased tremendously over the last decade. The Society for Assisted Reproductive Technologies reports over 146,000 assisted reproductive technique cycles were carried out in the United States in 2010.[8] "The success of modern assisted reproductive technologies has completely revolutionized both the evaluation and treatment of infertility."[9]

25.2 Factors affecting the success of ART

Many factors have been shown to contribute to the overall success of ART, which include, but are not limited to, the ages of the patients, the cause and duration of infertility, the number of embryos transferred, the day of embryo transfer, and the quality of transferred embryos.[9] Interestingly, data accumulated over the past two decades suggests the creation of an optimal environment for the culture of human embryos is indispensable for maintaining embryo viability, which inevitably improves pregnancy outcomes. To this end, the laboratory environment and air quality within ART centers have been identified as critically important and have been shown to influence the success of ART.[10,11]

25.2.1 Air pollution and environmental factors

Air pollution is a serious global public health problem that has been linked to an increased risk of acute and chronic adverse human health conditions.[12] Studies have shown that reductions in exposure at the population level significantly improve health outcomes.[13,14] More specific to human reproductive technologies, numerous studies provide compelling evidence of the negative effects of poor air quality on embryo development, which ultimately affects pregnancy rates and outcomes.[15–20] One such observation was made in Naples, Italy, in 1992, where an in vitro fertilization laboratory noted decreases in in vitro embryo development and pregnancy rates associated with the move from a suburban area to a more urban setting.

Volatile organic compounds (VOCs) are organic chemicals that are numerous and include both synthetic and naturally occurring chemical compounds (i.e., acetone, benzene, ethanol, formaldehydes, glutaraldehydes, styrenes, toluene, etc.). Many of these compounds have been shown to have harmful effects on human health and are regulated by local, state, and federal laws. Said laws are more stringent indoors where concentrations are highest. Sources of these VOCs in the laboratory setting include outside air, equipment, furniture, gases, personnel, and plastic ware. It is now well established that VOCs contained within the air of assisted reproductive centers are harmful to developing embryos.[15,21] Cohen et al. have demonstrated that the air inside an incubator contained significantly higher concentrations of VOCs than the external air.[16] Even at low levels in the circulating air of ART centers, these compounds have been shown to have deleterious effects on success rates and act by forming covalent bonds within DNA of developing embryos leading to inhibited growth and diminished pregnancy rates.[22] To this end, air quality improvements that include positive air pressure in the lab, high efficiency particulate air (HEPA) filtration of laboratory air, filtration of laboratory air for volatile and chemically active compounds via activated charcoal filters, and the use of laminar flow hoods were measures identified as a critical factors in top performing in vitro fertilization laboratories in the United States.[23]

25.2.2 Laboratory guidelines

In an effort to standardize laboratory conditions, the American Society for Reproductive Medicine (ASRM) in conjunction with recommendations from the Food and Drug Administration (FDA) and World Health Organization (WHO) published a series of committee opinions entitled "Recommended practices for the management of embryology, andrology, and endocrinology laboratories: a committee opinion" for assisted reproductive technology laboratories within the continental United States and its territories.[24–27] The committee opinions outline general principles and recommendations, which apply to the aforementioned laboratories. These documents recommend that all laboratories:

1. "Whether located in a university, hospital, or private setting should be registered, accredited, and certified at the national levels." In addition, if applicable, said laboratories should satisfy all state licensure requirements.
2. "Should document an ongoing quality control program for each test and piece of equipment contained within the laboratory."
3. "Required to maintain documentation of all activities conducted within the facility" to include current policy and procedure manuals as well as manuals or documentation of laboratory safety, infection control, disaster plans, Health Insurance Portability and Accountability Act (HIPAA) procedures, chemical hygiene, and laboratory personnel.
4. "Must maintain a system that provides proper patient preparation and identification; proper patient specimen collection, preservation, transportation, and processing; and accurate reporting of laboratory test and procedural results."
5. "Must have a director, or supervisor, who meets the qualifications defined in the Clinical Laboratory Improvement Act of 1988 (CLIA '88), who supervises the activities in all sections of the laboratory, including endocrinology, andrology, and embryology." Additional recommendations suggest that if the laboratory director/supervisor does not provide daily supervision, there should be a "general supervisor" who performs the aforementioned duties under the direction of the laboratory director.
6. The final general recommendation made within the document "requires all testing personnel to be licensed per the state requirements and must meet CLIA'88 standards."

Despite all the recommendations and guidance given in these documents, there still remains no specific language concerning air quality or air handling specifications or requirements.

25.3 Design of an assisted reproductive technology (ART) laboratory

25.3.1 Overall design

The authors' original ART clinic and laboratory was retrofit into an available tertiary care hospital operating room space in 1996. The ART laboratory, oocyte retrieval, and embryo transfer rooms were located in separate operating rooms and connected by two internal hallways. The internal air environment for the laboratory was provided by the hospital operating room air handling system and the facility often had negative pressure relative to outside common areas. The heating, ventilation, and air conditioning air intake was located on the roof of the hospital approximately 10 feet from the cafeteria exhaust port. Analysis of the air quality revealed the VOC level at the air intake was 184.6 $\mu g/m^3$. The entire assisted reproductive technique clinic and laboratory lacked a humidity control system; therefore, relative humidity was consistent with outside conditions. Ultimately, this unit was found to provide unreliable heating, ventilation, and air conditioning, and therefore it did not always maintain proper air balance, temperature, or humidity.

To circumvent the identified deficiencies and improve the air environment, four Coda® tower filter units (Life Global, Guelph, Canada) were installed in the laboratory and two Coda® Loboy filter units were installed in the oocyte retrieval space. No additional CODA® filter systems were installed in the embryo transfer room. Each of the newly installed filter systems was maintained according to Life Global's protocol with main stage filter changes occurring before each coordinated in vitro fertilization cycle. In addition, high efficiency particulate air (HEPA) filter changes occurred annually per the manufacture's recommendations.

The internal environment of the incubators and isolettes was maintained by individual gas cylinders that were housed in the hallway directly adjacent to the laboratory space or to the particular pieces of equipment using the gas. The gasses were fed to each piece of equipment using sterilized Tygon® tubing (Saint-Gobain Performance Plastics, Mickleton, NJ) that was run from one room to the next through a hole in the wall. Each line was filtered by Coda® Inline filter cartridges (Life Global, Guelph, Canada). Each filter unit was maintained according to the manufacturer's protocol with changes occurring before each in vitro fertilization series. Last, the procedural and laboratory areas were lit by surgical lamps and fluorescent lighting. The lighting level was kept low to minimize detrimental effects.

In 2006, the decision was made to close the tertiary treatment facility that housed the authors' original ART clinic and laboratory to move into a modernized facility approximately eight miles away. The move was seen as an opportunity to improve environmental conditions within the new ART suite by strategic engineering decisions during the planning phase for the construction of the new facility. Plans were made to create a new ART suite built floor to ceiling to create a sealed box environment to prevent contamination from inter-floor or wall sources. The original plan included an operating room, an ART laboratory, embryo transfer room, and andrology laboratory. Each room would be separated by magnetic lock controlled doors with sealing, designed to help maintain a positive pressure environment. The ART laboratory was to have the highest level of positive air pressure with a decreasing pressure gradient as the air flows to each subsequent space until the external portions of the suite were reached. All materials used within the ART suite were approved by an environmental specialist (Alpha Environmental, Jersey City,

NJ) to contain low, or no, VOCs. After completion of the suite, the unit was off-gassed by using a burn-off period of six weeks after construction was complete.

Access to the ART suite is now limited exclusively to assisted reproduction technique personnel to decrease contamination of the suite. During IVF cycles, only essential personnel in appropriate clean attire are permitted to enter the laboratory. All entrances are equipped with an adhesive mat to remove any dust and/or dirt from the soles of shoes. All personnel entering the laboratory spaces during in vitro fertilization cycles are required to wear clean scrubs, dedicated shoes or booties, and a scrub cap in accordance with best practice habits of high performing in vitro fertilization programs.[23]

25.3.2 *Air filtration system*

The new air filtration system included clean steam technology to control humidity, air that was passed through paper pre-filters, an ultraviolet light section, two chemical beds of activated carbon mixed with potassium permanganate (Purafil, Doraville, Georgia) and a bank of high efficiency filters. Ultimately, air entered the ART suite through a final set of HEPA filters. Air temperature and humidity within the ART suite were controlled before reaching the laboratory and procedure room environments by a programmed control system.

Plans were made for the entire ART suite to undergo 15 air changes per hour. The temperature is maintained at 22.0°C–25.0°C, and relative humidity is maintained at 30–35%. The air supply for the laboratory is maintained at 50% outside air and 50% recirculated air. The air supplied to the ART suite heating, ventilation, and air conditioning (HVAC) unit from the outside is provided from a region of the building that was previously determined to have the cleanest air (15.1 $\mu g/m^3$ total VOC content) around the hospital building. Recirculated air has been filtered by the hospital's HVAC system starting after the pre-filters. In the event of poor outside environmental conditions (i.e., construction, high pollution day), the air-handling unit can be "submarined" and adjusted to run on 100% recirculated air to significantly decrease contaminants.

Gas cylinders that supply incubators and isolettes used for embryology procedures were confined to a dedicated tank room outside the ART suite. This allowed the potentially unclean exteriors of the gas cylinders to be maintained separately from the laboratory environment. Gas was then transported from the cylinder banks to various pieces of equipment through fluorinated ethylene propylene tubing that was installed as continuous lines during construction. This prevented potential contamination of gassed environments because there are no entry points created by connections.

25.4 *Our experience*

25.4.1 *Study design*

As a result of the required lab move and resultant laboratory design and construction, the authors set out to compare patient cycle outcomes along with laboratory measures for the last year of IVF cycles at the old facility and the first year at the new facility.[10] An Internal Review Board (IRB) approved retrospective cohort analysis of all fresh, autologous, IVF and intracytoplasmic sperm injection (ICSI) cycles carried out at the old and new facilities between January 2011 and October 2012 was conducted. The last cycle at the old facility was conducted in August 2011 and the first cycle in the new facility was carried out in January 2012. It is important to note there were no changes in physician personnel, laboratory equipment, or protocols during the defined study period. Moreover, no donor oocyte or donor embryo cycles were performed at our facility.

The primary outcome was live birth with secondary outcomes including implantation, clinical pregnancy, multiple gestations, biochemical pregnancy, spontaneous abortion, number of embryos transferred, number of day 5 transfers, and number of embryos cryopreserved.

25.4.2 Outcomes

As referred to previously, air quality testing carried out at the new facility revealed improved air quality metrics and decreased environmental contaminations at the new ART site, as compare with the old site (total VOCs were 819.4 μg/m^3 vs. 32 μg/m^3). The average temperature and humidity in the in vitro fertilization suite at the old facility were 20°C and 51.8%, whereas the new air handling system conditions were 25°C and 30%.

A total of 820 fresh start cycles were included in the retrospective analysis. In 2011 there were 388 at the old facility and in 2012 there were 432 at the new facility that were identified for the study time period. There were no statistically significant differences noted in the baseline demographics (e.g., age, cycle number, day 3 FSH, or primary infertility diagnosis) between the cohorts.

Comparison of the average number of oocytes retrieved, mature oocytes, and fertilized oocytes revealed no difference between the two study years. However, when the mature and fertilized oocyte percentage per patient was analyzed, a higher percentage of fertilized oocytes per patient was observed at the new facility.

A total of 377 transfers were carried out at the old facility and 406 transfers carried out in the new facility. No differences were observed in the percentage of day 3 and day 5 transfers between the cohorts. One interesting finding was that more single blastocyst transfers were carried out at the new facility. No differences were observed in the total number of patients who had at least one embryo available for cryopreservation, but in patients with embryos available, there were more embryos vitrified per patient at the new facility, as compared to the old facility.

Implantation, clinical pregnancy, and live births were all significantly increased in the new facility, while the percentage of biochemical pregnancies and spontaneous abortions were consistent between the two facilities. The incidence of multiple gestation pregnancies was decreased by 40%.

Comparison of day 3 embryology was conducted to assess any difference in laboratory embryology metrics between the two facilities. A total of 2548 embryos at the old facility and 2955 at the new facility were analyzed and no differences were noted in the number of embryos with six or more cells with 20% or more fragmentation on day 3.

No differences were found between the two cohorts when comparing the number of transfers of blastocysts (blastocyst, expanded blastocyst, hatching blastocyst); comparing inner cell mass (ICM) grade between transferring embryos; fertilization rates; or intracytoplasmic sperm injection rates when comparing the two facilities. Of note, improved trophectoderm cell grading was seen at the new facility.

25.5 Expert commentary

At this point, most authorities recognize the negative ramifications poor air quality and laboratory conditions exhibit on developing embryos in the in vitro setting. There can be profound consequences on IVF success using identifiable and quantifiable measures to include embryo quality, implantation, and pregnancy.

The literature is growing with evidence suggesting that improvements in air quality and laboratory conditions improve in vitro fertilization outcomes. Boone et al. published a retrospective cohort study that revealed an improvement in air quality and IVF success rates after constructing a class 100 clean room.[15] Cohen et al. examined the effect of ambient air in the IVF laboratory and showed that outside air may actually be a better source than laboratory air because of the accumulation of VOCs in outside air.[16] Off-gassing from sterile Petri dishes, incubators, cleaning supplies, monitors, microscopes, and furniture all contribute compounds, which may negatively affect air quality. Esteves et al. compared IVF outcomes after intracytoplasmic sperm injection between 1999 and 2010 in an in vitro fertilization laboratory after the implementation of Brazilian national clean room standards. These investigators showed an improvement in live births with a decrease in spontaneous abortions between the defined study periods.[11] Khoudja et al. reported improved in vitro fertilization outcomes with air quality improvements.[19] In their study, the authors compared two filtration systems (carbon vs. a honeycomb matrix media aligned in the Landson™ series system) and found the new technology significantly improved air and embryo quality, ultimately improving implantation and pregnancy rates. Taken together, these studies make the argument for systems to improve air handling and filtration to minimize negative effects of VOCs.

25.6 Conclusion

Analysis of data from the new ART laboratory facility, built with consideration of environmental factors and a state of the art air handling system, reveal an increase in both implantation and live birth without an increase in biochemical pregnancies or spontaneous abortions. Most importantly, the improvements observed with regard to pregnancy were seen in conjunction with an increased use of single blastocyst transfer. While commonly understood to be a critical aspect of the ART program, evidence supporting the importance of the laboratory environment is underreported in the literature. Our program's experience helps to reinforce the evidence of improved IVF outcomes after improvement in air quality and environmental conditions.

References

1. Practice Committee of the American Society for Reproductive Medicine. Diagnostic evaluation of the infertile female: A committee opinion. *Fertility and Sterility* 2015; **103**(6): e44–50.
2. Practice Committee of the American Society for Reproductive Medicine. Diagnostic evaluation of the infertile male: A committee opinion. *Fertility and Sterility* 2015; **103**(3): e18–25.
3. Healy DL, Trounson AO, and Andersen AN. Female infertility: Causes and treatment. *Lancet* 1994; **343**(8912): 1539–44.
4. Stanford JB. What is the true prevalence of infertility? *Fertility and Sterility* 2013; **99**(5): 1201–2.
5. Macaluso M, Wright-Schnapp TJ, Chandra A et al. A public health focus on infertility prevention, detection, and management. *Fertility and Sterility* 2010; **93**(1): 16 e1–0.
6. Warner L, Jamieson DJ, and Barfield WD. CDC releases a national public health action plan for the detection, prevention, and management of infertility. *Journal of Women's Health* 2015; **24**(7): 548–9.
7. Trantham P. The infertile couple. *American Family Physician* 1996; **54**(3): 1001–10.
8. Sunderam S, Kissin DM, Crawford S et al. Assisted reproductive technology surveillance—United States, 2010. *Morbidity and Mortality Weekly Report Surveillance Summaries* 2013; **62**(9): 1–24.

9. Fritz MA and Speroff L. *Clinical Gynecologic Endocrinology and Infertility*. Philadelphia, PA: Lippincott Williams & Wilkins, a Wolters Kluwer business; 2011.
10. Heitmann RJ, Hill MJ, James AN et al. Live births achieved via IVF are increased by improvements in air quality and laboratory environment. *Reproductive Biomedicine Online* 2015.
11. Esteves SC and Bento FC. Implementation of air quality control in reproductive laboratories in full compliance with the Brazilian Cells and Germinative Tissue Directive. *Reproductive Biomedicine Online* 2013; **26**(1): 9–21.
12. Laumbach R, Meng Q, and Kipen H. What can individuals do to reduce personal health risks from air pollution? *Journal of Thoracic Disease* 2015; **7**(1): 96–107.
13. Pope CA, 3rd, Ezzati M, and Dockery DW. Fine-particulate air pollution and life expectancy in the United States. *The New England Journal of Medicine* 2009; **360**(4): 376–86.
14. Laden F, Schwartz J, Speizer FE, and Dockery DW. Reduction in fine particulate air pollution and mortality: Extended follow-up of the Harvard Six Cities study. *American Journal of Respiratory and Critical Care Medicine* 2006; **173**(6): 667–72.
15. Boone WR, Johnson JE, Locke AJ, Crane MM, and Price TM. Control of air quality in an assisted reproductive technology laboratory. *Fertility and Sterility* 1999; **71**(1): 150–4.
16. Cohen J, Gilligan A, Esposito W, Schimmel T, and Dale B. Ambient air and its potential effects on conception in vitro. *Human Reproduction* 1997; **12**(8): 1742–9.
17. Cohen J, Gilligan A, and Willadsen S. Culture and quality control of embryos. *Human Reproduction* 1998; **13 Suppl 3**: 137–44; discussion 45–7.
18. Hall J, Gilligan A, Schimmel T, Cecchi M, and Cohen J. The origin, effects and control of air pollution in laboratories used for human embryo culture. *Human Reproduction* 1998; **13 Suppl 4**: 146–55.
19. Khoudja RY, Xu Y, Li T, and Zhou C. Better IVF outcomes following improvements in laboratory air quality. *Journal of Assisted Reproduction and Genetics* 2013; **30**(1): 69–76.
20. Legro RS, Sauer MV, Mottla GL et al. Effect of air quality on assisted human reproduction. *Human Reproduction* 2010; **25**(5): 1317–24.
21. Ritz B and Wilhelm M. Ambient air pollution and adverse birth outcomes: Methodologic issues in an emerging field. *Basic & Clinical Pharmacology & Toxicology* 2008; **102**(2): 182–90.
22. Dadvand P, Rankin J, Rushton S, and Pless-Mulloli T. Association between maternal exposure to ambient air pollution and congenital heart disease: A register-based spatiotemporal analysis. *American Journal of Epidemiology* 2011; **173**(2): 171–82.
23. Van Voorhis BJ, Thomas M, Surrey ES, and Sparks A. What do consistently high-performing in vitro fertilization programs in the U.S. do? *Fertility and Sterility* 2010; **94**(4): 1346–9.
24. Practice Committee of American Society for Reproductive Medicine, Practice Committee of Society for Assisted Reproductive Technology. Revised guidelines for human embryology and andrology laboratories. *Fertility and Sterility* 2008; **90**(5 Suppl): S45–59.
25. Practice Committee of the American Society for Reproductive Medicine, Society for Assisted Reproductive Technology. Revised guidelines for human embryology and andrology laboratories. *Fertility and Sterility* 2004; **82**(6): 1736–53.
26. Practice Committee of the American Society for Reproductive Medicine, Practice Committee of the Society for Assisted Reproductive Technology. Revised guidelines for human embryology and andrology laboratories. *Fertility and Sterility* 2006; **86**(5 Suppl 1): S57–72.
27. Practice Committee of the American Society for Reproductive Medicine, Practice Committee of the Society for Assisted Reproductive Technology, Practice Committee of the Society of Reproductive Biologists and, Technologists. Recommended practices for the management of embryology, andrology, and endocrinology laboratories: A committee opinion. *Fertility and Sterility* 2014; **102**(4): 960–3.

chapter twenty-six

Clean room technology and IVF outcomes: Brazil

Sandro C. Esteves and Fabiola C. Bento

Contents

Abstract

The Brazilian Cells and Tissue Directive (BCTD) established common standards of quality and safety for the donation, procurement, testing, processing, preservation, storage, and distribution of human tissues and cells across Brazil. The BCTD requires ART units to provide air quality control with chemical and particle filtration for gamete/embryo processing. The new requirements led many clinics, including ours, to modify their laboratories to improve air quality. This chapter describes how we designed our facility at Androfert Center in compliance with the BCTD with regard to air quality standards. We also describe how we monitor air quality within the clean room areas, and present data of air monitoring and intracytoplasmic sperm injection outcomes performed in our controlled environments. Our experience with the handling of human gametes and culturing embryos in full compliance with the Brazilian directive air quality standards has been reassuring. According to our data, performing assisted reproductive technology in controlled environments not only optimizes IVF outcomes but also ensures the highest safety standards.

26.1 Introduction

The Brazilian National Agency for Sanitary Surveillance (ANVISA) has established specific recommendations for air quality standards in reproductive laboratories since 2006.[1] This directive, namely, the Brazilian Cells and Tissues Directive (BCTD), is a legal document setting standards of quality and safety for the donation, procurement, testing, processing, preservation, storage, and distribution of human reproductive tissues and cells. In brief, the BCTD aims at increasing quality through the mandatory implementation of a quality management system that involves the presence of adequately trained and certified staff, full documentation and formulation of standard operating procedures, and quality control and quality assurance at all units performing assisted reproduction. Its aims are to safeguard public health by preventing the transmission of infectious diseases via transplanted tissues and cells, according to the premises of the precautionary principle.[2] Assisted reproductive technology (ART) is under the coverage of this directive. It means all Brazilian Fertility Centers performing ART should comply with this legal document.

The Brazilian Cells and Tissues Directive was amended in 2011. It included specific air quality recommendations for rooms where gametes are collected in addition to the existing standards for reproductive laboratories.[3] With respect to laboratory ambient air, the BCTD dictates that it should be at least equivalent to ISO class 5 in the critical areas where tissues or cells are exposed to the environment during processing, and recommends one of the following methods to achieve such conditions: (1) biological safety cabinet class II type A; (2) unidirectional laminar flow workstation; or (3) at least equivalent ISO 5 clean room.[4] Whenever biological safety cabinets and unidirectional laminar flows are used, background air (clean areas for carrying out less critical stages) should be pressurized. Specifically, minimum standards include an outside and total air volume of 15 and 45 $[m^3/h]/m^2$. In addition, supplied air from outside should be filtered for particulates using at least G3 + F8 dust filtration.

Areas in which gametes are surgically retrieved (oocytes, reproductive tissue, and epididymal/testicular sperm) should have the ambient air pressurized (outside and total air volume of 6 and 18 $[m^3/h]/m^2$ or higher) and filtered for particulates (at least G4 class dust filtration). In addition, cryostorage rooms should be equipped with systems to monitor oxygen in ambient air and to exhaust air under negative pressure equivalent to at least 75 $m^3/h/m^2$. Last, ventilation systems should be equipped with filters embedded with activated charcoal to remove volatile organic compounds (VOCs). A detailed discussion about the BCTD and how it compares with the European Union directive is presented in Chapter 18.

In this chapter, we describe how we implemented an embryology laboratory and related areas with air quality control in full compliance with the Brazilian Cells and Germinative Tissue Directive. We also present results from monitoring air quality within the clean room areas, and retrospective data from handling and culturing human embryos in our clean room facilities. At large, the information presented here has been published elsewhere.[5,6]

26.2 Design and implementation of clean room areas

26.2.1 Overall air filtration system design

In order to comply with the BCTD air quality requirements, we opted for a clean room model. This system was applied not only to the embryology laboratory but also to related areas, including the operating theater where oocytes and sperm are retrieved, and embryo transfer and sperm processing rooms (Figure 26.1). Our system was designed to supply pressurized air, cleaned by chemical and particulate filters, with adequate heating, cooling, and humidification capacity to meet daily needs. Lock-controlled doors with sealing, designed to maintain a positive pressure environment, separate each room. The embryology lab has the highest level of positive air pressure with a decreasing pressure gradient as the air flows to each subsequent room. At the end of the construction, we waited three months to allow off-gassing before occupying the new facilities. During this period, the air handling ventilation unit, described below, was set up to continuously bring in fresh air. After this period, testing was carried out by a third party company to validate our areas, both "at rest" and "at operational" states. Validation procedures confirmed that our facility was built according to the design of the engineers and met the standards required by both the user and regulatory authorities.

26.2.2 Construction details

Our clean room facility was designed and constructed following the ISO 14644-4 standards.[7] Constructive materials, including internal finishes, doors, air vents/diffusers, floor and ceiling elements, were selected based on their cleanability, durability, maintainability, and low VOC emission. Specifically, exposed materials were suitable for effective and frequent cleaning. All surfaces, including ceilings, walls, and floors, were made of smooth, impervious, and nonshedding materials that offered no surface asperities or porosity which might allow retention of particulate and chemical contamination, or the development of microbiological contamination. Wall surfaces are covered with low odor epoxy-based paint, and floors are made of sheet vinyl with heat-welded seams and a coved base, with the exception of the embryology laboratory in which polyurethane-based coatings were used for walls and floor finishes.

The junctures of the ceiling to the walls are coved. Lighting fixtures are flush-mounted within the ceiling and sealed, and there are no sinks or floor drains in the clean room areas. We selected materials with reduced VOC off-gassing potential in accordance with the United States Environmental Protection Agency specifications on the environmental impact of materials.[8] As examples, fiberglass, wood, and plastic-based materials were not used, and prefabricated site-assembled construction materials were avoided. Instead, in situ wet construction with applied surface finishes was preferred. Stainless steel and anodized aluminium were used in doors, windows, air vents, and diffusers, as well as in workstations. Water-based low VOC adhesives were used when needed.

26.2.3 Air handling ventilation unit (AHVU) room

The AHVU room (2.1 m width × 3.9 m length × 2.5 m height [20.5 m^3]) included a rooftop air-handling unit (model UAECA-300, Veco, Campinas, Brazil) that draws outside air through coarse (G4) and activated carbon pre-filters before it enters the main ventilation unit. A free-standing main ventilation unit (model UVCA-3000; Veco, Campinas, Brazil) pulls pre-filtered outside air and clean rooms' return air through coarse (G3) filters (first

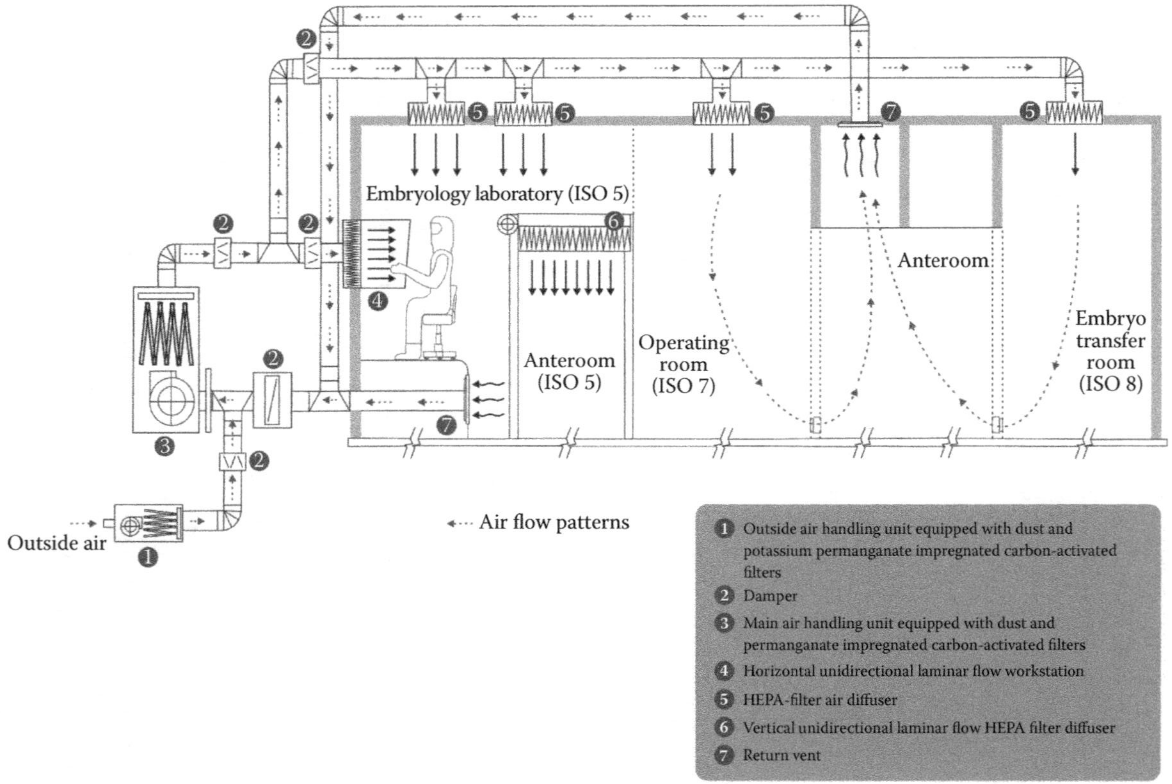

Figure 26.1 Schematic representation of clean rooms (embryology suite, operating theater, and embryo transfer suite). Airflow patterns and filtration units are also depicted. The air-handling ventilation unit is located in a separate room. An external rooftop subunit draws outside air that goes through coarse and activated carbon prefilters before entering into the main unit. The main ventilation unit pulls pre-filtered outside air and the clean rooms' return air through coarse filters, past a 16-unit potassium permanganate-impregnated pelletized coconut shell-based activated carbon filter and then through fine dust filters. Last, filtered air enters the clean rooms through a set of high efficiency particulate air (HEPA) filters. Floor- and ceiling-level vents in the clean rooms return air to the main ventilation unit to be remixed with the existing air. Differential positive pressure is maintained between rooms. The embryology laboratory/anteroom is positive to the operating room, which is positive to both the embryo-transfer room and the dressing room/hallways. (Reprinted from Esteves SC and Bento FC, *Reprod Biomed Online* 2013; 26(1): 9–21, with permission from Elsevier.)

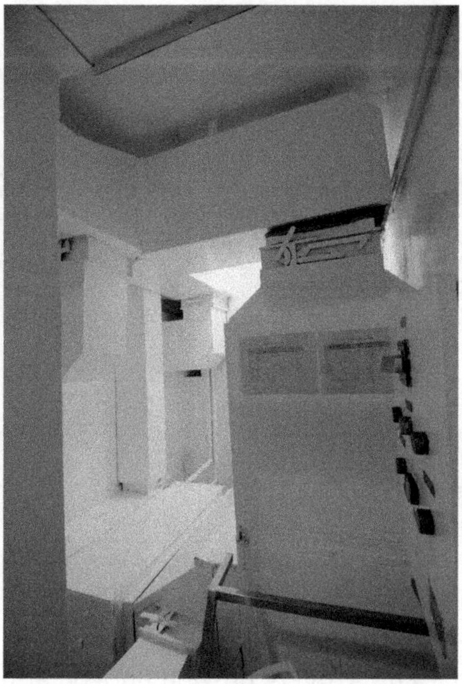

Figure 26.2 Air handling ventilation unit room depicting the free-standing main ventilation unit.

stage filtration), past a 16-unit pelletized coconut shell-based activated carbon impregnated with potassium permanganate filters (second-stage filtration), and then through fine (F8) dust filters (third-stage filtration) (Figure 26.2). Last, filtered air enters clean rooms through high efficiency particulate air (HEPA) filter diffusers. Floor- and ceiling-level vents return air to the main ventilation unit, to be remixed with the existing air. The air supply for the clean rooms is maintained at 20% outside air and 80% recirculated air. The temperature and humidity of air supplied to the clean rooms are controlled.

Filter beds (593 × 593 × 22 mm; mesh size 4 × 8), containing potassium permanganate impregnated zeolite plus activated carbon, are utilized. Chemical filters, located downstream of the cooling and heating coils, were arranged in a "Z" configuration with the airflow nearly perpendicular through each bed. Nominal bed residence times of chemical air cleaners are 0.082 second. Activated-carbon lifetime estimates were determined by sampling in service filters at three-month intervals over a one-year period by carbon tetrachloride activity (CTC) method.[9] A reduction of 50% of the original filter activity was observed after 12 months and determined filter-working capacity. The replacement schedule was set at six- to eight-month intervals. This estimation was considered to be adequate to avoid reaching breakthrough capacity due to the moderate polluted urban nonindustrial area where our facility is located. Type G3 filters are primary filters that collect coarse dust with a dust spot efficiency of 80–90%, while type F8 are secondary filters that collect and retain small particle dust with a spot efficiency of 90–95%.

26.2.4 *Embryology laboratory suite*

Air enters the embryology lab suite (3.5 m width × 3.9 m length × 2.5 m height [34.1 m^3]) through a final set of ceiling-mounted high efficiency particulate air (HEPA) filters (Figure 26.3).

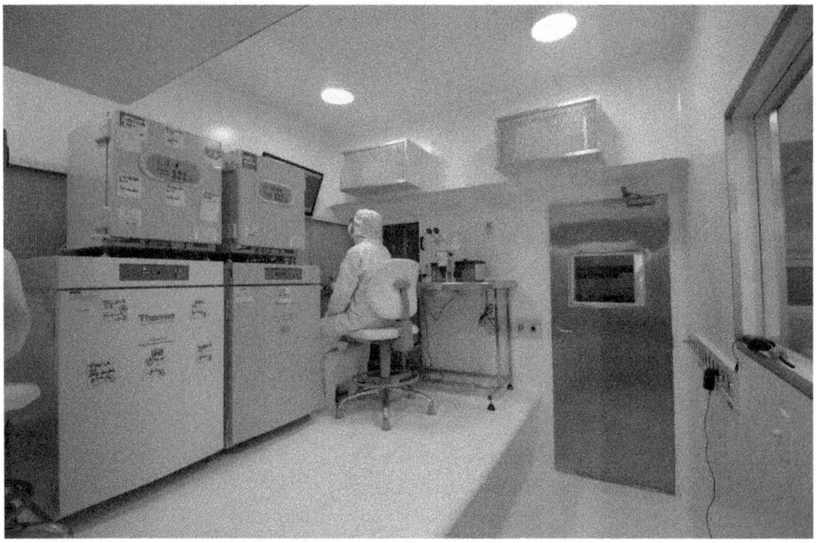

Figure 26.3 **(See color insert.)** Overview of embryology laboratory suite.

Wall-mounted terminal HEPA filters provide horizontal unidirectional laminar air flow to the incoming oocytes and outgoing embryos and micromanipulation workstations (Figures 26.4 and 26.5).

Four vents at the floor level return the air to the main air handling ventilation unit (Figure 26.6). Gas cylinders that supply incubators are confined to a dedicated tank room outside the lab suite.

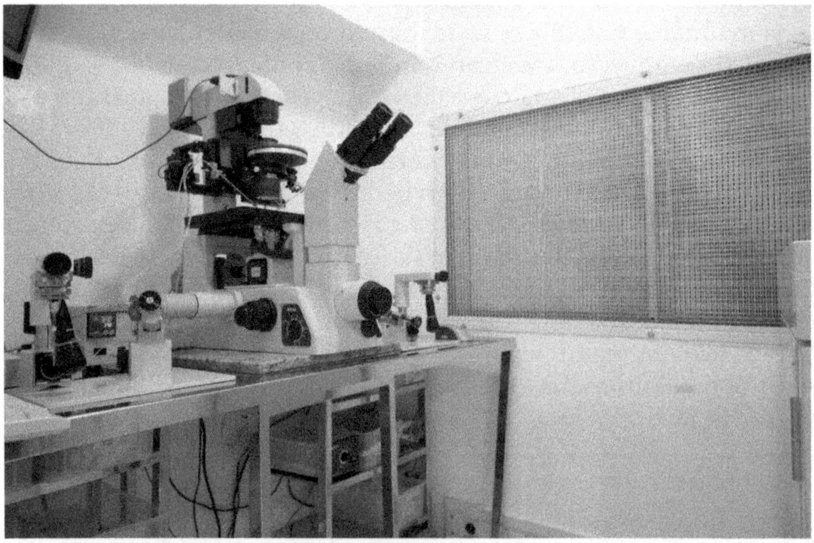

Figure 26.4 **(See color insert.)** Overview of a workstation for micromanipulation of oocytes, sperm, and embryos. A wall-mounted frame with a terminal high efficiency particulate air (HEPA) filter supplies unidirectional airflow within the work area.

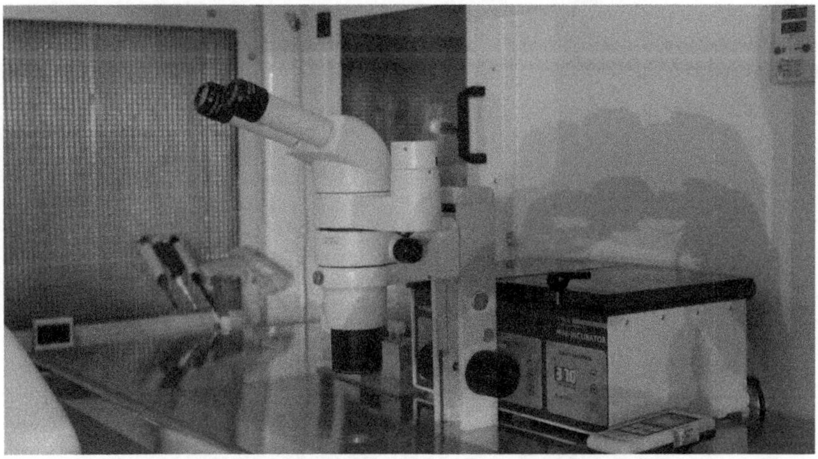

Figure 26.5 **(See color insert.)** Overview of a workstation for handling oocytes and embryos. A wall-mounted frame with a terminal high efficiency particulate air (HEPA) filter supplies unidirectional airflow within the work area.

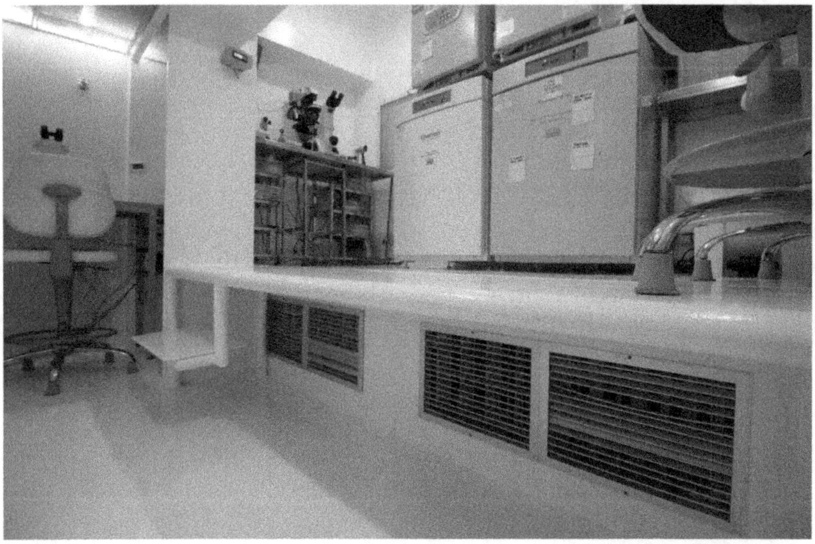

Figure 26.6 **(See color insert.)** Overview of floor level return vents in the embryology laboratory suite.

Access to the clean room is made through an anteroom equipped with two ceiling HEPA filter air diffusers that draw clean room air and provide vertical unidirectional laminar airflow to the entire anteroom. This room has a clean closet to store face masks, safety glasses, hoods, coveralls, boots, and a few disposable laboratory supplies for daily use, and is used as a gowning room (Figure 26.7).

The anteroom and clean room IVF lab undergo 499 and 103 air exchanges per hour, respectively. The anteroom is a transitional area that maintains a differential air pressure relationship between the embryology laboratory and andrology laboratory. The embryology lab is an ISO 5 clean room where temperature is maintained at 22–25°C and relative humidity at 30–55%.

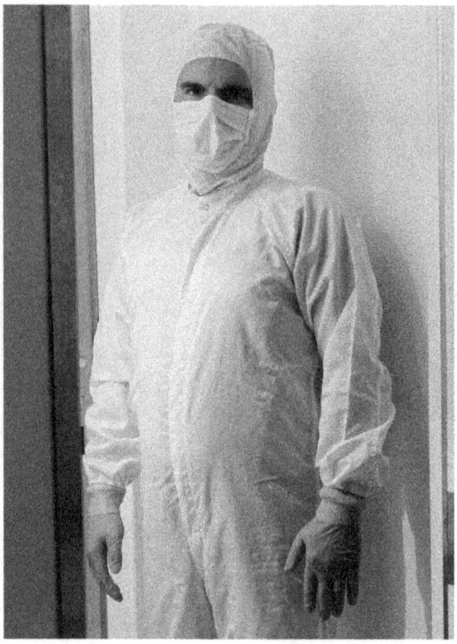

Figure 26.7 Gowned staff.

26.2.5 Andrology laboratory suite

The andrology laboratory (3.5 m width × 5.1 length × 2.8 m height [50.0 m^3]) has a rooftop air-handling unit (model UAECA-300, Veco, Campinas, Brazil) that draws outside air through coarse (G3 and F8) and activated carbon filters before it enters a ceiling-mounted HEPA-filter air diffuser that distributes filtered air to the laboratory under positive pressure at 721 m^3/h, as depicted in Figure 26.8. The andrology lab is an ISO 7 clean room where the temperature is maintained at 22–25°C and the relative humidity at 30–55%.

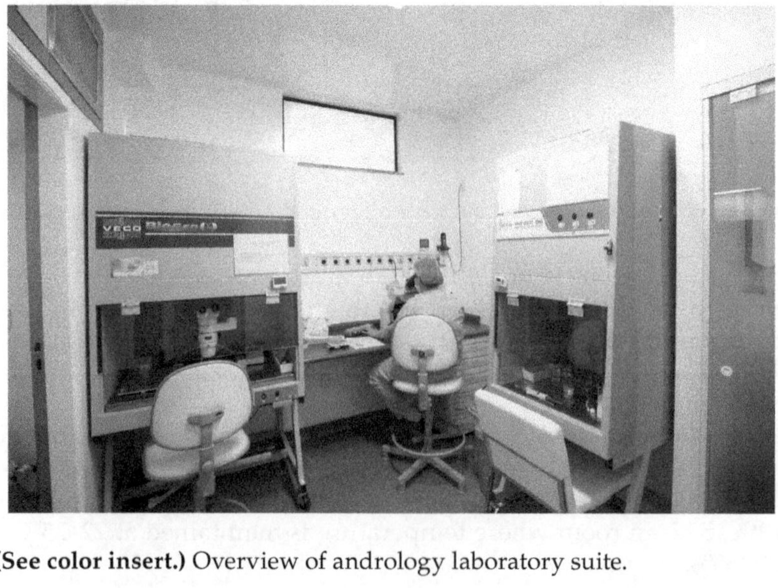

Figure 26.8 **(See color insert.)** Overview of andrology laboratory suite.

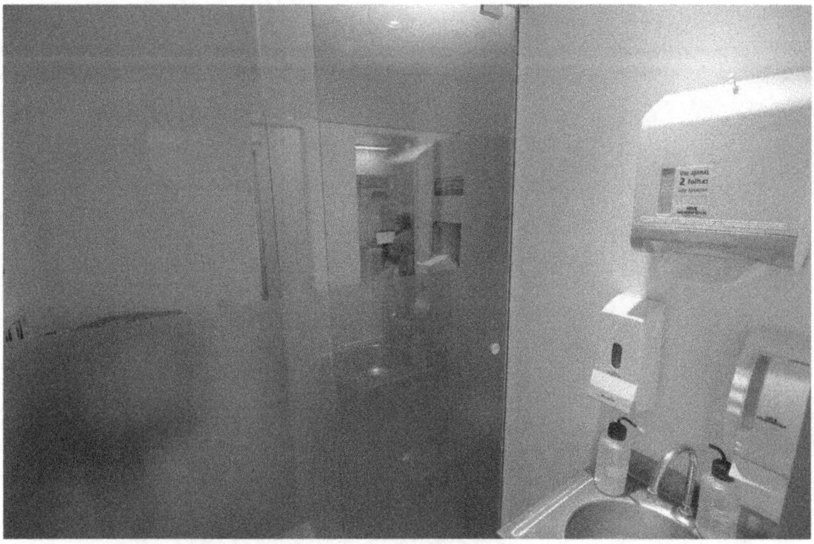

Figure 26.9 Overview of andrology laboratory suite anteroom.

The andrology lab is used for sperm processing, and for thawing gametes, embryos, and reproductive tissue. The laboratory is equipped with class II type A1 biological safety cabinets (model Bioseg-09, Veco, Campinas, Brazil) where handling of biological material takes place. This type of cabinet is appropriate for the aforementioned activities due to the absence of hazard vapors/gases and low contamination risk of reproductive cells/tissues to personnel and the ambient air. Access to the andrology laboratory suite is made through an anteroom where personnel dress and perform hand hygiene (Figure 26.9).

26.2.6 *Operating theater*

Air enters the operating theater (4.7 m width × 3.6 length × 2.8 m height [47.4 m^3]) through a final set of ceiling-mounted high efficiency particulate air (HEPA) filters. Return vents are located at wall level (Figures 26.1 and 26.10). Using these passageways, the air in the room undergoes 12 exchanges per hour. The operating theater is an ISO 7 clean room.

The operating theater is equipped with a mobile cabinet (model DM-66, Veco, Campinas, Brazil) that provides HEPA-filtered, vertical, and unidirectional airflow to the work area where tubes are uncapped during oocyte collection (Figure 26.11).

Access to the operating room is made through an anteroom where personnel perform hand hygiene. Also, this anteroom is a transitional area that maintains the air pressure relationship between the operating and gowning rooms, ensuring air flows from clean to dirty areas, reducing the need for the HVAC control system to respond to significant disturbances.

26.2.7 *Embryo transfer suite*

Air enters the embryo transfer suite (3.0 m width × 3.2 length × 2.6 m height [24.9 m^3]) through a terminal ceiling-mounted HEPA filter. The embryo transfer room, located

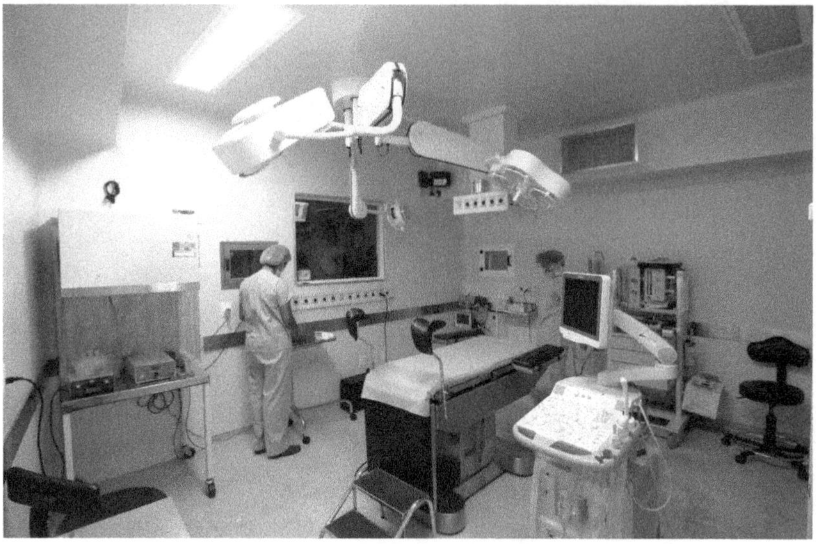

Figure 26.10 **(See color insert.)** Overview of operating theater.

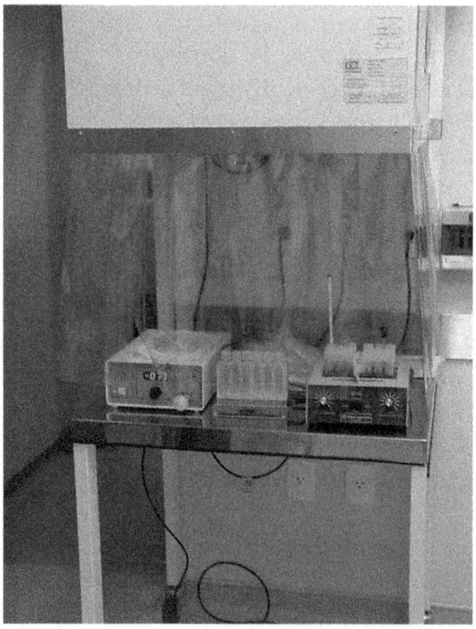

Figure 26.11 **(See color insert.)** Cabinet in which tubes to collect follicular fluid are handled during oocyte pick-up. A ceiling-mounted high efficiency particulate air (HEPA) filtration system provides vertical unidirectional airflow to the work area.

adjacent to the operating room (Figure 26.1), undergoes nine air exchanges per hour. The embryo transfer room is an ISO 8 clean room.

26.2.8 Positive pressure

Differential positive pressure is maintained among rooms. The embryology lab has the highest level of positive air pressure with a decreasing pressure gradient as the air flows to each subsequent room. The embryology laboratory/anteroom is positive to the andrology laboratory (2.1 mm water column differential [mmWC]), which is positive to both the andrology laboratory anteroom and hallways (1.5 mmWC). The operating theater is positive to both the transfer room and the dressing room/hallways (0.5 mmWC).

26.2.9 Cryostorage suite

Liquid nitrogen tanks containing cryopreserved specimens are stored in the cryopreservation room (3.1 m width × 3.5 length × 3.0 m height [32.5 m^3]). The cryoroom is equipped with an oxygen depletion alarm unit and a ventilation system (model UE 500, Veco, Campinas, Brazil) to exhaust ambient air under negative pressure at 150 cubic meters per hour per square meter (Figure 26.12).

Table 26.1 provides a summary of how we set up our facility in compliance with the Brazilian Cell and Tissue Directive requirements regarding air quality control.

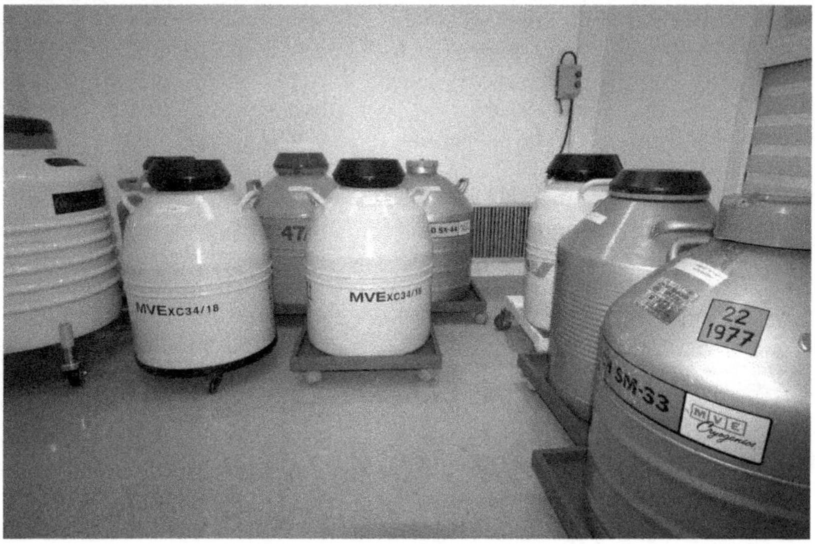

Figure 26.12 Overview of cryostorage suite.

Table 26.1 Air quality requirements as per the Brazilian Cell and Tissue Directive and how Androfert Center has complied with these requirements

Air quality control	Directive requirements (Anvisa RDC33/2006; RDC23/2011)	How we implemented at Androfert
Particulate matter	At least equivalent to ISO class 5 (NBR/ISO 14644-1) in the critical areas where tissues or cells are exposed to the environment during processing, and one of the following methods should be used to achieve such conditions: (1) biological safety cabinet class II type A; (2) unidirectional laminar flow workstation; (3) at least equivalent ISO 5 clean room.	A dedicated room holds a free-standing air handling ventilation unit (AHVU) that insufflates a combination of outside and recirculated indoor filtered air to the embryology laboratory. The system comprises three filtration stages, including coarse (G3) filters (first stage filtration), activated carbon impregnated with potassium permanganate filters (second stage filtration), and fine (F8) dust filters followed by high efficiency particulate air (HEPA) filters (third stage filtration). The AHVU provides 30 and 268 $[m^3/h]/m^2$ outside and total air volume, respectively, and the embryology lab undergoes 103 air exchanges per hour. As a result, the embryology laboratory is equivalent to an ISO 5 clean room.
	Whenever biological safety cabinets and unidirectional laminar flows are used, background air (clean areas for carrying out less critical stages) should be pressurized. Minimum standards include an outside and total air volume of 15 and 45 $[m^3/h]/m^2$. In addition, supplied air should be filtered for particulates using at least G3 + F8 dust filtration.	The andrology laboratory is equipped with class II type A1 biological safety cabinets where sperm processing and related-activities takes place. An independent AHVU air-handling unit draws outside air that is pushed through coarse filters (type G3; first-stage filtration), activated carbon filters containing potassium permanganate impregnated zeolite (second-stage filtration), and then F8 + HEPA filters (third-stage filtration). Filtered air is distributed to the lab under positive pressure with 15 and 51 $[m^3/h]/m^2$ outside and total air volume, respectively. As a result, the andrology laboratory is equivalent to an ISO 7 clean room.
	Areas in which gametes are surgically retrieved should have ambient air pressurized. Minimum standards include an outside and total air volume of 6 and 18 $[m^3/h]/m^2$. In addition, supplied air should be filtered for particulates using at least G4 filters.	Air supplied to the operating theatre, where oocytes and surgically retrieved sperm are collected, comes from the main AHVU that supplies air to the embryology lab. Filtered air is distributed to the room under positive pressure with 8 and 34.8 $[m^3/h]/m^2$ outside and total air volume, respectively. As a result, the operating theatre laboratory is equivalent to an ISO 7 clean room.

(*Continued*)

Table 26.1 (Continued) Air quality requirements as per the Brazilian Cell and Tissue Directive and how Androfert Center has complied with these requirements

Air quality control	Directive requirements (Anvisa RDC33/2006; RDC23/2011)	How we implemented at Androfert
Volatile organic compound	Ventilation systems are equipped with filters imbedded with activated carbon.	A 16-filter beds containing pelletized coconut shell based activated carbon impregnated with potassium permanganate comprises a second stage filtration. Chemical filters, arranged in a "Z" configuration with the airflow nearly perpendicular through each bed, were located downstream of the cooling and heating coils.
Cryopreservation storage room	Cryostorage rooms are equipped with systems to monitor oxygen in ambient air and to exhaust air under negative pressure equivalent to at least 75 $m^3/h/m^2$.	Cryorooms are equipped with oxygen depletion alarms and a ventilation system that exhausts ambient air under negative pressure at 150 $m^3/h/m^2$.

26.3 Additional mechanisms to reduce contamination

In addition to the construction details, several measures are taken to reduce contamination. Only the minimum amount of furniture, equipment, and supplies are brought into the clean rooms. Furniture and equipment are nonpermeable, nonshedding, cleanable, and resistant to frequent cleaning and disinfecting. Personnel access to reproductive laboratories is limited, and is made through anterooms equipped with a gowning chamber and hand-hygiene area. All personnel entering the clean rooms are required to gown up properly. Embryology laboratory personnel wear nonshedding Dacron coveralls, hoods, and shoe covers as well as masks and nitrile gloves. In addition, personnel are required to step on adhesive covered mats that remove dirt and dust from the soles of shoes. Wall-mounted pass-throughs between the embryology laboratory and operating room, and between the andrology lab and operating room allow for passage of gametes and embryos between these locations, thus minimizing air pressure differential loss. Care is taken to select and use commodity items in the embryology laboratory. Lint-free wipes, clean room paper, and pencils only are allowed. Cosmetics are banned. Ultra high-purity (UHP) medical grade compressed carbon dioxide is supplied to incubators, and dedicated gas lines are fitted with particulate and chemical filters (GenX, US).

A list of cleaning tasks is performed on a daily basis in all clean rooms, including wiping of all work surfaces as well as equipment and vents, and mopping floors and walls. For this, clean room tissue and isopropyl alcohol are used. Cleaning activities are carried out at the end of working days. On a monthly basis, incubators are "term-cleaned." Annually, rooms are sanitized with 2% sodium hypochlorite solutions. As part of quality control, rooms' and incubators' temperature and humidity values are obtained twice a day. Quarterly, an inhibitive mold agar Petri dish (for molds/fungus) and a blood agar

Petri dish (for bacteria) are labelled with the room, location, and date, and sent to microbiological analysis.

26.4 Air-quality monitoring

Initial testings were performed before occupation ("as built"), "at rest" and "at normal operation." Assessed parameters included determination of air volume flow rate, air exchange rate, room air pressure differential, filter integrity leak testing, airborne particle cleanliness counts, recovery performance testing, lighting and noise level measurements, temperature, and humidity monitoring. Particle counts were performed in various locations within the embryology laboratory and other critical areas. We monitored the embryology suite, the operating room, anterooms, laminar flow cabinets, embryo transfer room, andrology laboratory, and the gowning room (Figure 26.13).

Ten-particle-count cycles were performed at each of the nine sites, and the results were pooled to provide mean counts for different particle sizes (0.3, 0.5, and 5.0 μm) in each site. Determination of VOC levels in the embryology laboratory was carried out by active sampling on Tenax TA sorbent, followed by thermal desorption and gas chromatography employing a mass spectrometric detector, in accordance with the US EPA method TO-1.[10] The presence of aldehydes was determined by active sampling using adsorbent cartridges coated with 2,4-dinitrophenylhydrazine (DNPH) and subsequent analysis of the hydrazones formed by high performance liquid chromatography with detection by ultraviolet absorption, in accordance with the ISO 16000-3 standards.[11] The embryology laboratory was selected as the appropriate room for sampling because it is the place where gametes and embryos are exposed to ambient air. Incubators were not checked since 90–95% of chamber air consists of ambient air, and the remaining comes from chemical and particulate-filtered CO_2.

After initial validation, a third-party certification company has been carrying out monitoring to ensure compliance with the ISO 14644-1 norm. The schedule of testing to demonstrate compliance with limits of airborne particle concentration, airflow volume, air pressure difference, number of air exchanges per hour, ambient air humidity, and room temperature was set at six-month intervals, in accordance to the ISO 14644 (parts 2 and 3) specifications.[12,13] Physical inspection of the ventilation and filtration mechanical system is also performed. Annually, additional testing within the testing schedule includes HEPA filter integrity leak testing, recovery performance testing, and containment leakage and noise levels. A detailed analysis of clean room monitoring and validation is provided in Chapter 16.

Routine determination of VOC levels is not performed. Instead, we check the remaining activity of activated-carbon filters by the CTC method at every other carbon replacement to determine whether our schedule of filter changing is adequate for safe operating life cycles.[9] Filters attached to incoming CO_2 gas lines are replaced at three-month intervals in accordance with manufacturer specifications (GenX, US). The temperature and humidity levels of incoming air are checked on a daily basis, and kept within the limits of 22–25°C and 40–60% relative humidity, respectively, as values above these limits may interfere with filter de-absorption capacity.[14] In addition, chemical filters are inspected monthly for plugging of activated carbon pellet beds due to particulate matter.

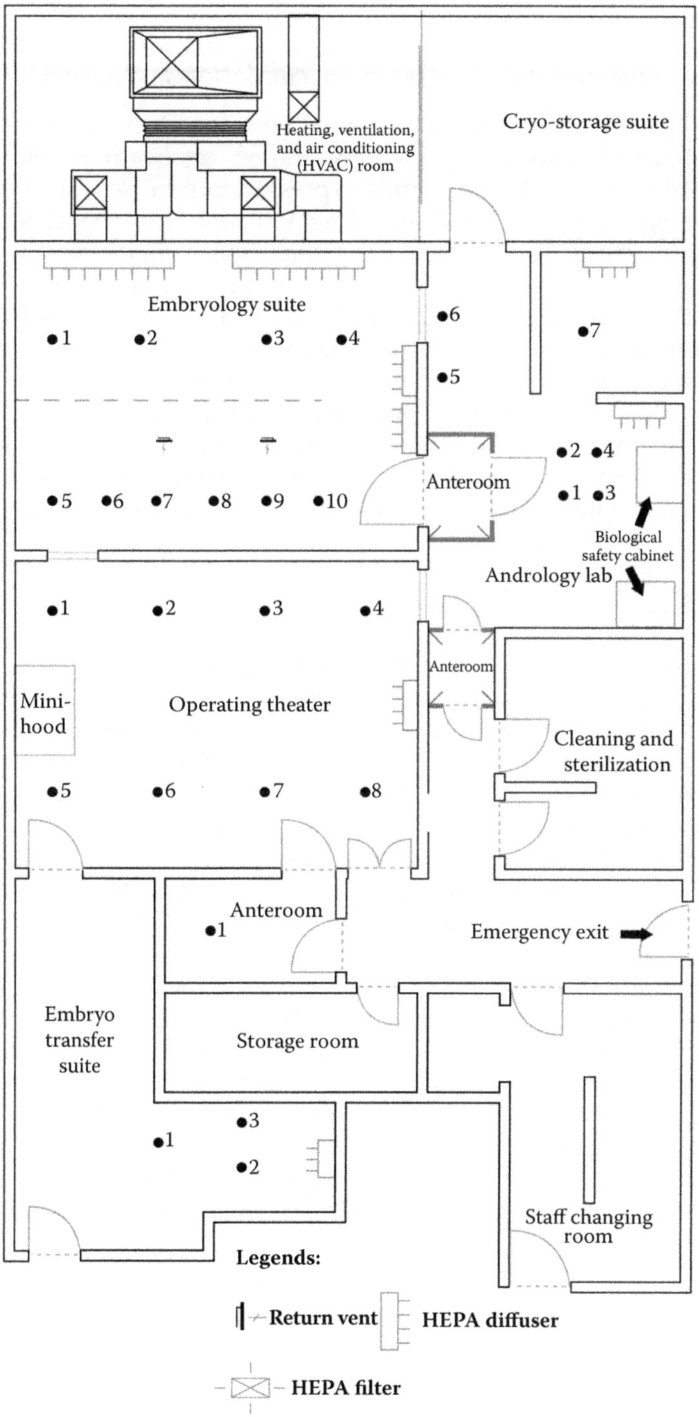

Figure 26.13 Diagrammatic layout depicting sampling locations of airborne particle count within clean rooms.

26.5 Our experience

26.5.1 Particle count monitoring and other validation measurements

Air quality validation testing results confirmed that the clean room facility was built according to design and in compliance with regulatory agency requirements. Total VOC levels, defined as the sum of all compounds expressed in toluene equivalents that appear in the gas chromatogram between and including n-hexane and n-hexadecane, were below 2 μg/m^3 of air. Aldehyde levels were below the detectable limit of 1 μg/m^3.

The results of air quality monitoring within clean rooms and associated areas are shown in Table 26.2. There was a significant location effect for each of the three particle sizes ($p = 0.001$). In the 0.5- and 5.0-μm particle groups, counts for the embryology facility and its anteroom were not different from one another, respectively, while the 0.3-μm particle group was lower in the latter ($p = 0.0008$). Mean particle counts (sizes 0.3, 0.5, and 5.0 μm) differed for the embryology facility and associated areas ($p < 0.001$). No major fluctuations were observed in the validation measurements which included air particle count, air volume flow rates, number of air exchange per hour, ambient air humidity, room temperature, and noise levels.

26.5.2 Case series

The authors compared patient cycle outcomes along with key performance laboratory indicators between the last triennium of IVF cycles at their old facility and the subsequent triennium (2002–2010) at the new facility.[5] A total of 2060 consecutive in vitro fertilization (IVF)/intracytoplasmic sperm injection (ICSI) cycles involving fresh embryo transfers were performed in the new clean room facility between 2002 and 2010. Outcome measures were compared to a historical cohort of consecutive IVF/ICSI cycles performed by the same staff in an older facility located in a different building within the same institution between 1999 and 2001. The aforementioned old facility was equipped with a Coda Tower filter unit (Life Global, Canada) installed inside the embryology lab. No additional filter systems were installed in the andrology lab, embryo transfer suite, and operating theater. Ovarian stimulation, oocyte and sperm retrieval, sperm processing, and sperm injections were carried out as previously reported.[15,16] Fertilization was considered normal when oocytes with 2PN and 2 polar bodies were observed 16 to 18 hours after ICSI. Fertilized oocytes were cultured until embryo transfer to the uterine cavity, which was guided by abdominal ultrasound on day 3 or 5 of embryo culture. Embryos were graded morphologically using a light inverted microscope on days 2, 3, and 5 as appropriate. Clinical pregnancy was confirmed by a gestational sac with an embryo showing cardiac activity on ultrasound at weeks 6 to 7. Miscarriage was considered when nonviable clinical pregnancy was noted on ultrasound follow-up. The live birth rate was defined as the ratio between the number of deliveries resulting in at least 1 live birth and the number of embryo transfers.

26.5.3 Clinical results

A total of 2315 fresh cycles were included in this retrospective analysis.[5] Cycles involving egg donation and frozen-thawed embryo transfers were excluded. There were no statistically significant differences in the proportion of patients undergoing IVF/ICSI for male and female factor infertility between the cohorts. The mean ± SD female patient age was significantly lower in the group treated in the old facility (30.8 ± 5.2 vs. 36.5 ± 4.1 years; $p < 0.001$).

Table 26.2 Validation testing results for reproductive laboratories and associated critical areas

Area	ISO 14644-1 clean room classification	Air particle count μm/m³ 0.3	0.5	5.0	Ambient air relative humidity (%)	Room temperature (°C)	Noise level (dBA)[b]	Air volume flow rate (m³/h)	No. of air exchanges per hour	No. personnel in daily activities
Embryology suite	ISO 5	2767 ± 1231	621 ± 299	0 ± 0	45.0 ± 6.9	23.5 ± 0.5	63 ± 11	3523 ± 201	102 ± 4	3
Embryology anteroom	ISO 5	1329 ± 1105	527 ± 507	0 ± 0	NR	NR	60 ± 6	1583 ± 112	489 ± 16	1
Operating theater	ISO 7	98,231 ± 26,607	1567 ± 496	81 ± 59	46.1 ± 5.8	23.8 ± 0.8	65 ± 22	589 ± 96	12 ± 2	4
Operating theater anteroom	ISO 7	80,042 ± 11,822	2008 ± 412	2221 ± 116	NR	NR	67 ± 12	NR	NR	1
Embryo transfer suite	ISO 8	83,261 ± 10,023	1213 ± 782	1711 ± 601	49.0 ± 4.9	24.2 ± 1.6	59 ± 9	234 ± 27	9 ± 1	3
Andrology laboratory suite	ISO 7	NR	312,812 ± 38,175	332 ± 80	47.3 ± 6.9	23.1 ± 1.9	69 ± 14	721 ± 88	14 ± 2	2
P-value	–	0.001	<0.001	<0.001	0.23	0.34	0.04	0.003	<0.001	–

Source: Adapted from Esteves SC and Bento FC, Reprod Biomed Online 2013; 26(1): 9–21, with permission from Elsevier. Values are mean ± SD or n. Validation measures were obtained "at operation." Data pooled from semi-annual validation testing performed by a third-party company (CCL, Campinas, Brazil) from 2002–2010. NR, not reported.

[a] Air particle counts pairwise comparisons not significant for: operating room anteroom versus embryo transfer at 0.3 μm/m³; embryology versus embryology anteroom; and operating room versus embryo transfer at 0.5 μm/m³.

[b] Noise level pairwise comparisons significant for only andrology versus embryo transfer suites.

Embryologic outcomes were compared between cohorts. No differences were noted in the total number of retrieved and mature oocytes between the groups. The mean rate of 2PN zygotes was not statistically different. However, the proportion of high quality embryos was significantly higher in the new facility (51.2% vs. 36.4%, $p < 0.001$). The mean number of transferred embryos was significantly lower in the group treated in the new facility ($p < 0.001$), which reflected the change in our center's policy and compliance with regulatory requirements.

Clinical pregnancy (47.9% vs. 36.2%, $p = 0.02$) and live birth rates (38.5% vs. 25.8%, $p = 0.01$) were significantly increased during the first triennium after moving to the new facility, whereas miscarriage rates were decreased (28.7% vs. 14.2%, $p = 0.01$). Embryo development also improved significantly ($p < 0.001$). These results were achieved by transferring lower numbers of embryos and treating women at older age compared with the group of patients treated before the implementation of clean rooms. During these same years, the mean number of embryos transferred significantly decreased (3.3 vs. 2.6; $p < 0.001$) while the mean age of females who sought IVF increased (36.4 vs. 30.8 years-old, $p = 0.01$). A significantly higher proportion of embryos were classified as having 8-cell stage and grades 1–2 cytoplasmic fragmentation on day 3 of embryo culture after clean room implementation (52% vs. 78%, $p = 0.01$). On average, one additional high quality embryo was obtained, either for a fresh transfer or cryopreservation, in treatment cycles performed in the clean room facilities (3.4 vs. 2.3; $p = 0.01$).

26.6 Expert commentary

In this chapter, we presented a detailed description on how we implemented an embryology laboratory and related areas with air quality control in full compliance with the Brazilian Cells and Germinative Tissue Directive, and the results of monitoring air quality within the clean room areas. The cleanliness of our facilities was periodically validated and no major variation was noted over a 12-year period. Furthermore, we presented retrospective data of sperm injection cycles performed in our IVF facilities before and after the implementation of the clean rooms. Our results showed that it is not only feasible to implement air quality standards but also possible to operate and comply with such standards while maintaining sustainable results of an ongoing assisted reproduction program.

Outcomes were analyzed on an overall basis before and after the implementation of clean rooms, and thereafter stratified by different time periods. This stratification was important to appreciate the overall impact of air quality control in the face of important changes that occurred over time. For example, the mean age of women who sought IVF at our institution increased steadily while the mean number of embryos transferred significantly decreased. Nevertheless, there were no major changes in culture media, catheters, and other disposable products used in the laboratory. Moreover, embryologists performing procedures were practically unchanged over these time periods. The mean number of oocytes retrieved, mature oocytes, and normal fertilization rates after ICSI were not statistically different. Furthermore, the reasons patients underwent IVF/ICSI did not significantly change after installation of the clean rooms. These factors did not seem to have impacted on the events, although other uncontrolled factors rather than air quality may have influenced IVF outcomes. After 2004, there was a change of practice in terms of the number of embryos transferred to the uterine cavity. Our policy of transferring up to four embryos regardless of female age was changed to a maximum of two in the younger group (35 years old or less). Later in 2010, Brazilian regulatory authorities enforced this practice.

As a result, the mean number of embryos transferred significantly decreased from 3.4 to 2.1 while the mean age of females who sought IVF increased significantly during these same years from 30.8 to 36.4. In spite of that, the proportion of cleavage-stage embryos classified as high-quality at the day of transfer steadily increased over all periods after implementation of clean rooms. Interestingly, we noted that the net effect of applying clean room technology on embryo development was an additional high quality embryo, on average, per treatment cycle.

Installation of centralized air filtration such as the one presented in this chapter involves significant investment. The cost for implementing clean room technology to our facilities was estimated at $150,000 USD. Operational costs, including filter changing, certification, maintenance, and purchase of clean room disposable supplies are approximately $10,000 USD per year. A less expensive but yet to be proven effective alternative, particularly for existing IVF laboratories, would be to incorporate compact or portable freestanding commercial units. However, it is unlikely that these systems provide the same air quality as a robust, centralized air filtration system. Notwithstanding, considering that our program performed approximately 6000 IVF cycles from 2002 to 2013, the additional cost per cycle to pay off the investment and cover maintenance costs over this 12-year period was approximately $45 USD. Our data indicate that performing IVF in controlled environments is beneficial to embryo development, and confirm our previous observations.[5,17,18]

Increasing evidence indicates that laboratory air quality plays a significant role in IVF outcome.[19] Implementation of air quality control by the combination of particulate matter and chemical filtration seems sound, but guidelines on the target limits and best practice statements on how to implement air quality control to IVF are still lacking. At present, built-in systems supplying filtered air to the IVF lab and adjacent areas seems to be the best alternative to mitigate the risks of poor IVF outcomes related to laboratory air.[19,20]

26.7 Conclusions

Implementation of clean room standards to reproductive laboratories, which include air quality control through filtration of airborne particles and VOCs, and the adoption of good laboratory practices, offers adequate conditions for contamination control and risk management. Our data demonstrated that it is feasible to handle human gametes and to culture embryos in clean room environments in full compliance with air quality standards directives, as the one imposed by the Brazilian regulatory authorities, and suggest that performing IVF in controlled environments may optimize its outcomes.

Acknowledgments

The authors thank Danielle T. Schneider and Sidney Verza Jr. for their help in data collection, and Raul A. Sadir for providing technical support with regard to air filtration.

References

1. ANVISA. Brazilian National Agency for Sanitary Surveillance, 2006. Resolução no. 33 da Diretoria colegiada da Agência Nacional de Vigilância Sanitária (amended by RDC23 of 27 May 2011 on setting standards of quality and safety for the donation, procurement, testing, processing, preservation, storage and distribution of human tissues and cells). http://www.uberlandia.mg.gov.br/uploads/cms_b_arquivos/8262.pdf. Accessed June 27, 2015.

2. Commission of the European Union Communities, 2000. Communication from the Commission on the precautionary principle. http://eur-lex.europa.eu/smartapi/cgi/sga_doc?smartapi!celexplus!prod!DocNumber&lg=en&type_doc=COMfinal&an_doc=2000&nu_doc=1. Accessed February 14, 2015.
3. ANVISA. Brazilian National Agency for Sanitary Surveillance, 2011. Resolução no. 23 da Diretoria colegiada da Agência Nacional de Vigilância Sanitária of May 27, 2011 on setting standards of quality and safety for the donation, procurement, testing, processing, preservation, storage and distribution of human tissues and cells). http://portal.anvisa.gov.br/wps/wcm/connect/d3f7c4804986e29a8e51ff4ed75891ae/RDC_23_2011.pdf?MOD=AJPERES. Accessed June 27, 2015.
4. International Organization for Standardization, 1999. ISO NBR 14644-1:2005 on cleanrooms and associated controlled environments. Associação Brasileira de Normas Técnicas (ABNT), Brasilia, DF, Brasil.
5. Esteves SC and Bento FC. Implementation of air quality control in reproductive laboratories in full compliance with the Brazilian Cells and Germinative Tissue Directive. *Reprod Biomed Online* 2013; 26: 9–21.
6. Esteves SC and Agarwal A. Explaining how reproductive laboratories work. In: Bento F, Esteves SC, and Agarwal A. (eds.), *Quality Management in ART Clinics: A Practical Guide*. 1st ed., Springer Science+Business Media, New York, pp. 79–127, 2013.
7. International Organization for Standardization, 2001. ISO NBR 14644-4:2004 on cleanrooms and associated controlled environments—Part 4: Design, construction and start-up. Associação Brasileira de Normas Técnicas (ABNT), Brasilia, DF, Brasil.
8. United States Environmental Protection Agency, 2014. Specifications on the environmental impact of materials (EPA 01120). http://www2.epa.gov/about-rtp/greening-epa-sustainable-design-epas-campus-research-triangle-park-nc-environmental-0. Accessed June 8, 2015.
9. American Society for Testing and Material, 2009. Test Method D3467-99: Standard test method for carbon tetrachloride activity of activated carbon (ASTM D3467-04). http://www.astm.org/Standards/D3467.htm. Accessed August 8, 2012.
10. United States Environmental Protection Agency, 1984. Method for determination of volatile organic compounds in ambient air using TENAX® adsorption and gas chromatography/mass spectrometry (GC/MS) (EPA Method TO-1). http://www.epa.gov/ttn/amtic/files/ambient/airtox/to-1.pdf. Accessed August 8, 2012.
11. International Organization for Standardization, 2001. ISO 16000-3:2001 on determination of formaldehyde and other carbonyl compounds—Active sampling method. Associação Brasileira de Normas Técnicas (ABNT), Brasilia, DF, Brasil.
12. International Organization for Standardization, 2000. ISO NBR 14644-2:2006 on cleanrooms and associated controlled environments—Part 2: Specifications for testing and monitoring to prove continued compliance with ISO 14644-1. Associação Brasileira de Normas Técnicas (ABNT), Brasilia, DF, Brasil.
13. International Organization for Standardization, 2005. ISO NBR 14644-3:2009 on cleanrooms and associated controlled environments—Part 3: Test methods. Associação Brasileira de Normas Técnicas (ABNT), Brasilia, DF, Brasil.
14. Worrilow KC, Huynh HT, Gwozdziewicz JB, Schillings W, and Peters AJ. A retrospective analysis: The examination of a potential relationship between particulate (P) and volatile organic compound (VOC) levels in a class 100 IVF laboratory cleanroom (CR) and specific parameters of embryogenesis and rates of implantation (IR). *Fertil Steril* 2001; 76 (Suppl. 1): S15–6.
15. Esteves SC, Schertz JC, Verza S Jr, Schneider DT, and Zabaglia SFC. A comparison of menotropin, highly-purified menotropin and follitropin alfa in cycles of intracytoplasmic sperm injection. *Reprod Biol Endocrinol* 2009; 7: 111.
16. Esteves SC and Agarwal A. Sperm retrieval techniques. In: Gardner DK, Rizk BRMB, and Falcone T, eds. *Human Assisted Reproductive Technology: Future Trends in Laboratory and Clinical Practice*. 1st ed, Cambridge University Press, Cambridge, pp. 41–53, 2011.

17. Esteves SC, Gomes AP, and Verza S Jr. Control of air pollution in assisted reproductive technology laboratory and adjacent areas improves embryo formation, cleavage and pregnancy rates and decreases abortion rate: Comparison between a class 100 (ISO 5) and a class 1.000 (ISO 6) cleanroom for micromanipulation and embryo culture. *Fertil Steril* 2004; 82 (Suppl. 2): S259–60.
18. Esteves SC, Verza S Jr, and Gomes AP. Comparison between International Standard Organization (ISO) type 5 and type 6 cleanrooms combined with volatile organic compounds filtration system for micromanipulation and embryo culture in severe male factor infertility. *Fertil Steril* 2006; 86: S353–4.
19. Esteves SC and Bento FC. Air quality control in the ART laboratory is a major determinant of IVF success. *Asian J Androl* 2015 Nov 10.
20. Esteves SC and Bento FC. Implementation of cleanroom technology in reproductive laboratories: The question is not why but how. *Reprod Biomed Online* 2016; 32: 9–11.

chapter twenty-seven

Clean room technology and IVF outcomes: United Kingdom

Paul Knaggs

Contents

Abstract

The European Union Tissues and Cells Directive (EUTCD) established common standards of quality and safety for the donation, procurement, testing, processing, preservation, storage, and distribution of human tissues and cells across all member nations of the European Union, including the United Kingdom. The EUTCD requires ART units to have designated air quality with a Grade A environment for gamete/embryo processing and a background of Grade D. The new requirements led many clinics, including ours, to modify their laboratory to improve air quality. The data indicates that there is no detrimental effect from operating under EU Tissue Directive/GMP conditions; in fact, operating under such stringent air quality standards may be responsible for increased success. The main driver for building clean room IVF facilities is to improve results and indeed the author has seen improvements in overall pregnancy rates in the laboratories he has been involved in building in the region.

Table 27.1 Classes of air cleanliness and microbial control

	Maximum permitted number of particles/m³, equal to or above			
	At rest		**In operation**	
Grade	0.5 µm	5 µm	0.5 µm	0.5 µm
A	3500	1	3500	1
B	3500	1	350,000	2000
C	350,000	2000	3,500,000	20,000
D	3,500,000	20,000	Not defined	Not defined

		Recommended limits for microbial contamination		
Grade	**Air sample CFU/m²**	**Settle plate (diam. 90 mm), CFU/4 hours**	**Contact plate (diam. 55 mm), CFU/plate**	**Glove print 5 fingers CFU/glove**
A	<1	<1	<1	<1
B	10	5	5	5
C	100	50	25	–
D	200	100	50	–

27.1 Introduction

Directive 2004/23/EC, commonly referred to as the European Union Tissues and Cells Directive (EUTCD) together with its additional technical directives (Directive 2006/17/EC and Directive 2006/86/EC) established common standards of quality and safety for the donation, procurement, testing, processing, preservation, storage, and distribution of human tissues and cells across all member nations of the European Union.[1–3]

From a laboratory point of view, one of the main challenges of the EUTCD was the requirement to have designated air quality with a Grade A environment being required for gamete/embryo processing and a background of Grade D (Table 27.1).

The new requirements led many clinics to modify their laboratories to improve air quality. Some clinics took a step further and built entirely new clean room facilities often with air quality that exceeded the air quality standards set out by the EUTCD. The decision to do this was often based on future proofing the new facility against potential tightening of regulation and the fact that the increased build costs were relatively modest over a facility that would meet the current requirements. Once you have decided to build a new laboratory, there are several key stages that you will need to be involved with.

27.2 Preparing your user requirement specification (URS)

Once the decision to build a new laboratory has been made, you can begin to prepare the "User Requirement Specification" (URS). The URS will form the basis of your new build and will help organize thoughts and ideas about the new build. A good place to start is to decide on the quality of air that will be required. Do you want or need to build a facility with Grade B background air quality or would Grade C or D be more appropriate/acceptable (Table 27.1)? This decision can heavily influence the size of the facility, the way personnel and materials enter the laboratory, and how the workspace is used, so it is critically important to understand your current and future needs. The reality is that the higher the air quality, the more time, effort, and money are required to maintain it. Remember too that it is much easier to run a facility designed to produce a high air quality at a lower quality than it is to try to modify a lower air quality facility to produce a high air quality environment.

Once you have decided on air quality, try to assess your current and future workload and the way that gametes and embryos will move through the laboratory. Do you want the sperm preparation and cryostorage areas integrated into the main IVF laboratory or do you want a separate laboratory? Now that you have a rough idea of what your ideal lab should look like, it is time to get the measurements of the space you have available. There are a number of free to use interior design programs available via the Internet and these can be useful in helping decide whether your design is feasible. Measure the dimensions of your equipment or obtain them from manufacturers to get an idea whether everything will fit for the workflow you want. Alternatively, drawing your design on graph paper and using paper cut-outs to represent your equipment works just as well. You will probably go through several different versions of your design until you find one that you're happy with but this is time well spent. It is better to have a clear idea of what you want from the very start.

Once you have finished the outline design it's time to look at the space in more detail. Imagine you are in each room in your laboratory space and look at the floor, ceiling, and each wall in turn. Will they be painted, what type of floor covering will you have? What type of lighting do you want? How many power outlets will you require for all the equipment in each location, will they require gas outlets (assuming you have room to build a separate gas store), data points, and so on? The one piece of advice I was given when I started designing clean rooms is that you can never have too many power outlets, gas outlets, or data points. Once a clean room is up and running, it is very disruptive and often very expensive to add more services so it is best to install them during the initial build even if they will not be used for some time after the facility becomes operational. Transcribe your ideas for each wall, ceiling, and floor onto separate sheets of paper to create your first draft of room data sheets.

27.3 Getting professional help

Once the in-house specifications have been finalized, it is now time to call on some professional help to build the new laboratory as it is unlikely that all the expertise required will be found in your organization.

Specialist IVF clean room companies often offer full turn-key solutions from design and build through to validation and equipping. They will deal with every aspect of the project but calculating value for money can be difficult if a single price is quoted for the job (where possible ensure they agree to open book accounting so that it is possible to analyze costs). There can also be a tendency to recycle some of their designs, resulting in different projects looking very similar.

Employing architects and separate contractors can offer the opportunity to design a truly bespoke facility. Opportunities exist to seek out experts for each stage of the process and also to get the most competitive pricing. This approach requires a higher degree of involvement than employing a specialist company; however, this can be greatly reduced by employing the services of a professional project manager.

Whichever approach is taken, it is advisable to seek recommendations from other colleagues who have undertaken similar projects and if possible obtain quotes from at least three different companies before signing contracts. Also ensure that the professionals that you deal with really understand the specialist nature of IVF and its requirements. For example, the author has seen a number of labs where heating, ventilation, and air conditioning (HVAC) vents were placed directly above planned intracytoplasmic sperm injection (ICSI)/biopsy stations. Clean rooms operate with considerable air movement, which can cause surface cooling on work benches and microscope stages and have negative effects on the gametes and embryos placed in these areas.

Once the design/build team has been contracted, the design will be further discussed and refined. It is important that these changes are documented clearly on plans and other paperwork and each new revision given a unique reference. The new documentation should then be issued from a central point in a format that does not allow unauthorized modifications. Without such an approach it is easy for different people or groups to be working from different drawings or specifications. This stage of planning/build results in the production of the "Design Qualification" (DQ) that describes the functional and operation specifications of the facility.

27.4 Preparing for the build

For a brand new build, hopefully there is little for the end user (you) to think about. All building permissions, etc., will have been taken care of by the professionals that you have contracted for the build.

The most challenging situation occurs when the new facility is to be housed in an existing space, for example, in the case of a full laboratory upgrade. Decisions will need to be made about how this process is managed from a clinic operational point of view. Does the clinic close for the duration of the build? Can the laboratory be temporarily moved to another room and if it can, what is the likely outcome in terms of pregnancy rates, etc.? There is no one correct answer for this and all the available options should be risk assessed well in advance of any building work taking place.

27.5 After the build

Once building work is complete, the first task will be the "Installation Qualification" (IQ). Put simply, the IQ is the process of checking that everything that forms part of the facility has been installed correctly from making sure that electrical outlets work to having the appropriate filters fitted in the HVAC system.

The IQ is closely followed by "Operational Qualification" (OQ); this entails checking that the facility operates in the specified manner. In an IVF laboratory the most obvious OQ job is checking that the HVAC system delivers the required air quality. Once the OQ is performed and has parameters judged to be satisfactory, the facility would then be formally handed over from the contractors to the end users. The OQ is often performed with all the equipment in situ, for example, safety cabinets, centrifuges, etc., as patterns of airflow can be drastically changed once the laboratory space is occupied.

Ongoing checks of the facility are often referred to as the "Performance Qualification" (PQ) and are done on a regular basis—daily, weekly, or monthly in order to prove that the facility is still operating according to the designed specifications.

27.6 Equipment validation

Once you have a new shiny clean laboratory, the equipment (new or already owned) can be moved in. Safety cabinets, centrifuges, refrigerators, etc., should all undergo a process of validation to ensure that they operate according to the manufacturer's specifications. Some laboratories may choose to do these validations in-house and have access to equipment such as temperature measurement equipment whose calibration can be traced back to an accredited standard. Other laboratories may prefer to hire a specialist validation company to do this work. Many laboratories validate all of their equipment on an annual basis and after periods of maintenance or repair.

27.7 Process validation

All laboratory processes should be validated (in the United Kingdom it is a Human Fertility and Embryology Authority [HFEA] requirement) to ensure the best outcome of that particular process. In new laboratories, process validation can be done on a retrospective basis or based on current scientific literature/best practice. Scientific literature can also be used as a guide to deciding on the key performance indicators (KPIs) for each process, for example, fertilization rates for IVF and ICSI. In an established laboratory, existing processes (such as insemination concentration) can be benchmarked against historical data or other IVF units that are willing to allow access to their data. In this way, changes to processes can be analyzed and continuous improvements made.

27.8 Benefits of clean room IVF

The main driver for building clean room IVF facilities is to improve results and indeed the author has seen improvements in overall pregnancy rates in the laboratories he has been involved in building in the region of almost 40% (30.2–42.2% fetal heart/embryo transfer).[4] It should be noted that such improvements are not always accompanied in improvements in other laboratory KPI such as fertilization rates or even embryo quality. While it is tempting to ascribe any improvements purely to air quality, it is unlikely to be the only factor affecting laboratory performance.

It is highly likely that many procedures and processes will be reassessed, modified, or changed altogether before and after the clean room build. Clean room installation allows workflow in the laboratory to be optimized with the result that environmental exposure is decreased, which can improve temperature and pH control, both of which are of positive benefit to human embryo culture. Indeed, if improvements in outcomes are not seen after a clean room build, workflow should be one of the first things to be investigated.

27.9 Maintaining an IVF clean room

Once built, a major challenge is keeping the facility at the desired level of cleanliness. To know that the laboratory is clean requires a comprehensive testing strategy that at least covers particulates and microbiological testing. Additional testing may be required for VOCs. Testing frequency should ideally be established for individual laboratories depending on usage. After commissioning, testing will be more frequent, perhaps weekly. Once up and running and trends become apparent, it may be possible to scale back the frequency of testing to fortnightly, monthly, or even longer periods.

The two ways of reducing contaminants in the IVF laboratory are reducing the number of products/items that are taken into the laboratory and cleaning the laboratory.

When choosing products that are taken into the lab, care should be taken when not only assessing the product itself but also its packaging. There are an increasing number of products that are clean room compatible. Items such as wipes for cleaning and spillages can be made of low shedding materials (and so do not add to the particulate count in the lab) and can be supplied sterile and double bagged in plastic rather than paper. This means that the outer packaging can be cleaned before being removed and the inner sterile package taken into the lab. This then decreases the amount of cleaning products taken and used in the lab and decreases the particulate and microbial load inside the lab. The choice of laboratory clothing can be treated the same way with low shedding materials being chosen over traditional cotton theater scrub suits.

Cleaning the lab itself, much like the testing regime, will be more frequent after the initial commissioning and depending on the results of testing may be able to be scaled back once enough testing data have been accumulated to inform those decisions. There are a number of systems that can be used to clean clean rooms and encompass large double or triple bucket systems which are economical and perhaps best suited to larger facilities, to pre-dosed mopping systems which can include detergents, biocides, and alcohols depending on the regime the laboratory wishes to use.

References

1. Directive 2004/23/EC of the European Parliament and of the Council. Official Journal of the European Union; March 31, 2004: L012/48-58.
2. Directive 2006/17/EC of the European Parliament and of the Council. Official Journal of the European Union; February 8, 2006: L38/40-52.
3. Directive 2006/86/EC of the European Parliament and of the Council. Official Journal of the European Union; February 8, 2006: L294/32-50.
4. Knaggs P, Birch D, Drury S, Morgan M, Kumari S, Sriskan-dakumar R, and Avery S. Full compliance with the EU directive air quality standards does not compromise IVF outcome. *Hum Reprod* 2007; 22, Suppl 1, i164–5.

Index

Page numbers followed by f and t indicate figures and tables, respectively.

D

I

N

S

T